2015
The Year Book of PATHOLOGY AND LABORATORY MEDICINE®

Editor-in-Chief

Stephen S. Raab, MD

Professor of Pathology, University of Washington, Seattle, Washington, and Memorial University of Newfoundland/Eastern Health Authority, St John's, Newfoundland, Canada

Editors

M. Sherif Said, MD, PhD, FCAP

Associate Professor of Pathology, University of Colorado Denver; Associate Director of Pathology, Denver Health, Denver, Colorado

Maxwell L. Smith, MD

Assistant Professor, Department of Laboratory Medicine and Pathology, Mayo Clinic, Scottsdale, Arizona

ELSEVIER
MOSBY

VP Global Content: Judith Fletcher
Publisher: Adrianne Brigido
Supervisor, Electronic Year Books: Donna M. Skelton
Electronic Article Manager: Mike Sheets
Illustrations and Permissions Coordinator: Dawn Vohsen

2015 EDITION

Composition by TNQ Books and Journals Pvt Ltd, India

Editorial Office:
Elsevier
Suite 1800
1600 John F. Kennedy Blvd.
Philadelphia, PA 19103-2899

International Standard Serial Number: 1077-9108
International Standard Book Number: 978-0-323-35550-6

Contributing Editor

Dana Marie Grzybicki, MD, PhD
Quality Systems Research Manager, Department of Quality, Patient Safety and Risk Management, Eastern Health, St. John's, NL, Canada

Table of Contents

Journals Represented vii

ANATOMIC PATHOLOGY 1
1. Outcomes Analysis 3
2. Hepatobiliary System and Pancreas 27
3. Cytopathology 51
4. Head and Neck 61
5. Kidney 97
6. Female Genital Tract 121
7. Breast 129
8. Lung and Mediastinum 139
9. Cardiovascular 165
10. Gastrointestinal System 167
11. Hematolymphoid 179
12. Neuropathology 185
13. Soft Tissue and Bone 189
14. Pediatrics 195
15. Techniques/Molecular 199
16. Urinary Bladder and Male Genital Tract 209

LABORATORY MEDICINE 217
17. Clinical Chemistry 219
18. Clinical Microbiology 223
19. Cytogenetics and Molecular Pathology 229
20. Hematology and Immunology 231
21. Laboratory Management and Outcomes 233

Article Index 239

Author Index 247

Journals Represented

Journals represented in this Year Book are listed below.

Acta Cytologica
American Journal of Clinical Pathology
American Journal of Gastroenterology
American Journal of Kidney Diseases
American Journal of Pathology
American Journal of Surgical Pathology
American Journal of Transplantation
Annals of Diagnostic Pathology
Annals of Internal Medicine
Annals of Laboratory Medicine
Annals of Transplantation
AORN Journal
Applied Immunohistochemistry & Molecular Morphology
Archives of Pathology & Laboratory Medicine
Biochemia Medica
BioMed Research International
British Journal of Cancer
Cancer Treatment Reviews
Case Reports in Otolaryngology
Clinica Chimica Acta
Clinical Chemistry
Clinical Kidney Journal
Clinical Microbiology and Infection
Clinical and Translational Gastroenterology
Clinics in Laboratory Medicine
Cytopathology
Diagnostic Pathology
Endocrine Pathology
Esophagus
Fetal and Pediatric Pathology
Head and Neck Pathology
Histopathology
Human Pathology
International Cardiovascular Research Journal
International Journal of Clinical and Experimental Pathology
International Journal of Infectious Diseases
International Journal of Surgery Case Reports
International Journal of Surgical Pathology
Journal of Clinical Pathology
Journal of Neuro-ophthalmology
Journal of Pathology Informatics
Journal of Surgical Research
Kidney International
Liver Transplantation
Modern Pathology
Oral & Maxillofacial Surgery Clinics of North America
Otology & Neurotology

Pathology Research and Practice
Pediatric and Developmental Pathology
Polish Journal of Pathology
Public Library of Science One
Sarcoma
Seminars in Diagnostic Pathology
Virchows Archiv
World Journal of Gastrointestinal Surgery
World Journal of Nephrology

Standard Abbreviations

The following terms are abbreviated in this edition: acquired immunodeficiency syndrome (AIDS), cardiopulmonary resuscitation (CPR), central nervous system (CNS), cerebrospinal fluid (CSF), computed tomography (CT), deoxyribonucleic acid (DNA), electrocardiography (ECG), health maintenance organization (HMO), human immunodeficiency virus (HIV), intensive care unit (ICU), intramuscular (IM), intravenous (IV), magnetic resonance (MR) imaging (MRI), ribonucleic acid (RNA), ultrasound (US), and ultraviolet (UV).

Note

The Year Book of Pathology and Laboratory Medicine is a literature survey service providing abstracts of articles published in the professional literature. Every effort is made to assure the accuracy of the information presented in these pages. Neither the editors nor the publisher of the Year Book of Pathology and Laboratory Medicine can be responsible for errors in the original materials. The editors' comments are their own opinions. Mention of specific products within this publication does not constitute endorsement.

To facilitate the use of the Year Book of Pathology and Laboratory Medicine as a reference tool, all illustrations and tables included in this publication are now identified as they appear in the original article. This change is meant to help the reader recognize that any illustration or table appearing in the Year Book of Pathology and Laboratory Medicine may be only one of many in the original article. For this reason, figure and table numbers will often appear to be out of sequence within the Year Book of Pathology and Laboratory Medicine.

PART I

ANATOMIC PATHOLOGY

1 Outcomes Analysis

The Modern Pathologist: Lab Data Deliverer, Interpreter, and Diagnostician

Brat DJ (Emory Univ Hosp, Atlanta, GA)
J Neuroophthalmol 34:1-2, 2014

Background.—The modern pathologist contributes to patient management through the provision of expertise and testing of patient biospecimens that leads to a pathological diagnosis and influences treatment. A definitive, accurate diagnosis is critical to correct patient care and relies heavily on the results of laboratory-based tests performed under the supervision of a pathologist. A recent estimate found that laboratory results account for 70% to 90% of the data in patients' electronic medical records. In addition, some believe that nearly 70% of all medical decisions depend on laboratory test results. Thus the pathologist plays a vital role in tissue-based diagnoses, provides laboratory test results that guide patient management, and establishes an infrastructure for clinically relevant research to aid in understanding and managing disease.

Case Examples.—Man, 18, was diagnosed with cerebral hemispheric lesion extending to involve the optic chiasm and nerve. An infiltrative disease process was suggested by magnetic resonance imaging (MRI), but the differential diagnosis was too broad, so a tissue-based diagnosis was required. Biopsy revealed an anaplastic astrocytoma, grade III, with a pattern of brain involvement on MRI that was consistent with gliomatosis cerebri. Histologic section showed neoplastic cells with astrocytic differentiation invading through the brain neuropil. Further laboratory testing to indicate the prognosis included assessment of *isocitrate dehydrogenase 1 (1DH1)* mutational status and a MIB-1 proliferation index. Pathologists were able to interpret the histological findings and contribute to the definitive diagnosis.

Three patients had initial symptoms that ranged from visual field defect to cortical blindness plus significant cognitive decline and psychiatric manifestations. All experienced rapid clinical deterioration. The presumptive diagnosis was Heidenhain variant of Creutzfeldt-Jakob disease (HvCJD). Tests ordered to accompany the clinical examination were diffusion-weighted imaging, electroencephalography, and testing of the cerebrospinal fluid (CSF) for proteins 14-3-3 and neuron-specific enolase (NSE). The cumulative results provided enough evidence to support the diagnosis and institute medical care to address the expected rapid clinical decline of the patients. Currently, neuropathologists are investigating HvCJD through molecular testing, disease tracking, research, and education on prion diseases to advance the understanding of this disease and its variants.

Man, 29, had flu-like symptoms, headaches, and retinopathy, with a diagnosis of acute multifocal placoid pigment epitheliopathy based on the results of fundoscopy and fluorescein angiography. However, the disease progressed rapidly, with new-onset seizures and multiple cerebral infarcts occurring within 2 weeks. Several infectious and autoimmune etiologies were possible, so clinical laboratory tests were used extensively to eliminate possibilities. The patient died within 2 weeks, but postmortem brain evaluation noted multiple cerebral infarctions of variable ages, consistent with a progressively evolving disease. Leptomeningeal vessel section revealed striking giant cell arteritis involving large-caliber vessels, indicating an underlying vasculopathy of the brain that led to the fatal ischemic course. Cases such as this increase clinicians' awareness of potential pathophysiological problems underlying clinical syndromes and can influence patient management.

Conclusions.—The pathologist establishes an accurate tissue-based diagnosis, with clinical laboratory testing generating important results that can guide the clinician to specific treatment decisions. As laboratory-based testing becomes more complex, pathologists will play an increasingly important role in data delivery and interpretation.

▶ In this essay, Brat provides a good summary of the near future, in which the pathologist provides accurate information in the era of proteomics and genomics and interprets, educates, assists in patient management, and performs research.

S. Raab, MD

Anatomic and Clinical Pathology Boot Camps: Filling Pathology-Specific Gaps in Undergraduate Medical Education

Naritoku WY, Vasovic L, Steinberg JJ, et al (Keck School of Medicine of the Univ of Southern California, Los Angeles; Albert Einstein College of Medicine, Bronx, NY; et al)
Arch Pathol Lab Med 138:316-321, 2014

Context.—The Liaison Committee on Medical Education began an initiative to change medical education across the United States in the early 2000s. With the explosion in medical science knowledge, the need arose to teach selected fundamental information both in a contextual and in an active learning manner.

Objective.—To identify ways to address gaps in training and knowledge that became apparent following implementation of learner-centered teaching methods, with devotion of more time to Internet-based learning and less emphasis on face-to-face lecture time. There was a dramatic departure from or de-emphasis of many traditional courses, such as embryology, gross anatomy, microscopic anatomy, and pathology, to the integration of these sciences into system-based active learning courses. This change in medical school curricula produces a medical graduate who hopefully thinks differently but certainly lacks subject-specific knowledge for a variety of medical specialties.

Data Sources.—Pathology residency programs have developed "boot camps" for the initial months of residency training both to provide the necessary foundation of pathology-specific medical science and to introduce basic skills and processes required for practice of anatomic pathology and laboratory medicine. The College of American Pathologists Graduate Medical Education Committee sent a questionnaire out on the Program Directors Section Listserv; the results are discussed and 3 boot camp programs are described.

Conclusions.—Boot camps have 2 purposes: (1) to teach or strengthen knowledge required to practice pathology and (2) to introduce basic skills and processes that will be used during the practitioner's career.

▶ This article describes the emerging development of first-year pathology trainee boot camps, which have been found to be helpful if not necessary for early trainees. The underlying reason for the necessity of these boot camps is the gradual elimination of basic science content, including basic pathology, from many medical school curricula. In essence, pathology training programs are now feeling the need to provide educational content that once was provided during the initial stages of medical school. This state of affairs is highly disappointing and frustrating. One can only hope that at some time in the future the pendulum will start swinging the other way, and fundamental knowledge of the basic sciences will be seen as a priority for students training to become physicians of any specialty.

S. Raab, MD

A clinician's perspective on laboratory utilization management

Yeh DD (Massachusetts General Hosp, Boston)

Clin Chim Acta 427:145-150, 2014

Background.—Excessive laboratory utilization is a common problem in the hospital setting. Physicians control up to 80% of healthcare costs and wield great influence.

Methods.—This review article describes reasons for overutilization of labs and recommends interventional strategies to change clinician ordering behavior.

Results.—Powerful factors exist that encourage overutilization, including fear of missing a diagnosis, provider inexperience, peer pressure, financial rewards, practice inertia, and fear of legal punishment. Features of automated order entry, such as bundling and "daily until discontinued" options contribute to wasteful ordering behavior.

Conclusion.—The most successful and long-lasting interventions are multi-faceted and have included a combination of education, feedback and audit, and administrative changes. The support of senior physicians and top administration is critical to the success of any initiative and ideally, interventions should be original from a multi-disciplinary committee of respected individuals.

▶ Although this article is a review rather than a research study, it is enormously interesting and important for pathologists to read. It is important because, as the title indicates, it summarizes reasons and thinking behind laboratory test overutilization and provides views about the various ways that are used by pathology laboratories to limit utilization, from the clinician's viewpoint. No one argues with the fact that extensive laboratory test overutilization is a major quality and cost issue for laboratory medicine, but varying levels of success in decreasing overutilization currently are reported. In addition, these reports have essentially exclusively been written from the pathologist's viewpoint and have focused on banning the ordering of tests by clinicians. Although banning testing definitely will curb overutilization, it does not take into consideration the multiple reasons for clinician overutilization, as articulated in this report. A broader consideration of this problem, in collaboration with clinician colleagues, may, as this author advocates "foster a return to the culture of critical reasoning coupled with conscientious and thoughtful investigation." For further reading, see reference list below.[1,2]

D. M. Grzybicki, MD

References

1. Grossman RM. A review of physician cost-containment strategies for laboratory testing. *Med Care.* 1983;21:783-802.
2. Squires DA. Explaining high health care spending in the United States: an international comparison of supply, utilization, prices, and quality. *Issue Brief (Commonw Fund).* 2012;10:1-14.

Cancer Tracking: Clinician Compliance and Program Outcome

Layfield LJ, Schnabel JL (Univ of Missouri, Columbia)

Am J Clin Pathol 142:773-776, 2014

Objectives.—Certain laboratory tests are critical for patient care and must be communicated rapidly. Professional societies have developed guidelines for reporting of "critical values" and significant or unexpected surgical pathology findings. Urgent diagnoses requiring rapid reporting include new or unexpected diagnoses of malignancy. The University of Missouri established a "cancer-tracking" protocol in which all diagnoses of malignancy require acknowledgment by the responsible clinician.

Methods.—We reviewed 5 months of compliance with the cancer-tracking protocol. The protocol requires the Department of Pathology to send a letter to the responsible clinician requesting acknowledgment of the report. In total, 1,155 confirmation requests were sent to the physicians named on the request form.

Results.—Following the first letter, 692 acknowledgments were received, and 356 acknowledgments followed the second letter. In 107 (9%) cases, no response was received.

Conclusions.—Confirmation that the physician caring for a patient receives a pathology diagnosis is important for patient management and quality assurance. While the surgical pathology report was placed in the chart, it was impossible to confirm that the responsible physician had reviewed the report in 9% of cases. Techniques for communication and confirmation of transmission of anatomic pathology diagnoses need to be developed.

▶ The hand-off of a cancer diagnosis from the pathologist to the clinician is critical to ensure that a patient receives appropriate cancer follow-up. Layfield and Schabel reported that a failure in receiving notification from the clinician that the cancer diagnosis was received was significantly high. Additional study is necessary to determine whether the clinician actually received the notification but did not respond, so that a true gap in notification occurred. The next step would then be to determine how this gap could be addressed. Rare cases anecdotally are missed, and the methods to bridge this gap will need an improved system design, which would involve both clinical and laboratory teams. This article sets the stage for moving in this direction.

S. Raab, MD

RP Implementation: Specimen Management

Graybill-D'Ercole P (Integra LifeSciences Corp, York, PA)

AORN J 100:626-633, 2014

Effective specimen management in the perioperative setting is essential for accurate patient diagnosis and intervention. AORN's "Recommended practices for specimen management" provides guidance to help perioperative nurses, in collaboration with a multidisciplinary team, implement a specimen management process that includes a needs assessment, site identification, collection and handling, transfer from the sterile field, containment, specimen identification and labeling, preservation, transport, disposition, and documentation. Accurate specimen management requires effective multidisciplinary communication and an awareness of the potential opportunities for error. Specimens discussed in the recommended practices document include breast cancer specimens, amputated digits and limbs to be reattached, forensic and radioactive specimens, and explanted medical devices and orthopedic hardware. The recommendations are applicable to both hospital and ambulatory settings.

▶ Graybill-D'Ercole provides a nursing point of view on how to handle and transport surgical pathology specimens to the laboratory. The article discusses 10 recommendations that encompass specimen handling in the preanalytic phase. Because errors happen more frequently in this phase (compared with the analytic phase), pathologists should participate (as a an active consultant) in this phase to ensure adequate specimen quality.

S. Raab, MD

Are Amended Surgical Pathology Reports Getting to the Correct Responsible Care Provider?

Parkash V, Domfeh A, Cohen P, et al (Yale Univ School of Medicine, New Haven, CT; et al)

Am J Clin Pathol 142:58-63, 2014

Objectives.—Amended reports (AmRs) need to follow patients to treating physicians, to avoid erroneous management based on the original diagnosis. This study was undertaken to determine if AmRs followed the patient appropriately.

Methods.—AmRs with diagnostic changes and discrepancies between ordering and treating physicians were tracked. Chart reviews, electronic medical report (EMR) reviews, and interviews were conducted to establish receipt of the AmR by the correct physician.

Results.—Seven of 60 AmRs had discrepancies between the ordering and treating physicians, all with malignant diagnoses. The AmR was present in the treating physician's chart in only one case. Ordering physicians indicated that AmRs were not forwarded to treating physicians when corrected results arrived after patient referral, under the assumption that the new physician was automatically forwarded pathology updates. No harm was documented in any of our cases. In one case with a significant amendment, the correct information was entered in the patient chart based on a tumor board discussion. A review of two electronic health record systems uncovered significant shortcomings in each delivery system.

Conclusions.—AmRs fail to follow the patient's chain of referrals to the correct care provider, and EMR systems lack the functionality to address this failure and alert clinical teams of amendments.

▶ Many information systems are not designed to deal with a "change" that needs to be added to previous documentation, such as an amended report. In these situations, relying on the electronic medical record to provide a correct connection is, unfortunately, often unreliable. These situations actually represent compounded errors (the first being the error in the original report that was corrected and the second being the failure to notify the correct individuals). Some pathology groups mandate that pathologists call their clinical colleagues for any "major" amended report. Ensuring that the correct people are called may still be a problem because in the age of specialization and fractured care, the entire care team is not always known to all its members. The concept of building an entire team is relatively new to health care and will require input from a large number of stakeholders. This article shows that this is a necessary endeavor.

S. Raab, MD

Analysis of Addenda in Anatomic Pathology as a Quality Monitoring Initiative

Babwah JP, Khalifa M, Rowsell C (Univ of Toronto, Ontario, Canada)
Arch Pathol Lab Med 138:1514-1519, 2014

Context.—Along with the integration of immunohistochemical markers and molecular techniques into routine practice, addenda in surgical pathology reporting have not only increased in frequency but also evolved to include prognostic and therapeutic information. Because of the lack of uniform practice with respect to issuing addenda, information that can significantly change the diagnosis, prognosis, or treatment plan may be issued as an addendum as opposed to an amendment.

Objective.—To audit addenda and identify instances of amendments masquerading as addenda.

Design.—All addenda during a 36-month period were reviewed. Each addendum report was classified by accession class, issuing pathologist, subspecialty category, indication for addendum, whether the addendum constituted a change in diagnostic meaning, whether a change in prognosis occurred, and if a change in treatment plan was necessary.

Results.—All cytology and autopsy addenda were deemed appropriate. Thirty-three of 5028 (6.5 of 1000) surgical pathology addenda were deemed to have changes: Among the 33 faux addenda, 30 (91%) contained supplemental diagnostic information that would alter patient management and 31 (94%) contained additional information that would change the prognosis from that entailed by the original diagnosis.

Conclusions.—Our study demonstrates that not infrequently, surgical pathology addenda contain information that significantly alters the report and thus merit an amendment. Quality monitoring initiatives that evaluate pathologist and departmental performance should assess both addenda and amendments.

► As the name suggests, an amended report represents a change in some aspect of the report, whereas an addended report represents the addition of supplementary information to the report. Although clinicians may not know the difference, an amended report may include a change in the interpretation (diagnosis), which could markedly affect patient outcome and treatment. The article by Babweh et al indicates that some pathologists may not fully distinguish or appreciate the difference between amended and addended reports. The gap between pathologist reporting and clinician interpretation of the report findings has been shown to vary, with some misunderstandings between pathologists and clinicians. Ideally, pathologists must assess the best means by which information regarding a patient report is transferred to the clinician to optimize patient care. For further reading, see reference list below.[1,2]

S. Raab, MD

References

1. Meier FA, Zarbo RJ, Varney RC, et al. Amended reports: development and validation of a taxonomy of defects. *Am J Clin Pathol.* 2008;130:238-246.
2. Nakhleh RE, Zarbo RJ. Amended reports in surgical pathology and implications for diagnostic error detection and avoidance: a college of American pathologists Q-probes study of 1,667,547 accessioned cases in 359 laboratories. *Arch Pathol Lab Med.* 1998;122:303-309.

Communicating diagnostic uncertainty in surgical pathology reports: Disparities between sender and receiver

Lindley SW, Gillies EM, Hassell LA (The Univ of Oklahoma Health Sciences Ctr)

Pathol Res Pract 210:628-633, 2014

Surgical pathologists use a variety of phrases to communicate varying degrees of diagnostic certainty which have the potential to be interpreted differently than intended. This study sought to: (1) assess the setting, varieties and frequency of use of phrases of diagnostic uncertainty in the diagnostic line of surgical pathology reports, (2) evaluate use of uncertainty expressions by experience and gender, (3) determine how these phrases are interpreted by clinicians and pathologists, and (4) assess solutions to this communication problem. We evaluated 1500 surgical pathology reports to determine frequency of use of uncertainty terms, identified those most commonly used, and looked for variations in usage rates on the basis of case type, experience and gender. We surveyed 76 physicians at tumor boards who were asked to assign a percentage of certainty to diagnoses containing expressions of uncertainty. We found expressions of uncertainty in 35% of diagnostic reports, with no statistically significant difference in usage based on age or gender. We found wide variation in the percentage of certainty clinicians assigned to the phrases studied. We conclude that non-standardized language used in the communication of diagnostic uncertainty is a significant source of miscommunication, both amongst pathologists and between pathologists and clinicians.

▶ Lindley et al detail the frequency of indeterminate diagnoses used in surgical pathology. It is not surprising that clinicians have different interpretations of expressions of uncertainty (such as "consistent with"), and Lindley et al propose a variety of solutions. In 1981, Schwartz et al published an article in the *New England Journal of Medicine* that offered a Bayesian solution. One can reason that as pathology is a diagnostic test, every interpretation is probabilistic because it changes the clinician's pretest probability of disease. Schwartz et al argued that pathologists could just report probabilities that then could be used by the clinician to calculate the posttest probability of disease. For example, a pathologist diagnosis could be 99% probability of cancer and 1% probability of benign. If the clinician's pretest probability of cancer is 90%, then the posttest probability would increase and essentially confirm the diagnosis. The problem, then as now, is that many physicians choose only to act in a semi-Bayesian manner and want certainty. In fact, pathologists are requested to be certain in surgical pathology (not so in cytopathology!), which leads to pathologist "hedging" of diagnoses to express their uncertainty. For further reading, see reference list.[1-3]

S. Raab, MD

References

1. Galway M, Taiyeb T. The interpretation of phrases used to describe uncertaintyin pathology reports. *Pathol Res Int.* 2011;2011:656079.
2. Foucar E. "Individuality" in the specialty of surgical pathology: self-expressionor just another source of diagnostic error? *Am J Surg Pathol.* 2000;24:1573-1576.
3. Schwartz WB, Wolfe HJ, Pauker SG. Pathology and probabilities: a new approach to interpreting and reporting biopsies. *N Engl J Med.* 1981;305:917-923.

Surgical pathology and the patient: a systematic review evaluating the primary audience of pathology reports

Mossanen M, True LD, Wright JL, et al (Univ of Washington, Seattle; et al)
Hum Pathol 45:2192-2201, 2014

The pathology report is a critical document that helps guide the management of patients with cancer. More and more patients read their reports, intending to participate in decisions about their care. However, a substantial subset of patients may lack the ability to comprehend this often technical and complex document. We hypothesized that most literature on pathology reports discusses reports from the perspective of other physicians and not from the perspective of patients. An expert panel of physicians developed a list of search criteria, which we used to identify articles on PubMed, MEDLINE, Cochrane Reviews, and Google Scholar databases. Two reviewers independently evaluated all articles to identify for detailed review those that met search criteria. We identified the primary audience of the selected articles and the degree to which these articles addressed clarity of communication of pathology reports with patients. Of 801 articles identified in our search, 25 involved the formatting of pathology reports for clarity of communication. Recurrent themes in proposed improvements in reports included content standardization, variation in terminology, clarity of communication, and quality improvement. No articles discussed patients as their target audience. No study evaluated the health literacy level required of patients to comprehend pathology reports. In summary, there is a scarcity of patient-centered approaches to improve pathology reports. The literature on pathology reports does not include patients as a target audience. Limited resources are available to help patients comprehend their reports. Efforts to improve patient-centered communication are desirable to address this overlooked aspect of patient care.

▶ One of the domains of quality as described by the Institute of Medicine (IOM) is patient-centeredness. Although many pathologists hold the view that everything they do is patient-centered because they are rendering a diagnosis for a patient that will guide patient care, the definition of patient-centered care expressed by this view is not exactly the definition articulated by the IOM: "[H]ealth care that establishes a partnership among practitioners, patients, and their families (when appropriate) to ensure that decisions respect patients' wants, needs, and preferences and that patients have the education and support they need to make decisions and participate in their own care." For anatomic pathology practice, a large component of patient-centeredness is to ensure that the information provided in pathology reports may be understood directly by patients or at least easily translated by clinicians so they may make informed decisions about their care. A major focus of radiology quality improvement in the past few years has been to rethink the design and content of imaging reports to be more patient-friendly. This systematic review documents the fact that a major quality gap in anatomic pathology is in patient-centeredness—and specifically, in patient-centered pathology reporting. Although this article focuses on the gap, it highlights an area of pathology practice that is ripe for local quality improvement initiatives as well as for pathology practice quality improvement research. For additional reading, please view reference list.[1-3]

S. Raab, MD

References

1. Alba-Ruiz R, Bermudez-Tamayo C, Pernett JJ, Garcia-Gutierrez JF, Cozar-Olmo JM, Valero-Aguilera B. Adapting the content of cancer web sites to the information needs of patients: reliability and readability. *Telemed J E Health*. 2013;19:956-966.
2. Mallinger JB, Griggs JJ, Shields CG. Patient-centered care and breast cancer survivors' satisfaction with information. *Patient Educ Couns*. 2005;57:342-349.
3. Butow PN, Kazemi JN, Beeney LJ, Griffin AM, Dunn SM, Tattersall MH. When the diagnosis is cancer: patient communication experiences and preferences. *Cancer*. 1996;77:2630-2637.

A Team-Based Approach to Autopsy Education: Integrating Anatomic and Clinical Pathology at the Rotation Level

Hébert TM, Maleki S, Vasovic LV, et al (Albert Einstein College of Medicine, Bronx, NY)

Arch Pathol Lab Med 138:322-327, 2014

Context.—Pathology residency training programs should aim to teach residents to think beyond the compartmentalized data of specific rotations and synthesize data in order to understand the whole clinical picture when interacting with clinicians.

Objective.—To test a collaborative autopsy procedure at Montefiore Medical Center (Bronx, New York), linking residents and attending physicians from anatomic and clinical pathology in the autopsy process from the initial chart review to the final report. Residents consult with clinical pathology colleagues regarding key clinical laboratory findings during the autopsy. This new procedure serves multiple functions: creating a team-based, mutually beneficial educational experience; actively teaching consultative skills; and facilitating more in-depth analysis of the clinical laboratory findings in autopsies.

Design.—An initial trial of the team-based autopsy system was done from November 2010 to December 2012. Residents were then surveyed via questionnaire to evaluate the frequency and perceived usefulness of clinical pathology autopsy consultations.

Results.—Senior residents were the most frequent users of clinical pathology autopsy consultation. The most frequently consulted services were microbiology and chemistry. Eighty-nine percent of the residents found the clinical pathology consultation to be useful in arriving at a final diagnosis and clinicopathologic correlation.

Conclusion.—The team-based autopsy is a novel approach to integration of anatomic and clinical pathology curricula at the rotation level. Residents using this approach develop a more holistic approach to pathology, better preparing them for meaningful consultative interaction with clinicians. This paradigm shift in training positions us to better serve in our increasing role as arbiters of outcomes measures in accountable care organizations.

▶ Efforts to enhance pathology residency curricula for the purpose of increasing young pathologists' skills in synthesizing pathologic and clinical information into a meaningful and useful body of knowledge have been ongoing for many years. The ultimate purpose of improving residents' ability to integrate this information is to produce pathologists who are able and confident to act as true consultants to their clinical colleagues regarding all aspects of anatomic and clinical pathology testing and to produce collaborators in institutional decision making about all components of the testing pathway. This article describes an interesting method for promoting an increased understanding of clinical pathology testing in the context of performing autopsies. The need for sound integration of clinical and anatomic pathology knowledge and skills with the clinical knowledge required to perform meaningful autopsy reports is an interesting and unique method that pathology residency programs should consider for trial adoption into their own training. See reference list for further reading.[1,2]

D. M. Grzybicki, MD

References

1. Wells A, Smith BR. The goals of resident training in laboratory medicine in combined anatomic pathology/clinical pathology programs: an overview. *Clin Lab Med.* 2007;27:229-240.
2. Reeves S, Perrier L, Goldman J, Freeth D, Zwarenstein M. Interprofessional education: effects on professional practice and healthcare outcomes (update). *Cochrane Database Syst Rev.* 2013;(3):CD002213.

Recognition and Discrimination of Tissue-Marking Dye Color by Surgical Pathologists: Recommendations to Avoid Errors in Margin Assessment

Williams AS, Hache KD (Dalhousie Univ, Halifax, Nova Scotia, Canada)
Am J Clin Pathol 142:355-361, 2014

Objectives.—A variety of tissue-marking dye (TMD) colors can be used to indicate surgical pathology specimen margins; however, the ability of pathologists to differentiate between specific microscopic margin colors has not been assessed systematically. This study aimed to evaluate pathologists' accuracy in identifying TMD color and determine the least ambiguous combinations of colors for use in surgical pathology.

Methods.—Seven colors of TMD were obtained from three manufacturers and applied to excess formalin-fixed uterine tissue. Study blocks contained multiple tissue pieces, each marked with a different color from the same manufacturer. Slides were assessed by eight participants for color and color distinctness of each piece of tissue.

Results.—Black, green, red, and blue TMDs were accurately identified by most participants, but participants had difficulty identifying violet, orange, and yellow TMDs. Black, green, and blue TMDs were most commonly rated as "confidently discernable."

Conclusions.—Pathologists have difficulty identifying and distinguishing certain colors of TMDs. The combined use of certain colors of TMDs (yellow/orange/red, blue/violet, and red/violet) within the same specimen should be avoided to decrease the risk of inaccurately reporting specimen margins.

▶ This is an interesting and useful study to read, despite the fact that the topic may seem mundane or even unrequired for investigation. However, despite the use of a rainbow of tissue-marking dyes to indicate margins on surgical specimens, no one previously has systematically investigated which colors are the most useful, meaning those that pathologists can reliably see on specimens and distinguish from one another. It goes without saying that this ability is critical for patient safety. These authors' conclusions should serve to guide gross examination practice regarding dye marking of surgical margins. See reference list for additional reading.[1,2]

D. M. Grzybicki, MD

References

1. Paterson DA, Davies JD. Marking planes of surgical excision on breast biopsy specimens: use of artists' pigments suspended in acetone. *J Clin Pathol.* 1988; 41:1013-1016.
2. Milovancev M, Löhr C, Bildfell R, Gelberg HB, Heidel JR, Valentine BA. A comparison of microscopic ink characteristics of 35 commercially available surgical margin inks. *Vet Surg.* 2013;42:901-908.

Q-Probes Studies in Anatomic Pathology: Quality Improvement Through Targeted Benchmarking

Tworek JA, Volmar KE, McCall SJ, et al (St Joseph Mercy Health System, Ann Arbor, MI; Rex Healthcare, Raleigh, NC; Duke Univ Med Ctr, Durham, NC; et al)

Arch Pathol Lab Med 138:1156-1166, 2014

Context.—The Q-Probes program is a peer-comparison quality assurance service offered by the College of American Pathologists that was created in 1989.

Objective.—To establish national benchmarks around a specific quality metric at a specific point in time in anatomic pathology (AP).

Design.—Q-Probes are based on a voluntary subscription for an individual study. Hospital-based laboratories in the United States, Canada, and 16 other countries have participated. Approximately one-third of all Q-Probes studies address AP metrics. Each Q-Probes study has a primary quality indicator and additional minor indicators.

Results.—There have been 52 AP Q-Probes studies addressing process-, outcome-, and structure-related quality assurance issues. These Q-Probes studies often represented the first standardized national benchmark for specific metrics in the disciplines of cytopathology, surgical pathology, and autopsy pathology, and as such have been cited more than 1700 times in peer-reviewed literature. The AP Q-Probes studies that have been repeated over time demonstrate improvement in laboratory performance across an international spectrum.

Conclusions.—The Q-Probes program has produced important national benchmarks in AP, addressing preanalytic, analytic, and postanalytic factors in the disciplines of cytopathology, surgical pathology, and autopsy pathology. Q-Probes study data have been published, cited, and used in the creation of laboratory accreditation standards and other national guidelines.

▶ The College of American Pathologists Q-Probes studies have a long history of determining current state quality metrics in both anatomic and clinical pathology.[1] The article by Tworek et al described some of the seminal Q-Probes studies that are now considered benchmarks for the field. Tworek et al also discussed 2 Q-Probes studies that were repeated and assessed if the outcomes for these studies improved over time.[2] The first study was a repeated evaluation of the adequacy of surgical pathology reports for colorectal carcinoma, and the second was a study of compliance with the American Society of Clinical Oncology/College of American Pathologists guidelines for testing of HER2.[3,4] The adequacy of reporting of colorectal carcinoma improved considerably over time. The study of compliance with the guidelines for testing of HER2 showed more mixed results. Although some improvements were noted, it would be interesting to determine the degree of improvement in other Q-Probes activities.

S. Raab, MD

References

1. Zarbo RJ. Interinstitutional assessment of colorectal carcinoma surgical pathology report adequacy: a College of American Pathologists Q-Probes study of practice patterns from 532 laboratories and 15 940 reports. *Arch Pathol Lab Med.* 1992;116:1113-1119.
2. Idowu MO, Bekeris LG, Raab S, Ruby SG, Nakhleh RE. Adequacy of surgical pathology reporting of cancer: a college of American pathologists Q-Probes study of 86 institutions. *Arch Pathol Lab Med.* 2010;134:969-974.
3. Nakhleh RE, Grimm EE, Idowu MO, Souers RJ, Fitzgibbons PL. Laboratory compliance with the American society of clinical oncology/college of American pathologists guidelines for human epidermal growth factor receptor 2 testing: a College of American Pathologists survey of 757 laboratories. *Arch Pathol Lab Med.* 2010; 134:728-734.
4. Dyhdalo KS, Fitzgibbons PL, Goldsmith JD, Souers R, Nakhleh RE. Laboratory compliance with the American society of clinical oncology/college of American pathologists (ASCO/CAP) human epidermal growth factor receptor 2 testing guidelines: a 3-year comparison of validation procedures. *Arch Pathol Lab Med.* 2014;138:876-884.

A systematic analysis of commonly used antibodies in cancer diagnostics

Gremel G, Bergman J, Djureinovic D, et al (Uppsala Univ, Sweden; et al)
Histopathology 64:293-305, 2014

Aims.—Immunohistochemistry plays a pivotal role in cancer differential diagnostics. To identify the primary tumour from a metastasis specimen remains a significant challenge, despite the availability of an increasing number of antibodies. The aim of the present study was to provide evidence-based data on the diagnostic power of antibodies used frequently for clinical differential diagnostics.

Methods and Results.—A tissue microarray cohort comprising 940 tumour samples, of which 502 were metastatic lesions, representing tumours from 18 different organs and four non-localized cancer types, was analysed using immunohistochemistry with 27 well-established antibodies used in clinical differential diagnostics. Few antibodies, e.g. prostate-specific antigen and thyroglobulin, showed a cancer type-related sensitivity and specificity of more than 95%. A majority of the antibodies showed a low degree of sensitivity and specificity for defined cancer types. Combinations of antibodies provided limited added value for differential diagnostics of cancer types.

Tumour Site	N	Sensitivity [%]																									
		TG	PSA	MelanA	S100	GCDFP15	MGB	NapsinA	CHGA	CDX2	SYP	WT1	PR	HEPAR1	TTF1	ER	CK5	CK20	p63	VIL*	CEA	CA125	VIM	CK7	CK19	EMA	CK18	AE1/3
Colon	60	0	0	0	0	0	0	0	2	92	10	2	0	14	3	0	2	95	8	98	96	2	5	7	100	88	100	100
Stomach	60	0	3	0	0	0	0	0	5	37	15	0	2	37	7	0	2	57	12	90	88	22	5	76	98	93	100	100
Pancreas	60	0	0	0	0	0	0	0	4	8	14	4	0	16	6	0	24	80	49	80	88	82	31	100	100	100	98	100
Cholangiocarc.	44	0	0	0	0	0	0	0	5	15	10	2	0	15	10	0	5	51	27	93	64	56	13	100	100	100	100	100
Gall Bladder	8	0	0	0	0	0	0	0	0	0	0	0	0	0	13	0	13	63	38	88	25	63	13	88	100	88	100	100
Hepatocellular	30	0	0	0	0	0	0	0	0	0	0	0	3	100	0	3	0	7	3	52	0	0	0	28	4	7	100	100
Esophagus	22	0	0	0	0	0	0	5	0	0	5	5	0	9	9	0	91	5	100	0	27	32	50	55	86	95	64	100
Head and Heck	20	0	0	0	0	0	5	0	0	0	0	0	0	0	5	0	95	10	95	0	30	50	45	25	45	95	53	95
Lung Squamous	37	0	0	0	0	0	0	17	3	0	0	8	0	6	24	6	86	31	89	11	44	26	25	53	100	94	81	100
Lung Adenocarc.	63	0	0	0	0	0	2	81	0	0	10	5	3	16	84	13	7	25	52	36	70	66	39	100	100	100	100	100
Lung NOS	9	0	0	0	0	0	0	63	0	0	0	0	0	0	88	0	13	0	25	13	38	63	75	100	100	100	100	100
Breast	60	0	0	0	3	43	55	0	0	0	7	14	62	0	2	78	3	5	8	7	32	35	18	92	98	100	100	100
Ovary	60	0	0	0	3	2	0	0	2	0	2	98	35	7	3	63	48	7	28	15	0	98	45	100	100	100	100	100
Endometrium	60	0	0	0	0	2	14	12	31	0	2	17	61	8	5	64	36	14	31	19	14	93	84	95	93	100	98	98
Cervix	60	0	0	0	0	0	0	2	0	0	0	5	7	8	3	21	82	7	83	3	62	64	14	79	95	98	72	100
Renal Cell Carc.	40	0	0	0	0	0	3	5	0	0	0	5	0	5	3	0	0	3	0	31	0	10	95	25	46	85	87	98
Urothelial	20	0	0	0	0	0	0	0	0	0	5	5	0	0	5	0	55	75	90	0	35	30	20	85	95	90	100	100
Prostate	60	0	98	0	0	7	0	0	7	0	11	3	9	9	19	0	0	11	7	3	2	7	10	33	76	47	100	100
Testis	19	0	0	0	12	0	6	0	6	11	11	0	0	22	0	0	5	11	6	29	6	16	44	28	33	11	59	61
Thyroid	18	100	0	0	0	0	0	33	0	0	0	0	33	0	100	17	6	6	61	11	0	50	100	100	94	94	100	100
Melanoma	20	0	0	85	80	0	10	0	0	0	10	0	0	5	0	0	0	0	5	0	0	0	100	15	0	10	25	20
Lymphoma	20	0	0	0	0	0	0	0	0	0	0	0	0	5	0	0	0	0	60	0	0	0	90	5	0	25	0	0
Neuroendocrine	30	0	0	0	0	0	0	0	97	17	100	0	7	3	13	0	0	13	0	83	3	0	13	10	60	37	100	100
Sarcoma	60	0	0	0	7	0	2	0	2	0	2	25	15	2	10	8	0	2	14	3	0	0	100	5	2	32	10	17

FIGURE 1.—Marker sensitivities for all included tumours sites. A total of 940 tumor samples originating from 18 different tumours sites, and four non-localized cancer types were stained immunohistochemically with 27 clinically used antibodies (Compare Table 2). Cases with moderate and strong staining intensities and a fraction of stained cells equal to or higher than 2% were regards as positive. The percentage positively for each tumour site is equivalent to the market sensitivity. Darker shades of green represent higher sensitivity levels. *N*, Number of total samples: *for brush boarder pattern annotation of Villin, see Figure S4. (Reprinted from Gremel G, Bergman J, Djureinovic D, et al. A systematic analysis of commonly used antibodies in cancer diagnostics. *Histopathology.* 2014;64:293-305, with permission from Blackwell Publishing Lmt.)

TABLE 4.—Diagnostic Performance of Selected Antibody Panels

Tumour Site	Marker (Panel)	All Tumours (%) Sens.	All Tumours (%) Spec.	All Tumours (%) PPV	Adenocarcinomas Only (%) Sens.	Adenocarcinomas Only (%) Spec.	Adenocarcinomas Only (%) PPV
Lung adeno.	TTF1+	84	90	39	84	90	51
	NapsinA+	81	97	64	81	97	78
	TTF1+/NapsinA+	79	98	77	79	99	89
	TTF1+ or NapsinA+	85	89	36	85	88	48
	CK7+/CK20–	74	59	12	74	49	16
	TTF1+/CK7+/CK20–	65	95	47	65	94	60
	NapsinA+/CK7+/CK20–	60	97	63	60	97	76
	TTF1+/NapsinA+/CK7+/CK20–	60	98	73	60	99	88
	(TTF1+ or NapsinA+)/CK7+/CK20–	65	94	43	65	93	54
Colon	CK20+	95	79	24	95	71	29
	CDX2+	92	95	58	92	93	63
	CK20+/CDX2+	86	97	67	86	95	69
	CK20+ or CDX2+	100	77	23	100	69	29
	CK20+/CK7–	88	97	68	88	98	83
	CDX2+/CK7–	85	99	81	85	99	91
	CK20+/CDX2+/CK7–	80	99	89	80	99	92
	(CK20+ or CDX2+)/CK7–	93	99	81	93	97	82
Breast	MGB+	55	98	69	55	98	79
	GCDFP15+	43	99	81	43	99	81
	MGB+/GCDFP15+	27	100	94	27	100	94
	MGB+ or GCDFP15+	72	98	68	72	97	75
	ER+	78	87	31	78	82	35
	MGB+/ER+	49	99	77	49	99	90
	GCDFP15+/ER+	35	100	91	35	100	91
	MGB+/GCDFP15+/ER+	25	100	94	25	100	94
	(MGB+ or GCDFP15+)/ER+	60	99	84	60	99	84

+, Positive staining; –, Negative staining; /, and; sens., Sensitivity; spec., Specificity; PPV, Positive Predictive Value; adeno., Adenocarcinoma.

Reprinted from Gremel G, Bergman J, Djureinovic D, et al. A systematic analysis of commonly used antibodies in cancer diagnostics. *Histopathology.* 2014;64:293-305, with permission from Blackwell Publishing Lmt.

Conclusions.—The results from analysing 27 diagnostic antibodies on consecutive sections of 940 defined tumours provide a unique repository of data that can empower a more optimal use of clinical immunohistochemistry. Our results highlight the benefit of immunohistochemistry and the unmet need for novel markers to improve differential diagnostics of cancer (Fig 1 and Table 4).

▶ Gremel et al provide a fascinating look at the performance characteristics of antibody panels in cancer diagnostics. Fig 1 shows the sensitivity of individual antibodies for tumors of different origin; note that few antibodies achieve high levels of sensitivity and specificity for specific tumor types. Table 4 shows the performance characteristics of antibody panels. For example, for lung adenocarcinoma, the panel of TTF+ has a higher sensitivity and only a slightly lower specificity than the panel (TTF1+ or NapsinA+)/CK7+/CK20–. Larger antibody panels do not generally provide significantly added diagnostic value, which conflicts with a bias that greater discrimination may be added with more antibodies.

S. Raab, MD

Interpretive Diagnostic Error Reduction in Surgical Pathology and Cytology: Guideline From the College of American Pathologists Pathology and Laboratory Quality Center and the Association of Directors of Anatomic and Surgical Pathology

Nakhleh RE, Nosé V, Colasacco C, et al (Mayo Clinic, Jacksonville, FL; Massachusetts General Hosp, Boston; College of American Pathologists, Northfield, IL; et al)

Arch Pathol Lab Med, 2015 [Epub ahead of print]

Context.—Additional reviews of diagnostic surgical and cytology cases have been shown to detect diagnostic discrepancies.

Objective.—To develop, through a systematic review of the literature, recommendations for the review of pathology cases to detect or prevent interpretive diagnostic errors.

Design.—The College of American Pathologists Pathology and Laboratory Quality Center in association with the Association of Directors of Anatomic and Surgical Pathology convened an expert panel to develop an evidence-based guideline to help define the role of case reviews in surgical pathology and cytology. A literature search was conducted to gather data on the review of cases in surgical pathology and cytology.

Results.—The panel drafted 5 recommendations, with strong agreement from open comment period participants ranging from 87% to 93%. The recommendations are: (1) anatomic pathologists should develop procedures for the review of selected pathology cases to detect disagreements and potential interpretive errors; (2) anatomic pathologists should perform case reviews in a timely manner to avoid having a negative impact on patient care; (3) anatomic pathologists should have documented case review procedures that are relevant to their practice setting; (4) anatomic pathologists should continuously monitor and document the results of case reviews; and (5) if pathology case reviews show poor agreement within a defined case type, anatomic pathologists should take steps to improve agreement.

Conclusions.—Evidence exists that case reviews detect errors; therefore, the expert panel recommends that anatomic pathologists develop procedures for the review of pathology cases to detect disagreements and potential interpretive errors, in order to improve the quality of patient care (Table 3).

▶ Nakhleh and coauthors performed a literature review examining the frequency of error detected by secondary review of surgical pathology and cytopathology cases.[1] The median error detection frequency was 18.3% (n = 116 studies), and the major discrepancy frequency was 5.9% (n = 78 studies). The authors recommend performing secondary reviews as close in time as possible to case sign out

TABLE 3.—Summary of Studies That Express a Discrepancy or Major Discrepancy Rate

	Discrepancy Rates, %		Major Discrepancy Rates, %	
Study Type	No. of Studies	Median (25th-75th Percentile)	No. of Studies	Median (25th-75th Percentile)
All studies	116[c]	18.3 (7.5-34.5)	78[d]	5.9 (2.1-10.5)
Surgical pathology	84[e]	18.3 (7.5-37.4)	63[f]	6.3 (1.9-10.6)
Cytology	19[g]	24.8 (17.4-38.8)	11[h]	4.3 (2.8-7.5)
Both	13[i]	9.1 (6.7-15.8)	11[j]	5.9 (3.3-8.7)
Multiorgan	43[k]	9.1 (3.8-18.7)	42[l]	3.9 (1.1-7.4)
Single-organ[a]	73[m]	25.2 (14.0-43.7)	36[n]	8.0 (3.7-15.8)
Internal[b]	35[o]	10.9 (3.8-17.6)	22[p]	1.2 (0.30-3.1)
External	79[q]	23.0 (10.6-40.2)	56[r]	7.4 (4.6-14.7)

Editor's Note: Please refer to original journal article for full references.

[a]*Single-organ* refers to studies that focus on one organ or organ system; multiorgan refers to studies that are not limited with regard to organs studied.

[b]Internal refers to reviews of pathology reports within a single institution; external refers to reviews of cases given a diagnosis at a different institution.

[c]References 9-15, 19-22, 25, 29, and 35-129.

[d]References 7, 10, 11, 14, 15, 19, 21, 24-26, 29, 35, 36, 40, 42, 47, 48, 50-52, 54-57, 59, 63, 67-71, 73, 74, 76, 80, 82, 84-91, 94, 95, 97, 101, 102, 105, 106, 108, 113, 115, 117, 120-122, and 130-143.

[e]References 10-15, 19-21, 25, 29, 36, 37, 39, 40,43-9, 51, 53-64, 66, 70-81, 84, 87-89, 92-94,96-99, 101, 103-107, 112-115, 118-120, 122, and 124-128.

[f]References 10, 11, 14, 15, 19, 21, 25, 29, 36, 40, 47, 48, 51, 54-57, 59, 63, 70, 71, 73, 74, 76, 80, 84, 87-89, 94, 97, 101, 105, 106, 113, 115, 122, 130-137, and 139-143.

[g]References 38, 42, 50, 52, 82, 83, 85, 86, 95, 102, 109-111, 116, 117, 123, and 129.

[h]References 24, 42, 50, 52, 82, 85, 86, 95, 102, 117, and 138.

[i]References 9, 22, 35, 41, 65, 67-69, 90, 91, 100, 108, and 121.

[j]References 7, 26, 35, 67-69, 90, 91, 108, and 121.

[k]References 9, 14, 19-22, 25, 29, 35, 36, 42, 44, 47, 50, 52-54, 56, 59, 64-69, 71, 76, 80-82, 90, 91, 95, 100, 101, 108, 113, 116, 117, 120, and 121.

[l]References 7, 14, 19, 21, 24-26, 29, 35, 36, 42, 47, 50, 52, 54, 56, 59, 67-69, 71, 76, 80, 82, 90, 91, 95, 101, 108, 113, 117, 120, 121, 137, 140, 141, and 143.

[m]References 10-13, 15, 29, 37-41, 43, 45, 46, 48, 49, 51, 55, 57, 58, 60-63, 70, 72-75, 77-79, 83-89, 92-94, 96-99, 102-107, 109-112, 114, 115, 118, 119, and 122-129.

[n]References 10, 11, 15, 29, 40, 48, 51, 55, 57, 63, 70, 73, 74, 84-89, 94, 97, 102, 105, 106, 115, 122, 1.30-136, 138, 139, and 142.

[o]References 9, 19-22, 25, 29, 36, 38, 40, 42, 56, 57, 59, 61, 62, 65-69, 92, 95, 102, 110, 111, 115, 116, 120, 123, 125, and 126.

[p]References 19, 21, 24-26, 29, 36, 40, 42, 56, 57, 59, 67-69, 95, 115, 120, and 141.

[q]References 10-15, 35, 37, 39, 41, 43-55, 58, 60, 63, 64, 70-91, 93, 94, 96, 97, 99-109, 112-114, 117, 118, 121, 122, 124, and 127-129.

[r]References 7, 10, 11, 14, 15, 35, 47, 48, 50-52, 54, 55, 63, 70, 71, 73, 74, 76, 80, 82, 84-91, 94, 97, 101, 102, 105, 106, 108, 113, 117, 121, 122, 130-140, 142, and 143.

(thus reducing the potential impact of a diagnostic disagreement). I think the best option is to perform this before sign out, if at all possible.

S. Raab, MD

Reference

1. Nakhleh RE, Fitzgibbons PL, eds. Quality Management in Anatomic Pathology: Promoting Patient Safety Through Systems Improvement and Error Reduction. Northfield, IL: College of America Pathologists; 2005.

Utilization management in anatomic pathology

Lewandrowski K, Black-Schaffer S (Massachusetts General Hosp, Boston)

Clin Chim Acta 427:183-187, 2014

There is relatively little published literature concerning utilization management in anatomic pathology. Nonetheless there are many utilization management opportunities that currently exist and are well recognized. Some of these impact only the cost structure within the pathology department itself whereas others reduce charges for third party payers. Utilization management may result in medical legal liabilities for breaching the standard of care. For this reason it will be important for pathology professional societies to develop national utilization guidelines to assist individual practices in implementing a medically sound approach to utilization management (Table 1).

► The Institute of Medicine Committee on Utilization Management by Third Parties (1989) defined utilization management (UM) as "a set of techniques used by or on behalf of purchasers of health care benefits to manage health care costs by influencing patient care decision-making through case-by-case assessments of the appropriateness of care prior to its provision."[1] Lewandrowski and Black-Schaffer provide several examples in anatomic pathology (Table 1). UM describes proactive procedures (such as peer review) and is similar to the Donabedian health care quality assurance model. As in any quality assurance program, a UM program comprises roles, policies, processes, and criteria.[2] A criticism of UM is that it treats cost of care as an outcome metric, and many believe that the objectives of health care should be about patient quality

TABLE 1.—Potential Areas is for Utilization Management in Anatomic Pathology

1. Develop strategies to implement established national guidelines (e.g. frequency of PAP smears).
2. Not submitting selected specimens for pathologic examination.
3. Restricting low-risk pathology specimens to "gross-only" examination.
4. Develop protocols to limit the number of standard paraffin blocks taken from specific specimens.
5. Develop protocols to specify how many levels are required for specific specimen types.
6. Develop protocols that eliminate unnecessary sections from selected specimens (e.g. tumor margins remote from the primary tumor).
7. Develop protocols to specify how many tissue specimens can be included in one block (e.g. prostale needle biopsies).
8. Develop guidelines for when frozen sections are unnecessary.
9. Develop guidelines to specify appropriate special stains and immunohistochemistry studies for specific diagnoses.
10. Develop protocols to specify what molecular pathology studies are appropriate for specific tumors.
11. Review the necessity for internal review of outside pathology reports from institutions within a single health care network.
12. Develop a standardized evidence base for when cytopathology specimen acquisition may be more cost effective than surgical biopsy.
13. Develop a standardized evidence base for when a rapid on-site evaluation of cytopathology specimens is cost effective.

outcomes (safety, effectiveness, efficiency, timeliness, patient-centeredness, and equity).

S. Raab, MD

References

1. Field MJ. *Controlling Costs and Changing Patient Care?: The Role of Utilization Management*. National Academies Press; 1989.
2. Donabedian A. *An Introduction to Quality Assurance in Health Care*. Oxford University Press; 2003:92-93.

The Wonderful Colors of the Hematoxylin–Eosin Stain in Diagnostic Surgical Pathology

Chan JKC (Queen Elizabeth Hosp, Hong Kong, SAR China)
Int J Surg Pathol 22:12-32, 2014

The hematoxylin-eosin (H&E) stain has stood the test of time as the standard stain for histologic examination of human tissues. This simple dye combination is capable of highlighting the fine structures of cells and tissues. Most cellular organelles and extracellular matrix are eosinophilic, while the nucleus, rough endoplasmic reticulum, and ribosomes are basophilic. This review discusses the spectrum, intensity, and texture of colors observed in H&E-stained slides to illustrate their value in surgical pathology diagnosis. Changes in color of the nuclei occur in the presence of nuclear pseudoinclusions (such as papillary thyroid carcinoma) or inclusions (such as viral infection, surfactant, immunoglobulin, and biotin). The color of the cytoplasm of spindly cells can provide clues to their nature, such as basophilic (fibroblast), eosinophilic (smooth muscle and others), and amphophilic (myofibroblast). Eosinophilic globules have diagnostic value for sclerosing polycystic adenosis of salivary gland, low-grade B-cell lymphoma, solid pseudopapillary tumor of pancreas, and inclusion body fibromatosis. Eosinophilic granules are characteristic of granular cells (lysosome-rich), oncocytic cells (mitochondria-rich), and cells with secretory products (including neuroendocrine cells). Eosinophilic crystals can be diagnostic of lymphoma/plasmacytoma and crystal-storing histiocytosis. Basophilic granules or inclusions are diagnostic of acinic cell carcinoma and malakoplakia (Michaelis–Gutmann bodies). Yellow or brown inclusions are characteristic of hyalinizing trabecular adenoma of thyroid (yellow bodies), brown bowel syndrome, and malignant melanoma. Extracellular eosinophilic deposits can be produced by many conditions, but amyloid and monoclonal immunoglobulin deposition disease are important considerations. Extracellular basophilic deposits may be seen in small cell carcinoma and systemic lupus erythematosus, but they differ in that the former is blue (nuclear material) while the latter is purple (nuclear material plus immunoglobulin).

▶ Chan provided a great review article of the typical morphologic findings on the hematoxylin–eosin stain. For example, Table 2 from the original article points out the morphology, occurrence, and significance of nuclear pseudoinclusions and inclusions; classic (common and uncommon) pitfalls are described and shown in photomicrographs (such as biotin inclusions mimicking a pseudoinclusion). I think this review is of value for even the experienced pathologist, as the specific findings we see every day through our heuristic thinking patterns are rationally explained and depicted.

S. Raab, MD

Variable fidelity of tissue-marking dyes in surgical pathology

Williams AS, Dakin Haché K (Dalhousie Univ, Halifax, NS, Canada)
Histopathology 64:896-900, 2014

Aims.—Pathology specimens often contain important margins that must be identified from gross examination of specimens through to microscopic examination. Commonly, unique colours of tissue-marking dye (TMD) are applied to each margin, which facilitates both macroscopic and microscopic identification. Various techniques have been described, but the colour endurance and fidelity of TMDs following special tissue processing have not been addressed. The aim of this study was to evaluate the

TABLE 1.—Tissue-Marking Dye Endurance and Colour Fidelity

	Observed Microscopic Colour								
	DMS			CDI			Artists' Ink*		
TMD Colour	H&E	Decal.	IHC	H&E	Decal.	IHC	H&E	Decal.	IHC
Black	Black	Black	Black	Black	Black	Black	Black	Black	Black
Blue	Blue	Blue	Black	Blue	Blue	Blue	Blue	Blue	Blue
Green	Green	Green	Green	Green	Green	Green	Green†	Green†	Green†
Red	Grey‡	Grey‡	Grey‡	Red	Red	Red	Red§	Red§	Red§
Yellow	Yellow	Yellow	Yellow	Yellow	Yellow	Yellow	NA¶	NA¶	NA¶
Orange	Orange	Orange	Orange	Orange	Orange	Orange	Yellow	Yellow	Yellow
Violet	Violet	Grey**	Brown	Violet	Violet	Violet	Violet	Violet	Violet

CDI, Cancer Diagnostics Incorporated; Decal., pretreatment with decalcification solution (10% formic acid); DMS, Davidson Marking System; H&E, routine tissue processing and staining with H&E; IHC, immunohistochemistry protocol performed following routine tissue processing; TMD, tissue-marking dye.

*Daler-Rowney FW Artists' Acrylic Ink.

†Emerald Green (335) variably appeared black at low power (×25–×50), but was identifiable as green at higher power (×100–×400).

‡Two different lot numbers were tested several times, and both showed at least partial loss of colour, with a residual grey colourless material remaining at the margin.

§Only Crimson Red (513) survived tissue processing with a red microscopic colour.

¶A very minimal amount of colourless residue was present on microscopy; most yellow ink did not survive routine processing.

**Surface dye lost identifiable violet colour after 14 days of decalcification.

Reprinted from Williams AS, Dakin Haché K. Variable fidelity of tissue-marking dyes in surgical pathology. *Histopathology.* 2014;64:896-900, with permission from Blackwell Publishing Lmt.

performance of various TMDs through decalcification and immunohistochemistry (IHC) protocols.

Methods and Results.—Samples of TMDs from two manufacturers and acrylic artists' inks were obtained in seven colours and applied to excess non-diagnostic surgical pathology tissue. Tissues were subjected to a decalcification protocol or directly processed in a routine fashion. The presence and colour of TMD or ink were assessed on routine H&E sections and following IHC. Of the colours that reliably survived routine processing, loss of colour and colour change following decalcification and IHC protocols were seen with one manufacturer's product.

Conclusions.—TMD may lose or change its colour during special tissue processing. This previously unreported artefact may lead to potentially serious errors in margin assessment and reporting. Laboratories should evaluate TMDs and inks through routine processing, decalcification, and IHC protocols, to ensure colour endurance and fidelity (Table 1).

▶ Anatomic pathology laboratories always perform validation when a new immunohistochemical study is brought online. However, anatomic pathology laboratories often (or generally do not) perform a validation process when setting up a gross tissue inking procedure for tissue-marking dyes. Williams and Dakin Haché show the variability for different manufacturers and describe the potential pitfalls (Table 1). Needless to say, pathology laboratories spend a large amount of effort in assessing margin status, and variability of process may lead to improper assessment.

S. Raab, MD

Turnaround Time for Large or Complex Specimens in Surgical Pathology: A College of American Pathologists Q-Probes Study of 56 Institutions

Volmar KE, Idowu MO, Souers RJ, et al (Rex Pathology Associates, Raleigh, NC; Virginia Commonwealth Univ, Richmond; College of American Pathologists, Northfield, IL)

Arch Pathol Lab Med 139:171-177, 2015

Context.—Turnaround time (TAT) for large or complex surgical pathology specimens is an indicator of efficiency in anatomic pathology and may affect coordination of patient care.

Objective.—To establish benchmarks for TAT and to identify practice characteristics that may influence TAT.

Design.—Participants in a 2012 Q-Probes quality improvement program of the College of American Pathologists retrospectively reviewed all surgical pathology cases from the prior 6 months to identify up to 50 cases coded as Current Procedural Terminology (CPT) code 88307 (excluding biopsies) or 88309. Participants reported the times and dates of accessioning and final sign-out.

Results.—A total of 56 institutions reported on 2763 large or complex cases, which included 70% with CPT code 88307 and 30% with CPT code 88309. Cases requiring special handling comprised 51.5%, and 48.5% were routine. Among all institutions the median TAT was 2.72 calendar days (10th-90th percentile range, 6.23–1.22 days). Longer TAT occurred in governmental institutions (median, 6.06 versus 2.13 days; $P < .001$) and in institutions that mandate overnight fixation for some specimen types (median, 3.83 versus 2.07 days; $P = .03$). Longer TAT was associated with CPT code 88309 (median, 3.99 versus 2.82 days; $P < .001$), special handling (median, 4.13 versus 1.94 days; $P < .001$), frozen section (median, 3.38 versus 2.92 days; $P < .001$), radical cancer resection ($P < .001$), and malignant cases ($P < .001$). Turnaround time was not significantly affected by either pathology training programs or routine weekend sign-out.

Conclusions.—This study provides benchmark data for TAT in large or complex surgical pathology specimens. Turnaround time was good overall, but the range among participating institutions was wide.

▶ This Q-Probes study written by Volmar et al shows that participating laboratories generally had excellent turnaround times (TATs) for large specimens. The 10th percentile was only 6.23 days, which is only slightly longer than a workweek. Interestingly, a prior Q-Probes study from 1993 to 1994 reported the aggregate TAT for complex specimens was a mean 1.5 working days (range 0–5 days). I was particularly interested in the cases that laboratories mandated overnight fixation; breast specimens were the only case type that was mandated for overnight fixation in more than 50% of participating laboratories. The laboratories show a dedicated focus to the timeliness and patient-centeredness of patient care. For further reading, see reference list.[1,2]

S. Raab, MD

References

1. Zarbo RJ, Gephardt GN. *Surgical Pathology Complex Specimen Turnaround Time. Q-Probes 9309.* Northfield, IL: College of American Pathologists; 1993.
2. Patel S, Smith JB, Kurbatova E, Guarner J. Factors that impact turnaround time of surgical pathology specimens in an academic institution. *Hum Pathol.* 2012;43:1501-1505.

2 Hepatobiliary System and Pancreas

Acute Liver Allograft Antibody-Mediated Rejection: An Inter-Institutional Study of Significant Histopathological Features

O'Leary JG, Michelle Shiller S, Bellamy C, et al (Annette C. and Harold C. Simmons Transplant Inst, Dallas, TX; Baylor Univ Med Ctr, Dallas, TX; Edinburgh Univ, Scotland; et al)

Liver Transpl 20:1244-1255, 2014

Acute antibody-mediated rejection (AMR) occurs in a small minority of sensitized liver transplant recipients. Although histopathological characteristics have been described, specific features that could be used (1) to make a generalizable scoring system and (2) to trigger a more in-depth analysis are needed to screen for this rare but important finding. Toward this goal, we created training and validation cohorts of putative acute AMR and control cases from 3 high-volume liver transplant programs; these cases were evaluated blindly by 4 independent transplant pathologists. Evaluations of hematoxylin and eosin (H&E) sections were performed alone without knowledge of either serum donor-specific human leukocyte antigen alloantibody (DSA) results or complement component 4d (C4d) stains. Routine histopathological features that strongly correlated with severe acute AMR included portal eosinophilia, portal vein endothelial cell hypertrophy, eosinophilic central venulitis, central venulitis severity, and cholestasis. Acute AMR inversely correlated with lymphocytic venulitis and lymphocytic portal inflammation. These and other characteristics were incorporated into models created from the training cohort alone. The final acute antibody-mediated rejection score (aAMR score)—the sum of portal vein endothelial cell hypertrophy, portal eosinophilia, and eosinophilic venulitis divided by the sum of lymphocytic portal inflammation and lymphocytic venulitis—exhibited a strong correlation with severe acute AMR in the training cohort [odds ratio (OR) =2.86, $P < 0.001$] and the validation cohort (OR = 2.49, $P < 0.001$). SPSS tree classification was used to select 2 cutoffs: one that optimized specificity at a score >1.75 (sensitivity = 34%, specificity = 86%) and another that optimized sensitivity at a score >1.0 (sensitivity = 81%, specificity = 71%). In conclusion, the routine histopathological features of the aAMR score can be used to screen patients for acute AMR via routine H&E staining of indication liver transplant biopsy samples; however, a definitive diagnosis requires substantiation by DSA testing, diffuse C4d staining, and the exclusion of other insults.

▶ Aside from the new medications, which are leading to the clearance of chronic hepatitis C virus infection as an indication for liver transplantation, one of the major developments in the field of liver transplantation has been the recognition of acute antibody-mediated rejection in the liver. The 2013 Banff Conference on Liver Allograft Pathology was nearly exclusively dedicated to the discussion and proposal of criteria for hepatic antibody-mediated rejection. This article reviews some of the key histopathologic features of antibody-mediated rejection, several of which made their way into the proposed classification of acute antibody-mediated rejection in the liver. The keys to diagnosing antibody-mediated rejection in the liver is similar those of other organs in that the primary histologic finding is the presence of microvascular injury, including endothelial cell hypertrophy, capillaritis, and edema. However, it should be noted that a clinical pathologic diagnosis of acute antibody-mediated rejection requires evidence of graft dysfunction as well as the presence of donor-specific antibody by immunohistochemical staining. It is encouraging that simple screening of these biopsies before histologic features raising the possibility of antibody-mediated rejection is sufficient for selecting cases for additional analysis. Because of the infrequent nature of antibody-mediated rejection in hepatic allografts, it seems unreasonable to be performing routine C4d immunohistochemistry on all allograft biopsies.

For additional reading regarding specific antibodies in liver transplant patients, I refer the reader to O'Leary and Klintmalm.[1]

M. L. Smith, MD

Reference

1. O'Leary JG, Klintmalm GB. Impact of donor-specific antibodies on results of liver transplantation. *Curr Opin Organ Transplant.* 2013;18:279-284.

SALL4 Immunoreactivity Predicts Prognosis in Western Hepatocellular Carcinoma Patients but Is a Rare Event: A Study of 236 Cases

Liu T-C, Vachharajani N, Chapman WC, et al (Washington Univ School of Medicine, Saint Louis, MO)

Am J Surg Pathol 38:966-972, 2014

Prognostic biomarkers that stratify patients with cancer are needed. Recent studies from Asia have implicated SALL4, a stem cell marker, as useful in identifying aggressive cases of hepatocellular carcinoma (HCC), and >50% of the cases tested had upregulation by microarray or dense immunoreactivity. Given the differences in predominant etiologic factors between the Asian and Western HCC, we sought to determine the prevalence of SALL4 immunoreactivity and its clinical relevance in Western HCC patients. We constructed tissue microarrays from 236 adult HCCs. Two cores each of tumor and nontumor tissue were included for each case. SALL4 immunohistochemistry was scored in a semiquantitative manner and the results correlated with recurrence-free and overall survival, in addition to standard demographics. Among the 236 cases, 165 (70.0%) were male. The median age was 59 years (range: 19 to 83 y). The majority (78.4%) of patients were white, followed by African American (15.7%), Asian (3.8%), Hispanic (1.7%), and Native American (0.4%). The majority of patients had hepatitis C (42.8%), followed by alcoholic liver disease and hepatitis B (both 8.9%), and nonalcoholic steatohepatitis (3.8%). SALL4 immunoreactivity was detected in a total of 3 cases (1.3%), and nonreactivity was validated on tissue sections from 73 cases. By univariate analysis, the SALL4-positive cases had significantly higher tumor grade ($P = 0.0251$), more frequent lymphovascular invasion ($P = 0.0150$), and shorter recurrence-free survival (7.90 vs. 57.54 mo; $P = 0.0115$) and overall survival (7.90 vs. 64.87 mo; $P = 0.0018$). Although SALL4 immunoreactivity in Western HCC is correlated with higher grade and poor prognosis, this is a rare event. Therefore, universal application of SALL4 as a biomarker for HCC should be performed with caution.

▶ The use of SALL4, an immunohistochemical marker, has been increasing over the past decade. The primary use of SALL4 is the identification of a germ-cell tumor as SALL4 is positive in many germ-cell tumors including seminoma, dysgerminoma, embryonal carcinoma, yolk sac tumor, and intratubular germ-cell neoplasia. It also shows some reactivity for pre-B lymphoblastic leukemia/lymphoma. In addition, people have reported the use of SALL4 as a distinguishing stain of hepatoid gastric carcinoma versus hepatocellular carcinoma. However, the current study suggests SALL4 may not be a specific marker for gastric versus hepatocellular carcinoma as it is found in a minority of cases of hepatocellular carcinoma (1.3%). However, this study did find that, although it is a rare event, it is associated with poor prognostic features on univariate analysis. Unfortunately, multivariate analysis was not performed, likely due to the small number of SALL4-positive cases. Additional investigation into this transcriptional factor, which is required for embryonic development, is essential before widespread application of SALL4 from either a prognostic or a diagnostic perspective. As with many antibodies, the initial excitement over sensitivity and specificity usually wanes with additional studies.

For additional review of SALL4, I refer the reader to Liu et al.[1]

M. L. Smith, MD

Reference

1. Liu A, Cheng L, Du J, et al. Diagnostic utility of novel stem cell marker SALL4, OCT4, NANOG, SOX2, UTF1, and TCL1 in primary mediastinal germ cell tumors. *Am J Surg Pathol.* 2010;34:697-706.

Update on the New Classification of Hepatic Adenomas: Clinical, Molecular, and Pathologic Characteristics

Dhingra S, Fiel MI (Icahn School of Medicine at Mount Sinai, NY)

Arch Pathol Lab Med 138:1090-1097, 2014

Context.—Hepatic adenoma is an uncommon, benign, hepatic neoplasm that typically occurs in women of child-bearing age, often with a history of long-term use of oral contraceptive drugs. This is usually detected as an incidental mass lesion in a noncirrhotic liver during imaging studies. Pathologic evaluation by needle core biopsy remains the gold standard for diagnosis. Molecular studies have revealed that hepatic adenomas involve unique molecular pathways that are distinct from hepatocellular carcinoma. Based on these studies, a French collaborative group has recently proposed a molecular-pathologic classification for hepatic adenomas. In addition, advances in molecular studies have led to reclassification of the "telangiectatic variant of focal nodular hyperplasia" as "hepatic adenoma, inflammatory subtype."

Objective.—To review the proposed, new classification of hepatic adenoma and the changes in diagnostic workup in light of the abovementioned developments.

Data Sources.—Review of published literature and illustrations from clinical case material.

Conclusions.—Definitive diagnosis of liver mass lesion on needle core biopsies has a decisive role in clinical management. With the advent of the new classification of hepatic adenomas and its prognostic implications, it is vital for pathologists to be aware of the morphologic features seen in different subtypes and the available diagnostic tools, such as immunohistochemistry, to help identify the correct subtype (Table 1).

▶ This is an excellent review article to bring the reader up to date on the latest classification of hepatocellular adenomas and its clinical significance. Many pathologists have a relatively limited differential diagnosis for benign hepatocellular lesions of the liver, including focal nodular hyperplasia and hepatocellular adenoma. However, extensive studies over the last decade have studied hepatocellular adenomas and their additional subclassification with regard to risk for transformation to hepatocellular carcinoma. Of particular interest is the so-called β-catenin–mutated hepatocellular adenoma, which has an increased risk of hepatocellular carcinoma development and is seen in atypical settings, such as older patients, male patients, and with atypical histologic features. Fortunately, the β-catenin–mutated hepatocellular adenoma is fairly easily recognized with appropriate immunohistochemical stains, including β-catenin and glutamine synthetase. These hepatocellular adenomas show nuclear overexpression of β-catenin and strong nuclear and cytoplasmic overexpression of glutamine synthetase, a downstream enzyme in the β-catenin pathway. These adenomas are important to recognize because of the aforementioned clinical significance. A summary of the different types of hepatocellular adenomas is given in Table 1. It should be noted that if a pathologist were to

TABLE 1.—Hepatic Adenoma Subtypes, Frequencies, Molecular Findings, Pathologic Features, and Immunohistochemistry

HA Subtype	Frequency Range, %	Molecular Findings	Pathologic Features	Immunohistochemistry
HA-H	35–40	Somatic mutations of (85%) *TCF1* (*HNF1A*) gene; heterozygous germline mutations (<5%) of *CYP1B1* gene	Steatosis, lack of inflammation, and cytologic atypia	Decreased or absent L-FABP in neoplastic hepatocytes, compared with nonneoplastic liver; patchy CD34 expression; focal, interspersed CK7 positivity in small hepatocytes
HA-B	15–19	β-catenin gene–activating mutations	Pseudoacinar pattern, cytologic atypia, steatosis, and/or lack of inflammation	Increased nuclear β-catenin protein expression; strong diffuse glutamine synthetase positivity
HA-I	30–35	Gain-of-function mutations of the *IL6ST* gene; 10% with coexisting β-catenin gene mutations	Pseudoportal tracts with thick-walled arteries and lack of bile ducts or veins; inflammatory infiltrate; ductular reaction; sinusoidal dilatation; and peliosis	Diffuse, strong serum amyloid-A and C-reactive protein expression; CD34 reactivity around pseudoportal tracts; diffuse glutamine synthetase positivity if associated with β-catenin mutation
HA-U	10	No specific mutations	No distinctive morphology	No specific protein expression

Abbreviations: HA-B, β-catenin–mutated hepatic adenoma; HA-H, *HNF1A*-mutated hepatic adenoma; HA-I, inflammatory hepatic adenoma; HA-U, hepatic adenoma, not otherwise specified; L-FABP, liver-type fatty acid binding protein expression.

Reproduced with permission of College of American Pathologists from Dhingra S, Fiel MI. Update on the new classification of hepatic adenomas: clinical, molecular, and pathologic characteristics. *Arch Pathol Lab Med.* 2014;138:1090-1097; permission conveyed through Copyright Clearance Center, Inc.

consider working up one antibody for the evaluation of benign hepatocellular lesions, glutamine synthetase would be an ideal candidate, as it has several uses in the differential diagnosis of different hepatocellular adenomas, focal nodular hyperplasia, and diagnosing malignancy and hepatocellular carcinoma.

For additional reading on the classification of hepatocellular carcinoma, I refer the reader to Bioulac-Sage et al.[1]

M. L. Smith, MD

Reference

1. Bioulac-Sage P, Laumonier H, Couchy G, et al. Hepatocellular adenoma management in phenotypic classification: the bordeaux experience. *Hepatology*. 2009;50: 481-489.

Diagnostic utility and limitations of glutamine synthetase and serum amyloid-associated protein immunohistochemistry in the distinction of focal nodular hyperplasia and inflammatory hepatocellular adenoma.

Joseph NM, Ferrell LD, Jain D, et al (Univ of California, San Francisco; Yale Univ, New Haven, CT; et al)

Mod Pathol 27:62-72, 2014

Inflammatory hepatocellular adenoma can show overlapping histological features with focal nodular hyperplasia, including inflammation, fibrous stroma, and ductular reaction. Expression of serum amyloid-associated protein in inflammatory hepatocellular adenoma and map-like pattern of glutamine synthetase in focal nodular hyperplasia can be helpful in this distinction, but the pitfalls and limitations of these markers have not been established. Morphology and immunohistochemistry were analyzed in 54 inflammatory hepatocellular adenomas, 40 focal nodular hyperplasia, and 3 indeterminate lesions. Morphological analysis demonstrated that nodularity, fibrous stroma, dystrophic blood vessels, and ductular reaction were more common in focal nodular hyperplasia, while telangiectasia, hemorrhage, and steatosis were more common in inflammatory hepatocellular adenoma, but there was frequent overlap of morphological features. The majority of inflammatory hepatocellular adenomas demonstrated perivascular and/or patchy glutamine synthetase staining (73.6%), while the remaining cases had diffuse (7.5%), negative (3.8%), or patchy pattern of staining (15%) that showed subtle differences from the classic map-like staining pattern and was designated as pseudo map-like staining. Positive staining for serum amyloid-associated protein was seen in the majority of inflammatory hepatocellular adenomas (92.6%) and in the minority of focal nodular hyperplasia (17.5%). The glutamine synthetase staining pattern was map-like in 90% of focal nodular hyperplasia cases, with the remaining 10% of cases showing pseudo map-like staining. Three cases were labeled as indeterminate and showed focal nodular hyperplasia-like morphology but lacked map-like glutamine synthetase staining pattern; these cases demonstrated a patchy pseudo map-like glutamine synthetase

TABLE 2.—Histological Features of Focal Nodular Hyperplasia (FNH) and Inflammatory Hepatocellular Adenoma (IHA)

	FNH (n = 40)	IHA (n = 54)	*P*-value*	Indeterminate (n = 3)
Nodular architecture	34/40 (85)	4/54 (7.4)	< 0.001	1/3 (33)
Fibrous bands	36/40 (90)	14/54 (26)	< 0.001	1/3 (33)
Naked arterioles	8/36 (22)	30/50 (60)	0.001	1/3 (33)
Ductular reaction	33/40 (83)	23/54 (43)	< 0.001	1/3 (33)
Pseudo-portal tracts	8/36 (22)	36/50 (72)	< 0.001	0
Lymphocytic inflammation	19/40 (48)	32/53 (60)	0.08	1/3 (33)
Sinusoidal dilatation	7/39 (18)	44/53 (83)	< 0.001	1/3 (33)
Hemorrhage	2/39 (5)	35/50 (70)	< 0.001	0
Steatosis	8/39 (21)	31/54 (57)	< 0.001	0

**P*-values reflect comparison between focal nodular hyperplasia (FNH) and inflammatory hepatocellular adenoma (IHA); numbers in parentheses reflect percentages.

Reprinted from Joseph NM, Ferrell LD, Jain D, et al. Diagnostic utility and limitations of glutamine synthetase and serum amyloid-associated protein immunohistochemistry in the distinction of focal nodular hyperplasia and inflammatory hepatocellular adenoma. *Mod Pathol.* 2014;27:62-72.

pattern along with the expression of serum amyloid-associated protein. Our results highlight the diagnostic errors that can be caused by variant patterns of staining with glutamine synthetase and serum amyloid-associated protein in inflammatory hepatocellular adenoma and focal nodular hyperplasia (Table 2).

▶ The main finding from this study is that the maplike pattern of glutamine synthetase reactivity is not entirely specific for focal nodular hyperplasia and that overexpression of C-reactive protein (CRP) or serum amyloid A protein is not entirely specific for inflammatory hepatocellular adenoma. However, in my opinion, for the general surgical pathologist, the most important information from this study is found in Table 2, where the authors review the histologic features of a total of 94 focal nodular hyperplasia and inflammatory adenomas. Close inspection of this table reveals that a nodular architecture, fibrous bands, and a ductular reaction are fairly strong histologic indicators for focal nodule hyperplasia, particularly when all 3 are present. Alternatively, naked arterioles within the hepatoid parenchyma, pseudoportal tracts, sinusoidal dilation, and hemorrhage are fairly specific histologic indicators for inflammatory adenomas. Using these histologic criteria carefully, one can arrive at a presumptive diagnosis based on the histologic features alone. If the CRP, serum amyloid A protein, or glutamine synthetase staining is in keeping with that initial histologic presumptive diagnosis, a definitive diagnosis can be rendered. However, there will be some that remain indeterminate, both from a histologic and an immunohistochemical perspective. Interestingly, the indeterminate cases showed a pseudo-maplike staining pattern as well as overexpression of serum amyloid A protein. This does raise the possibility that there may be an overlap in the spectrum of focal nodular hyperplasia versus inflammatory hepatocellular adenoma.

For additional review on this topic, I refer the reader to Bioulac-Sage et al.[1]

M. L. Smith, MD

Reference

1. Bioulac-Sage P, Cubel G, Taouji S, et al. Immunohistochemical markers on needle biopsies are helpful for the diagnosis of focal nodular hyperplasia in hepatocellular adenoma subtypes. *Am J Surg Pathol.* 2012;36:1691-1699.

Different collagen types show distinct rates of increase from early to late stages of hepatitis C-related liver fibrosis

Chen W, Rock JB, Yearsley MM, et al (Ohio State Univ Wexner Med Ctr, Columbus; et al)

Hum Pathol 45:160-165, 2014

During progression from normal liver to cirrhosis, total collagen increases nearly 10-fold with an abnormal increase in fibril-forming collagen and other extracellular matrix molecules. However, little is known regarding the changes each collagen type undergoes during fibrogenesis. We assessed the different collagen types by immunohistochemistry at various stages of hepatitis C-related liver fibrosis in core biopsies and compared changes in each with trichrome stain to better understand fibrogenesis. The possible utility in staging fibrosis was investigated. We found collagens III, IV, V, VI, vitronectin, and trichrome all showed statistically significant increases from early to late stages of fibrosis, but with temporal and quantitative differences. During the transition from early to late fibrosis, trichrome (stains primarily collagen I) and collagen IV showed the steepest increase and appear to be the most useful discriminators between early and late stages of fibrosis. Collagens V and VI have strong reactivity even in stage 1, which may be helpful in identifying early fibrosis when trichrome is weak or negative. Collagen III and vitronectin showed the most gradual increase. Interestingly, collagen V also showed increased staining in areas around inflammation/edema, which may overestimate established fibrosis as compared with trichrome (Fig 4).

▶ In today's health care environment of cost cutting, surgical pathologists must continue to investigate ways to add diagnostic and prognostic utility to the general surgical pathology report. This article highlights the variations in collagen deposition as fibrosis progresses from early to late stage in chronic hepatitis C-infected livers. Several interesting findings are identified. Not unexpectedly there is a general increase in all the types of collagen from early- to late-stage fibrosis. However, it should be noted that the trichrome stain and collagen 4 staining seems to be the most useful discriminator between early- and late-stage fibrosis. Fig 4 highlights the increase in the different types of collagen, trichrome, and fibronectin staining throughout the stages of liver fibrosis. Notably, collagens 5 and 6 may have some clinical usefulness in the identification of early fibrosis, particularly in the setting of necroinflammatory activity. In the pulmonary fibrosis literature, there is significant interest recently on antifibrotic agents, such as pirfenidone. There have been some initial investigations in the use of antifibrotics in chronic liver disease as well. It would be interesting

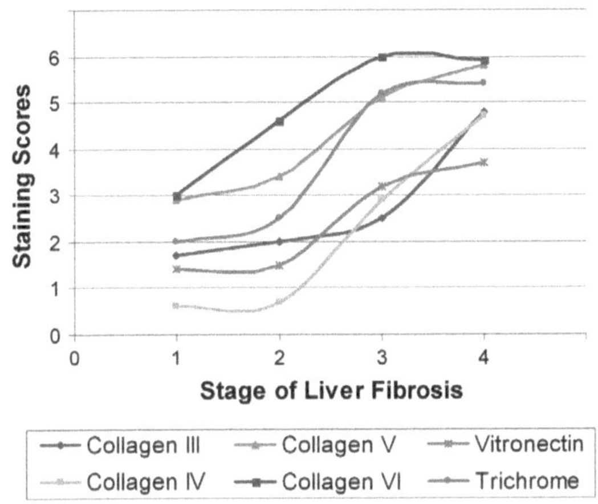

FIGURE 4.—Extracellular matrix staining scores at various stages of fibrogenesis. (Reprinted from Human Pathology. Chen W, Rock JB, Yearsley MM, et al. Different collagen types show distinct rates of increase from early to late stages of hepatitis C-related liver fibrosis. *Hum Pathol.* 2014;45:160-165, with permission from Elsevier.)

to better understand the role that antifibrotics such as pirfenidone play on the development of the different types of collagen fibrosis to better understand the pathophysiology of the development of fibrosis within the hepatic parenchyma.

For additional review of staining of different types of collagens in liver specimens, I refer the reader Ferrell and Greenberg.[1]

M. L. Smith, MD

Reference

1. Ferrell L, Greenberg MS. Special stains can distinguish hepatic necrosis with regenerative nodules from cirrhosis. *Liver International.* 2007;27:681-686.

Quantification of portal–bridging fibrosis area more accurately reflects fibrosis stage and liver stiffness than whole fibrosis or perisinusoidal fibrosis areas in chronic hepatitis C

Sandrini J, Boursier J, Chaigneau J, et al (Univ Hosp, Angers, France; LUNAM Univ, Angers, France; et al)

Mod Pathol 27:1035-1045, 2014

Morphometry provides an objective evaluation of fibrosis in liver diseases. We developed an image analysis algorithm using automated thresholding and segmentation to separately quantify the areas and the fractal dimensions of portal–bridging fibrosis and perisinusoidal fibrosis in chronic hepatitis C liver biopsies. We studied 427 digitized liver biopsies and compared the automated measures of the different fibrosis compartments with (1) the Metavir F (fibrosis) and A (activity) histological scores,

(2) the digitally assessed area of steatosis, and (3) the liver stiffness measured by elastography (Fibroscan). The perisinusoidal fibrosis area was higher than that of portal fibrosis in stages ≤F2; it reached its highest value in F2 stage and stabilized thereafter. The F3 stage was characterized by equal proportions of portal–bridging and perisinusoidal fibrosis, whereas portal–bridging area was predominant in cirrhosis. Measurement of portal–bridging fibrosis showed highly significantly different values between contiguous F stages; the ratio of portal–bridging fibrosis/perisinusoidal fibrosis displayed less overlap between Metavir stages than did the whole fibrosis area values. Fractal dimension showed that portal–bridging fibrosis tended to display a homogeneous surface-like spatial organization, whereas perisinusoidal fibrosis appeared more heterogeneous according to stage and curvilinear. The portal–bridging fibrosis area was low in cases with low Metavir activity and little steatosis, and became predominant with increasing activity and steatosis. Using stepwise multiple linear regression analysis, the liver stiffness was independently correlated to the portal–bridging fibrosis area (first step, $P < 0.001$), the steatosis area (second step, $P < 0.001$), and the Metavir A grade (third step, $P = 0.001$), but not to the perisinusoidal fibrosis area. Automated quantification in a large cohort of chronic hepatitis C showed that perisinusoidal fibrosis progressively grew in early fibrosis stages but did not increase in septal or cirrhotic stages and that the portal–bridging fibrosis area appeared as a more accurate tool to assess fibrosis progression than the whole fibrosis area.

▶ Because of the noninvasive nature of measuring liver fibrosis by elastography, Fibroscan has become increasingly used in clinical practice. We have observed a dramatic decrease in the number of liver biopsies we perform for staging of chronic hepatitis C virus infection due to the active use of elastography within our multidisciplinary practice. Elastography has the benefit of measuring the amount of fibrosis in a much larger area compared with a needle core biopsy. It is estimated that the elastography measures a core of liver tissue approximately 10 cm long and 1 cm in diameter, as opposed to a needle core biopsy, which is typically 0.2 cm in diameter and approximately 1.5 cm in length. Because of this disadvantage, it seems reasonable to go back to the surgical liver biopsy to investigate how the liver biopsy can be used to add further clinical value. This article correlates the different areas of liver fibrosis with the Metavir fibrosis stage and Fibroscan. Interestingly, the area of portal-to-portal bridging fibrosis correlated better with the degree of liver stiffness as measured by Fibroscan, when compared with the surface area of whole fibrosis, perisinusoidal fibrosis, and the ratio of portal–bridging fibrosis to perisinusoidal fibrosis. This suggests that it is the degree of portal-to-portal bridging fibrosis that contributes the most to liver stiffness, as measured by Fibroscan. One of the challenges associated with this case is that the measurements are not related to any outcomes data. Therefore, even though it is identified that the degree of portal-to-portal bridging fibrosis correlates best with Fibroscan, this may not necessarily relate to more advanced clinical disease. Further studies are required to investigate this relationship and to determine whether Fibroscan can supplant the biopsy in a wide variety of etiologic causes of liver disease.

For an additional review on elastography, I refer the reader to Castera et al.[1]

M. L. Smith, MD

Reference

1. Castera L, Forns X, Alberti A. Non-invasive evaluation of liver fibrosis using transient elastography. *J Hepatol.* 2008;48:835-847.

Discrepancy rates in liver biopsy reporting

Colling R, Verrill C, Fryer E, et al (Oxford Univ Hosps NHS Trust, UK; et al)

J Clin Pathol 67:825-827, 2014

Medical liver biopsy reporting is challenging, and maintaining competency with small case numbers is potentially difficult. This study evaluates the discrepancies identified in cases referred to a specialist centre between the specialist reports and those of the referring general departments. Fifty consecutive recently referred cases were selected, and original and final reports were compared. Discrepancies were classified as per the Royal College of Pathologists guidelines and scored for potential clinical impact. The overall rate of discrepancy was 38% with most of these due to differences in interpretation of morphology. Seventy per cent of these discrepancies were judged to have major clinical impact (26% of all referred cases). This study highlights the need for robust systems of quality control of liver biopsies in a general setting (Table 2).

▶ This article highlights the relative difficulties associated with nonneoplastic liver biopsy interpretation. Table 2 highlights the large number of discrepancies found from only 50 consecutive referred cases. One of the surprising aspects of this review is the large number of so-called B1 discrepancies. B1 discrepancies, according to the Royal College of Pathologists, are defined as a diagnosis that one is surprised to see from any pathologist (eg, an obvious cancer reported as benign). Approximately 10% of this group's recently referred liver biopsy specimens received a type B1 discrepancy designation. Two of the cases originally signed out as normal were found to have fairly significant disease. It is interesting that several of the referral report diagnoses on the cases that were discrepant have to do with biliary or vascular disease—9 of the 19 cases. Most liver pathologists recognize the fact that biliary disease can be focal and subtle, and if one is not trained specifically to look for biliary disease, it is easily missed. One of the main findings in chronic biliary disease is the presence of ductopenia. It is difficult for general surgical pathologists not familiar with liver pathology to recognize the absence of a structure as opposed to the presence of a pathologic finding. One of the take-home points from this article is that pathologists who see liver biopsies only rarely in their general pathology practice should have a low threshold for obtaining second opinions.

TABLE 2.—A Breakdown of Each Discrepancy Found and the Categorisation of this into Discrepancy Type and Potential Clinical Impact Score

Biopsy	Original Report	Referral Report	Discrepancy Type	Impact Score
Three cores, 14 portal tracts, 9 central veins*	Normal, no fibrosis	ASH/NASH, chronic hepatitis with mild fibrosis	B1	3
Two cores, 14 portal tracts, 14 central veins*	Granulomatous inflammation ? TB/sarcoid, no fibrosis	PBC added to differential, mild fibrosis	B1	3
Two cores, 16 and 6 mm, 14 portal tracts, 3 central veins	Chronic active inflammation	Steatohepatitis, and bile duct injury with CBP deposition? biliary disease	B1	3
Single 7 mm core, 2 portal tracts, 7 central veins*	Normal, no fibrosis	Ductopaenia, mild fibrosis and CBP deposition? biliary disease	B1	3
Four cores, 12 portal tracts, 17 central veins*	AIH, no fibrosis	Acute hepatitis with cholestasis and mild fibrosis, no evidence of AIH	B1	3
Two cores, 14 and 16 mm, 17 portal tracts, 17 central veins	Non-specific minor abnormalities	NRH and VO obstruction	B2	3
Single disrupted core, 7 portal tracts, 3 central veins	Cirrhosis	Cirrhosis with features of PSC	B2	3
Two cores, 20 and 21 mm, 9 portal tracts, 8 central veins*	PBC no fibrosis	PBC moderate fibrosis	B2	2
Two cores, 16 portal tracts, 12 central veins*	HBV mild fibrosis	HBV moderate fibrosis	B3	2
Two cores, 10 portal tracts, 8 central veins*	?PSC minor fibrosis	?PSC moderate fibrosis	B3	2
Multiple fragmented cores, 14 portal tracts, 9 central veins*	HBV fibrosis cannot be assessed	HBV mild fibrosis	B3	2
Three cores, 22 portal tracts, 9 central veins	PBC and AIH overlap	PBC no AIH	B3	3
One core, 9 portal tracts, 4 central veins*	Cirrhosis	Cirrhosis with resolving steatohepatitis	B3	3
Three cores, 22 portal tracts, 17 central veins*	AIH	?PSC	B3	2
Three cores	Lymphoma, no fibrosis	Chronic inflammation, mild fibrosis	B3	3
One core, 13 mm, 6 portal tracts, 5 central veins*	Non-specific minor abnormalities, no fibrosis	?PSC with mild fibrosis	B3	3
One core, 12 mm, 9 portal tracts, 3 central veins	ALD ?AIH	ALD possible biliary component	B3	2
One core, 15 portal tracts, 4 central veins	PSC with moderate fibrosis	Gallstone injury (high alk phos, gallbladder of same case showed chronic cholecystitis) with mild fibrosis	C	3
Two cores, 19 portal tracts	Cirrhosis ?cause	ALD (clinical history of high alcohol intake and raised GTT)	C	3

AIH, autoimmune hepatitis; ALD, alcoholic liver disease; ASH, alcoholic steatohepatitis; CBP, copper binding protein; HBV, hepatitis B virus; NASH, non-alcoholic steatohepatitis; NRH, nodular regenerative hyperplasia; PBC, primary biliary sclerosis; PSC, primary sclerosing cholangitis; TB, tuberculosis; VO, venous outflow obstruction.

*Cases reviewed due to transfer of clinical care.

Reproduced from Colling R, Verrill C, Fryer E, et al. Discrepancy rates in liver biopsy reporting. *J Clin Pathol.* 2014;67:825-827, with permission from the BMJ Publishing Group Ltd.

For additional reading on this topic, I refer the reader to Bejarano et al.[1]

M. L. Smith, MD

Reference

1. Bejarano PA, Koehler A, Sherman KE. Second opinion pathology in liver biopsy interpretation. *Am J Gastroenterol*. 2001;96:3158-3164.

Poorly differentiated neuroendocrine carcinomas of the pancreas: a clinicopathologic analysis of 44 cases

Basturk O, Tang L, Hruban RH, et al (Memorial Sloan-Kettering Cancer Ctr, NY; Johns Hopkins Univ, Baltimore, MD; et al)

Am J Surg Pathol 38:437-447, 2014

Background.—In the pancreas, poorly differentiated neuroendocrine carcinomas include small cell carcinoma and large cell neuroendocrine carcinoma and are rare; data regarding their pathologic and clinical features are very limited.

Design.—One hundred and seven pancreatic resections originally diagnosed as poorly differentiated neuroendocrine carcinomas were reassessed using the classification and grading (mitotic rate/Ki67 index) criteria put forth by the WHO in 2010 for the gastroenteropancreatic system. Immunohistochemical labeling for neuroendocrine and acinar differentiation markers was performed. Sixty-three cases were reclassified, mostly as well-differentiated neuroendocrine tumor or acinar cell carcinoma, and eliminated. The clinicopathologic features and survival of the remaining 44 poorly differentiated neuroendocrine carcinomas were further assessed.

Results.—The mean patient age was 59 years (range, 21–82) and the male/female ratio was 1.4. Twenty-seven tumors were located in the head of the pancreas, 3 in the body and 11 in the tail. The median tumor size was 4 cm (range, 2–18). Twenty-seven tumors were large cell neuroendocrine carcinomas and 17 were small cell carcinomas (mean mitotic rate, 37/10 HPF and 51/10 HPF; mean Ki67 index, 66% and 75%, respectively). Eight tumors had combined components, mostly adenocarcinomas. In addition, 2 tumors had components of well differentiated neuroendocrine tumor. Eighty-eight percent of the patients had nodal or distant metastatic disease at presentation and an additional 7% developed metastases subsequently. Follow-up information was available for 43 patients; 33 died of disease with a median survival of 11 months (range, 0–104); 8 were alive with disease, with a median follow-up of 19.5 months (range, 0–71). The 2-year and 5-year survival rates were 22.5% and 16.1%, respectively.

Conclusion.—Poorly differentiated neuroendocrine carcinoma of the pancreas is a highly aggressive neoplasm, with frequent metastases and poor survival. Most patients die within less than a year. Most (61%) are large cell neuroendocrine carcinomas. Well differentiated neuroendocrine tumor and acinar cell carcinoma are often misdiagnosed as poorly

TABLE 4.—Differential Diagnosis of Pancreatic Poorly Differentiated Neuroendocrine Carcinoma

	Poorly Differentiated Neuroendocrine Carcinoma	Well Differentiated Neuroendocrine Tumor	Acinar Cell Carcinoma*	Primitive Neuroectodermal Tumor
Histology	• Markedly cellular • Solid and nesting growth patterns • Acinar (glandular) units or pseudorosettes may be present. • Substantial necrosis	• Less cellular • Various organoid growth patterns • Limited or no necrosis	• Markedly cellular • Solid and acinar growth patterns • Necrosis may be extensive. • Eosinophilic granular cytoplasm	• Markedly cellular • Diffuse growth pattern • Pseudorosettes may be present.
Nuclei	• Hyperchromatic nuclei and inconspicuous nucleoli (small cell) • Vesicular chromatin or prominent nucleoli (large cell)	• Monotonous, round nuclei with vesicular chromatin • Nucleoli may be seen.	• Monotonous nuclei • Solitary large nucleoli	• Small, round monotonous nuclei • Inconspicuous nucleoli
Mitoses/10 HPF**	High (by definition >20 [1]; usually >30)	Low to intermediate (by definition ≤20 [1])	Variable but usually high (>20)	Variable but usually high (>20)
Ki67 Labeling Index	High (by definition >20%; usually >40%)	High (by definition ≤20%)	Variable but usually high (>20%)	Variable but usually high (>20%)
Immunohistochemistry				
Keratins	Positive	Positive	Positive	Usually positive [33]
Trypsin/Chymotrypsin	Rare, scattered cells may be positive.	Rare, scattered cells may be positive.	Positive	Negative
Chromogranin	Positive, may be weak or focal	Positive, usually strongly	Rare, scattered cells may be positive.	Usually negative [33]
Synaptophysin	Positive, may be weak or focal	Positive, usually strongly	Rare, scattered cells may be positive.	Usually negative [33]
CD99	Negative	May be positive (45% of cases) [38].	Negative	Positive (diffuse, membranous)

Editor's Note: Please refer to original journal article for full references.
*Mixed acinar-neuroendocrine carcinomas exhibit both acinar and neuroendocrine features.
**HPF High power field
Reprinted from Basturk O, Tang L, Hruban RH, et al. Poorly differentiated neuroendocrine carcinomas of the pancreas: a clinicopathologic analysis of 44 cases. *Am J Surg Pathol.* 2014;38:437-447.

differentiated neuroendocrine carcinoma, emphasizing that diagnostic criteria need to be clearly followed to ensure accurate diagnosis (Table 4).

▶ In 2010 the World Health Organization (WHO) classification of tumors of the digestive system issued a marked revision in how neuroendocrine neoplasms of the gastrointestinal and pancreaticobiliary tract are diagnosed. One of the overarching themes is the use of standardized diagnostic criteria across multiple organ systems. The grading classification for these neuroendocrine tumors is based primarily on mitotic count and Ki67 proliferation index. Lower-grade tumors show low mitotic counts and low Ki67 index, whereas grade-3 tumors show greater than 20 mitotic figures per 10 high-power fields and greater than 20% Ki67 index. They also clearly define how many high-power fields should be counted (50) and the size of a single high-power field (2 mm^2). Should Ki67 index be used, they suggest 2000 cells should be counted including the areas of strongest nuclear labeling, so-called hotspots. If there is discrepancy between the mitotic count and the Ki67 index, the higher grade is suggested to be assigned to the tumor. These changes in the classification system have led to fairly significant differences in diagnoses over time. This report highlights the changes in that of the 107 initially diagnosed pancreatic poorly differentiated neuroendocrine carcinomas, 63 cases were reclassified, and most were reclassified to well-differentiated neuroendocrine tumor or acinar cell carcinoma. This finding suggests that in the past, pathologists were overdiagnosing well-differentiated neuroendocrine tumors and acinar cell carcinomas as poorly differentiated neuroendocrine carcinomas. This may have had effects on past studies that evaluated the clinical aggressiveness of these tumors. When the cohort is purified, as in this study, based on 2010 WHO criteria, poorly differentiated neuroendocrine carcinomas of the pancreas have an exceedingly poor prognosis with most patients dying in less than 1 year. Table 4 is a nice guide to the differential diagnosis between poorly differentiated neuroendocrine carcinoma, well-differentiated neuroendocrine carcinoma, acinar cell carcinoma, and primitive neuroectodermal tumor.

For additional review of this topic, I refer the readers to Yang et al.[1]

M. L. Smith, MD

Reference

1. Yang Z, Tang LH, Klimstra DS. Gastroenteropancreatic neuroendocrine neoplasms: histological context and current issues. *Semin Diagn Pathol.* 2013;30:186-196.

Congestive hepatic fibrosis score: a novel histologic assessment of clinical severity

Dai D-F, Swanson PE, Krieger EV, et al (Univ of Washington School of Medicine, Seattle)

Mod Pathol 27:1552-1558, 2014

Chronic right heart failure predisposes to hepatic passive congestion and centrizonal necrosis that may lead to hepatic fibrosis (cardiac sclerosis).

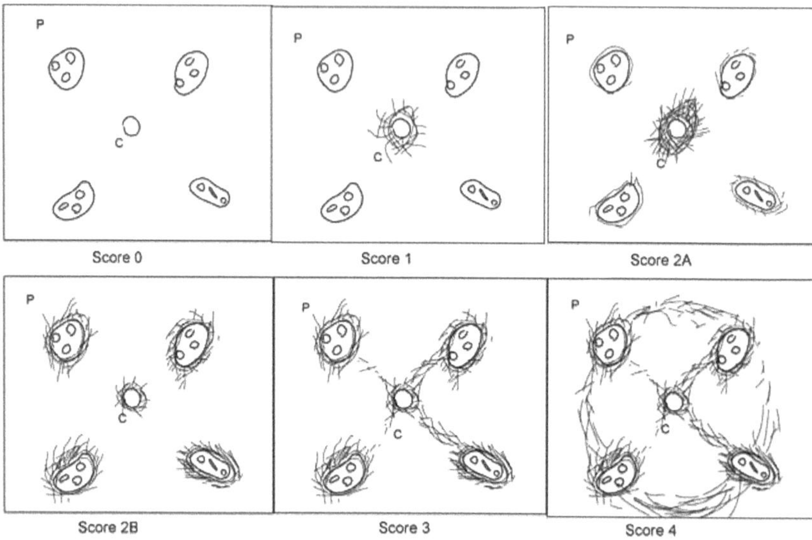

FIGURE 1.—Diagram of the proposed congestive hepatic fibrosis score: score 0, no fibrosis; score 1, central zone fibrosis only; score 2A, central zone and portal fibrosis, with accentuation of fibrosis in the central zone; score 2B, moderate portal fibrosis and central zone fibrosis, with accentuation of fibrosis in the portal zone; score 3, bridging fibrosis; and score 4, cirrhosis. (Reprinted by permission from Macmillan Publishers Ltd: Modern Pathology. Dai DF, Swanson PE, Krieger EV, et al. Congestive hepatic fibrosis score: a novel histologic assessment of clinical severity. *Mod Pathol.* 2014;27:1552-1558, Copyight 2014, by USCAP, Inc, http://www.nature.com/modpathol/.)

TABLE 1.—Proposed Scoring System for Congestive Hepatic Fibrosis

	Congestive Hepatic Fibrosis Score
0	No fibrosis
1	Central zone fibrosis
2A	Central zone and mild portal fibrosis, with accentuation at central zone
2B	At least moderate portal fibrosis and central zone fibrosis, with accentuation at portal zone
3	Bridging fibrosis
4	Cirrhosis

Reprinted by permission from Macmillan Publishers Ltd: Modern Pathology. Dai DF, Swanson PE, Krieger EV, et al. Congestive hepatic fibrosis score: a novel histologic assessment of clinical severity. *Mod Pathol.* 2014;27:1552-1558, by USCAP, Inc, http://www.nature.com/modpathol/.

Although there have been several studies on the histologic features of congestive hepatopathy, there is no available grading system. In this study we developed a novel grading system for congestive hepatic fibrosis. Liver biopsies were examined in patients with chronic heart failure of various etiologies including congenital heart disease, idiopathic cardiomyopathy, ischemic heart disease, and valvular heart disease. The cases with available echocardiography and/or right heart catheterization were included. Cases with other types of underlying chronic liver diseases, alcoholic liver disease, significant steatosis (>20%), malignant neoplasm, and acute heart failure or shock were excluded. After exclusion, 42 cases were included in the study. We herein proposed a novel congestive hepatic fibrosis score and correlated it with the right heart structure and function obtained by echocardiography and/or right heart catheterization. Our results showed that congestive hepatic fibrosis score is well correlated with the right atrial pressure (P for trend <0.001). The presence of portal fibrosis (congestive hepatic fibrosis scores 2 and 3) is associated with significantly higher right atrial pressure than those with no fibrosis ($P < 0.001$) or with centrizonal fibrosis only ($P = 0.02$). Congestive hepatic fibrosis score is also significantly associated with increasing severity of right atrial dilatation ($P = 0.03$) and right ventricular dilatation ($P = 0.02$), indicators for chronic volume and/or pressure overload. Other histopathologic features include sinusoidal dilatation and centrizonal hepatocyte atrophy. In summary, although sinusoidal dilatation and centrizonal fibrosis are the hallmarks of hepatic passive congestion, the presence of portal fibrosis is suggestive of more advanced disease, as it correlates with more severe impairment of right heart function, regardless of the etiologies of right heart failure. Congestive hepatic fibrosis score is a useful indicator of clinical severity (Fig 1, Table 1).

▶ One of the challenges in communicating the degree of fibrosis in various disease states within the liver is based on the fact that not all fibrosis is created by the same etiologic mechanism. Therefore, the progression of the fibrosis and the eventual development of cirrhosis may go through different morphologic forms, depending on the active pathologic insult. Therefore, when trying to stage the degree of fibrosis in patients with heart failure or other causes of suboptimal hepatic blood outflow, it is challenging to use staging systems, such as the Batts-Ludwig Fibrosis Staging System, which is based primarily on patients with chronic viral hepatitis. This report proposes a staging system for congestive hepatic fibrosis (Table 1) and has the benefit of comparing the fibrosis score with clinical parameters of the degree of heart dysfunction. One of the intriguing findings is that although most of the pathology in early heart failure-related liver disease is centrilobular in its distribution and consists of sinusoidal dilation with subsinusoidal fibrosis, it is the development of periportal fibrosis that is most suggestive of more advanced right heart dysfunction. Fig 1 highlights a schematic of the proposed staging system. Further studies are required to confirm the association of this staging system with the clinical parameters as well as the reproducibility of this staging system among pathologists and other institutions. Of critical importance is the stage cutoff for consideration of heart transplant. In many institutions, the presence of significant hepatic fibrosis related to heart failure precludes patients from undergoing evaluation for heart transplantation. It would be useful to have more well-defined criteria for the exclusion of these patients.

For additional review of cardiac sclerosis, I refer the readers to Myers et al[1] and Kendall et al.[2]

M. L. Smith, MD

References

1. Myers RP, Cerini R, Sayegh R, et al. Cardiac hepatopathy: clinical hemodynamic, and histologic characteristics and correlations. *Hepatology.* 2003;37:393-400.
2. Kendall TJ, Stedman B, Hacking N, et al. Hepatic fibrosis and cirrhosis in the fontan circulation: a detailed morphological study. *J Clin Pathol.* 2008;61:504-508.

Immunohistochemical distinction between intrahepatic cholangiocarcinoma and pancreatic ductal adenocarcinoma

Lok T, Chen L, Lin F, et al (Univ of California at Los Angeles; Geisinger Med Ctr, Danville, PA)

Hum Pathol 45:394-400, 2014

Distinction between primary intrahepatic cholangiocarcinoma (ICC) and metastatic pancreatic ductal adenocarcinoma (PDA) on a liver biopsy is essentially impossible histologically but has important clinical implications. In this study, 41 ICCs and 60 PDAs were immunohistochemically evaluated for the expression of S100P, pVHL, IMP3, maspin, MUC5AC, and CK17 proteins. The results showed pVHL expression in 29 (71%) ICCs but in only 3 (5%) PDAs. S100P, MUC5AC, and CK17 were frequently expressed in PDAs, seen in 57 (95%), 40 (67%), and 36 (60%) cases, respectively. In contrast, only 11 (27%), 5 (12%), and 5 (12%) ICC cases expressed these proteins. IMP3 was expressed in 37 (90%) ICC and 54 (90%) PDA cases with equal frequency. All 60 (100%) PDA and 30 (73%) ICC cases showed positive maspin immunoreactivity. A S100P−/pVHL+/MUC5A C−/CK17− staining pattern was essentially indicative of ICC, whereas the S100P+/pVHL−/MUC5AC+/ CK17+ and S100P+/pVHL−/MUC5AC−/CK17+ staining patterns were suggestive of PDA. These observations demonstrate that S100P, pVHL, MUC5AC, and CK17 are a useful immunohistochemical panel that may help distinguish primary ICC from metastatic PDA (Table 3).

▶ It is not uncommon to sign out an intrahepatic mass lesion that has undergone needle core biopsy as adenocarcinoma and in the comment section describe that

TABLE 3.—Comparison of Immunostaining Results Between ICCs and PDAs

Antibody	ICC (n = 41), n (%)	PDA (n = 60), n (%)	*P*
S100P	11 (27)	57 (95)	<.0001
IMP3	37 (90)	54 (90)	1.0000
pVHL	29 (71)	3 (5)	<.0001
Maspin	30 (73)	60 (100)	<.0001
MUC5AC	5 (12)	40 (67)	<.0001
CK17	5 (12)	36 (60)	<.0001

the differential diagnosis includes a primary intrahepatic cholangiocarcinoma as well as a metastatic pancreaticobiliary neoplasm. Many of these cases are resolvable by imaging studies. However, because there is a significant difference in clinical treatment options, including surgical approach, chemotherapy, and radiation, as well as a significant prognostic difference, the distinction between a primary intrahepatic cholangiocarcinoma and a metastatic pancreaticobiliary carcinoma to the liver is of clinical significance. Unfortunately, they show dramatic overlap from a histologic perspective as well as from an immunohistochemical staining profile perspective. This article evaluates several different immunohistochemical studies with regard to their staining characteristics in intrahepatic cholangiocarcinoma and pancreatic ductal adenocarcinoma. One of the strengths of this study is the large number of lesions evaluated (41 intrahepatic cholangiocarcinomas and 60 pancreatic ductal adenocarcinomas). It should be noted that these were all traditional adenocarcinomas, and histologic subtypes of mucinous, signet ring cell, and undifferentiated carcinomas were not included in this study. Table 3 highlights the comparative staining results and shows that, as is commonly the case, there is no perfect immunohistochemical stain. However, as a panel of immunohistochemical stains, excluding IMP3 and maspin, there may be clinical utility. One challenge to the implementation of this panel in clinical practice is the availability of the different immunohistochemical markers evaluated.

For additional review on the use of these different immunohistochemical studies, I refer the readers to Schmidt et al[1] and Liu et al.[2]

M. L. Smith, MD

References

1. Schmidt MT, Himmelfarb EA, Shafi H, Lin F, Xu H, Wang HL. Use of IMP3, S100P, and pVHL immunopanel to aid in the interpretation of bile duct biopsies with atypical histology or suspicious for malignancy. *Appl Immunohistochem Mol Morphol.* 2012;12:478-487.
2. Liu H, Shi J, Anandan V, et al. Reevaluation and identification of the best immunohistochemical panel (pVHL, maspin, S100P, IMP-3) for ductal adenocarcinoma of the pancreas. *Arch Pathol Lab Med.* 2012;136:601-609.

Aberrant Centrizonal Features in Chronic Hepatic Venous Outflow Obstruction: Centrilobular Mimicry of Portal-based Disease

Krings G, Can B, Ferrell L (Univ of California, San Francisco; Ondokuz Mayis Univ, Samsun, Turkey)

Am J Surg Pathol 38:205-214, 2014

Chronic hepatic venous outflow obstruction is characterized by centrizonal scarring but may also display features that can lead to portal tract mimicry and misdiagnosis as biliary disease, especially given elevated cholestatic liver profiles in these patients. However, these histopathologic features have not been systematically described. We graded the numbers of centrizonal arterioles, ductules, keratin 7$^+$ hepatocytes, CD34$^+$ microvessels, and capillarized sinusoids in 61 cases of chronic venous outflow obstruction and

TABLE 2.—Summary of Histopathologic Features in Chronic Venous Outflow Obstruction in Study Population

Sinusoidal dilatation/congestion (n = 61) (n [%])	58/61 (95.1)
Hepatocyte plate atrophy (n = 61) (n [%])	59/61 (96.7)
Hepatocyte necrosis/dropout (n = 61) (n [%])	7/61 (11.5)
Portal inflammation (n = 61) (n [%])	12/61 (19.7)
Periportal ductular reaction (n = 61)* (n [%])	
Grade 1	26/61 (42.6)
Grade 2	12/61 (19.7)
Grade 3	5/61 (8.2)
Total	43/61 (70.5)
Centrilobular ductular metaplasia (n = 61)* (n [%])	
Grade 1	29/61 (47.5)
Grade 2	7/61 (11.5)
Grade 3	8/61 (13.1)
Total	44/61 (72.1)
Centrizonal arterioles (n = 61)† (n [%])	
Grade 1	20/61 (32.8)
Grade 2	17/61 (27.9)
Grade 3	13/61 (21.3)
Total	50/61 (82.0)
Combined centrilobular ductular metaplasia and centrizonal arterioles (any grade) as a function of fibrosis stage (n = 61)*,†,‡	
Stage 1a	0/4 (0)
Stage 1b	10/18 (55.6)
Stage 2	10/15 (66.7)
Stage 3	16/20 (80.0)
Stage 4/cirrhosis	4/4 (100)
Total	40/61 (65.6)
Centrizonal microvessels (n = 27)*	
Grade 1	10/27 (37.0)
Grade 2	11/27 (40.7)
Grade 3	4/27 (14.8)
Total	25/27 (92.6)
Centrizonal sinusoidal capillarization (n = 27)*	
Grade 1	12/27 (44.4)
Grade 2	9/27 (33.3)
Grade 3	5/27 (18.5)
Total	26/27 (96.3)
Centrilobular intermediate-phenotype hepatocytes (n = 27)*	
Grade 1	8/27 (29.6)
Grade 2	12/27 (44.4)
Grade 3	5/27 (18.5)
Total	25/27 (92.5)
Aberrant GS zonation (n = 24)	
Absent or decreased	20/24 (83.3)
Reversed	2/24 (8.3)
Total	22/24 (91.7)
Fibrosis stage (n = 61)‡	
Stage 1a	4/61 (6.6)
Stage 1b	18/61 (29.5)
Stage 2	15/61 (24.6)
Stage 3	20/61 (32.8)
Stage 4/cirrhosis	4/61 (6.6)

*Semiquantitative grading of centrizonal capillarization and microvessels by CD34 immunohistochemistry, centrilobular ductular metaplasia, centrilobular intermediate-phenotype hepatocytes by CK7 immunohistochemistry, and periportal ductular reaction as follows: 0, none; 1, mild; 2, moderate; 3, marked.

†Grading of arterioles: 0, no arteriole in central zones; 1, 1 to 2 arterioles in 1 to 2 central zones; 2, >2 arterioles in <50% of central zones; and 3, >2 arterioles in >50% of central zones.

‡Fibrosis stage determined using the NASH CRN system.

Reprinted from Krings G, Can B, Ferrell L. Aberrant centrizonal features in chronic hepatic venous outflow obstruction: centrilobular mimicry of portal-based disease. *Am J Surg Pathol.* 2014;38:205-214, with permission from Lippincott Williams & Wilkins.

assessed changes in metabolic zonation by glutamine synthetase staining. Centrizonal arterioles and ductules were present in 82.0% and 72.1% of cases, respectively, and correlated with fibrosis. Centrizonal CD34$^+$ microvessels and sinusoidal capillarization were closely associated and present in 25 (92.6%) and 26 (96.3%) of 27 cases, respectively. Centrizonal capillarized sinusoids and microvessels, which were present in all cases with advanced fibrosis, were demonstrated in 90% and 80% of the cases without significant fibrosis, respectively. The results suggest that capillarization and/or microvessel formation precede and may contribute to centrizonal scarring, whereas arterialization likely reflects vascular remodeling associated with progressive fibrosis. Centrizonal ductules were often immature, being either keratin 7$^+$/keratin 19$^-$ (36.4%) or keratin 7$^-$/keratin 19$^-$ (10.0%). Centrizonal keratin 7$^+$ intermediate-phenotype hepatocytes were present in 25 (92.5%) of 27 cases. Lastly, 22 (91.7%) of 24 cases showed loss of metabolic zonation, with reversed zonation in 2 (8.3%) cases. Together, the findings indicate that vascular and lobular reorganization in chronic venous outflow obstruction may result in mimicry of central zones as portal tracts. Recognition of these changes is essential to prevent misdiagnosis of this condition as biliary tract disease (Table 2).

▶ In the majority of cases showing suboptimal hepatic blood outflow, the diagnosis is fairly straightforward. In addition, there is often a clinical/radiographic suspicion for the etiology of the liver disease such as congestive heart failure, Budd-Chiari syndrome, or veno-occlusive disease. However, simply because the patient has suboptimal hepatic blood outflow does not preclude the possibility of a second pathology affecting the hepatic parenchyma. The authors describe in detail the centrilobular changes in cases of chronic hepatic venous outflow obstruction, which often mimic chronic biliary disease. The differential diagnosis is further complicated by the fact that patients with suboptimal hepatic venous outflow often show a cholestatic pattern of liver function test abnormalities including elevated alkaline phosphatase and bilirubin studies. Therefore, the recognition of these potential pseudo portal tracks and pseudo biliary disease is important for the general surgical pathologist to avoid the possibility of additional unnecessary workup in these patients. Table 2 highlights the main pathologic findings in this cohort of 61 patients showing venous outflow obstruction. It is surprising to see the degree of ductular reaction, ductular metaplasia, centrizonal arterioles, centrizonal microvessel density, centrizonal sinusoidal capillarization, hepatocyte intermediate phenotype metaplasia, and aberrant glutamine synthetase zonation. The general result of these findings is that the development of pseudo portal tracks may show apparent bile duct dropout/ductopenia, which could be interpreted as a chronic biliary disease. The take-home message from this article for the general surgical pathologist is that in the setting of biopsies showing chronic venous outflow obstruction, the degree of portal-based biliary changes to suggest the possibility of a superimposed bile duct obstruction/stricturing process should be exceedingly high before making this diagnosis. In addition, some authors have suggested the use of glutamine synthetase as a tool for the identification of centrilobular regions to obtain a better sense of the architecture of a liver biopsy. This study highlights the fact that in some disease processes, such as suboptimal hepatic venous outflow, glutamine synthetase staining may not be representative of the true hepatic architecture.

For additional review of this topic, I refer the readers to the following reference Kakarg et al.[1]

M. L. Smith, MD

Reference

1. Kakar S, Batts KP, Poterucha JJ, Burgart LJ. Histologic changes mimicking biliary disease in liver biopsies with venous outflow impairment. *Mod Pathol.* 2004;17: 874-878.

Automatic classification of white regions in liver biopsies by supervised machine learning

Vanderbeck S, Bockhorst J, Komorowski R, et al (Univ of Wisconsin, Milwaukee; Med College of Wisconsin, Milwaukee; et al)

Hum Pathol 45:785-792, 2014

Automated assessment of histological features of non-alcoholic fatty liver disease (NAFLD) may reduce human variability and provide continuous rather than semiquantitative measurement of these features. As part of a larger effort, we perform automatic classification of steatosis, the cardinal feature of NAFLD, and other regions that manifest as white in images of hematoxylin and eosin-stained liver biopsy sections. These regions include macrosteatosis, central veins, portal veins, portal arteries, sinusoids and bile ducts. Digital images of hematoxylin and eosin-stained slides of 47 liver biopsies from patients with normal liver histology (n = 20) and NAFLD (n = 27) were obtained at 20× magnification. The images were analyzed using supervised machine learning classifiers created from annotations provided by two expert pathologists. The classification algorithm performs with 89% overall accuracy. It identified macrosteatosis, bile ducts, portal veins and sinusoids with high precision and recall (≥82%). Identification of central veins and portal arteries was less robust but still good. The accuracy of the classifier in identifying macrosteatosis is the best reported. The accurate automated identification of macrosteatosis achieved with this algorithm has useful clinical and research-related applications. The accurate detection of liver microscopic anatomical landmarks may facilitate important subsequent tasks, such as localization of other histological lesions according to liver microscopic anatomy (Fig 5B and Table 2).

▶ In the midst of today's technological revolution, it is compelling to look at how image analysis may be used to add further value to our present-day surgical pathology reports. Several studies in the past have looked at image analysis and its use in evaluating the degree of fibrosis of mature collagen within liver biopsies. The authors in this report sought to develop a supervised machine

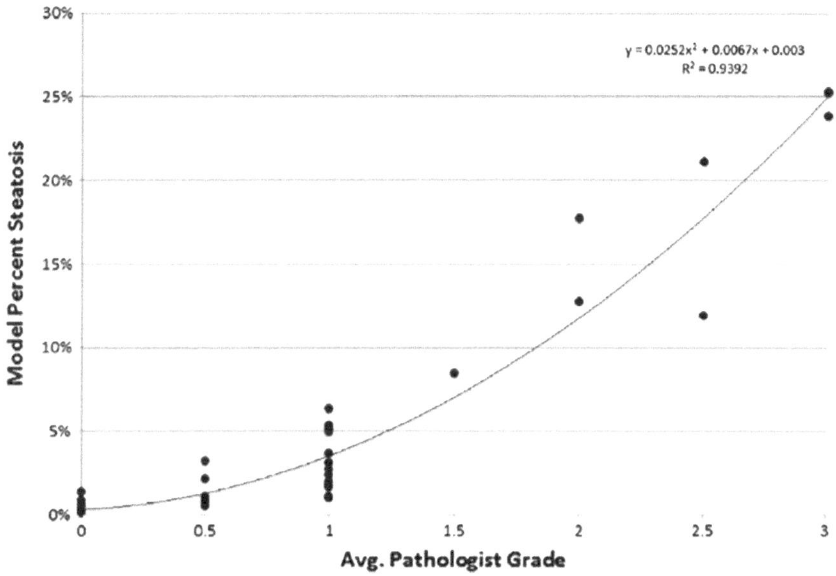

FIGURE 5.—(B) Relationships of computed percentage steatosis with the average of the two study pathologists' grades. (Reprinted from Human Pathology. Vanderbeck S, Bockhorst J, Komorowski R, et al. Automatic classification of white regions in liver biopsies by supervised machine learning. *Hum Pathol.* 2014;45:785-792, Copyright 2014, with permission from Elsevier.)

TABLE 2.—Confusion Matrix for Classified White Regions

	Predicted						
Actual	Bile Duct	Central Vein	Macrosteatosis	Other	Portal Artery	Portal Vein	Sinusoid
Bile duct	51	0	1	0	6	4	0
Central vein	0	72	8	2	2	13	17
Macrosteatosis	0	4	1072	4	1	3	16
Other	0	6	4	43	0	4	11
Portal artery	3	7	0	0	32	10	2
Portal vein	2	6	5	0	7	184	4
Sinusoid	0	12	30	1	0	5	305

NOTE. Classification performed using data from combined two-pathologists dataset created with support vector machine with a linear kernel.

Reprinted from Human Pathology. Vanderbeck S, Bockhorst J, Komorowski R, et al. Automatic classification of white regions in liver biopsies by supervised machine learning. *Hum Pathol.* 2014;45:785-792, Copyright 2014, with permission from Elsevier.

learning algorithmic approach to evaluate the degree of white regions as a surrogate marker for the degree of steatosis. This, of course, requires exclusion of other structures within the liver biopsy that appear white on standard microscopy (central veins, portal veins, portal arteries, sinusoids, and bile ducts). Table 2 shows the confusion matrix for the various classified white regions. What becomes obvious fairly quickly is the high rate of accurate classification of the different microscopic anatomic landmarks within the liver. However, close investigation shows that the distinction between sinusoids and other microscopic anatomic landmarks is of particular challenge. Fig 5B shows the relationship between the computed percentage of steatosis (solid line) and the average pathologist grade. Although these data are intriguing, there are still fairly substantial hurdles to clinical use. First, this was done, as best I can tell, on biopsies showing intact architecture without significant fibrosis. It is difficult to predict the impact of fibrosis and architectural distortion on the ability of the supervised learning to correctly classify different anatomic landmarks. In addition, it remains to be seen if the improved continuous variable data have any relationship to patient prognosis or outcome in the setting of fatty liver disease.

For further review of the assessment of hepatic steatosis, I refer the readers to Turlin et al.[1]

M. L. Smith, MD

Reference

1. Turlin B, Ramm GA, Purdie DM, et al. Assessment of hepatic steatosis: comparison of quantitative and semiquantitative methods in 108 liver biopsies. *Liver Int.* 2009;29:530-535.

3 Cytopathology

Increasing the sensitivity of endocervical curettings by performing ThinPrep® Pap on transport container fluid: is diagnostic material going down the drain?

Lastra RR, Meykler SE, Baloch ZW, et al (Hosp of the Univ of Pennsylvania, Philadelphia; Pennsylvania Hosp, Philadelphia)

Cytopathology 2014 [Epub ahead of print]

Objective.—The sensitivity of endocervical curettage (ECC) can be suboptimal because of limited epithelial tissue. The false-negative rate for ECC in patients with cervical intraepithelial neoplasia involving the endocervical canal has been reported to be 45%. ECC samples are transported to pathology in formalin- or saline-filled containers; this fluid is discarded after the specimen has been submitted. We evaluated the utility of performing liquid-based cytological preparations from ECC transport container fluid as a way to increase the sensitivity of ECC specimens.

Methods.—Consecutive ECC specimens received at one of the two participating institutions were selected prospectively. A surgical pathology mesh bag was placed over a ThinPrep® CytoLyt® solution container, and the specimen was filtered through the bag, collecting the transport fluid in the container. The CytoLyt® was processed to obtain a container fluid ThinPrep® (CF-TP) liquid-based Papanicolaou (Pap) slide. The CF-TP slides were reviewed and the findings were compared with those from the ECC and follow-up specimens.

Results.—The cohort included 53 patients. Discrepancies between CF-TP and ECC were seen in 14 of the 53 patients (26%); a more significant lesion was identified in CF-TP relative to ECC in 13 of these cases. CF-TP diagnosis was confirmed in eight of 11 cases with histological follow-up. A positive CF-TP result was confirmed by histology in six of nine cases with negative ECC.

Conclusions.—Combining the pathological evaluation of ECC specimens with liquid-based cytology performed on the transport container fluid can increase the diagnostic sensitivity of the ECC procedure for the detection of cervical lesions.

▶ The clinical utility of examination of endocervical curettings is currently being scrutinized based on reports of a high false-negative rate, a failure to improve diagnostic accuracy in the face of adequate colposcopy, and the addition of unnecessary procedural risks and discomfort for patients. This study convincingly shows that the sensitivity of examination of endocervical curettings increases significantly when the fluid in which curettings are submitted are also prepared and examined, including containing lesion material not identified in multiple curettings examined alone. Although these findings strongly support that the preparation and examination of the tissue and fluid in parallel significantly reduces false negatives, clinician preferences as well as laboratory resource availability will affect the degree of adoption of this method. For further reading, please see reference list.[1,2]

D. M. Grzybicki, MD

References

1. Solomon D, Stoler M, Jeronimo J, Khan M, Castle P, Schiffman M. Diagnostic utility of endocervical curettage in women undergoing colposcopy for equivocal or low-grade cytologic abnormalities. *Obstet Gynecol.* 2007;110:288-295.
2. Saslow D, Solomon D, Lawson HW, et al. American Cancer Society, American Society for Colposcopy and Cervical Pathology, and American Society for Clinical Pathology screening guidelines for the prevention and early detection of cervical cancer. *Am J Clin Pathol.* 2012;137:516-542.

Role of endoscopic ultrasound fine-needle aspiration evaluating adrenal gland enlargement or mass

Martinez M, LeBlanc J, Al-Haddad M, et al (Indiana Univ School of Medicine, Indianapolis)
World J Nephrol 3:92-100, 2014

Aim.—To report the clinical impact of adrenal endoscopic ultrasound fine-needle aspiration (EUS-FNA) in the evaluation of patients with adrenal gland enlargement or mass.

Methods.—In a retrospective single-center case-series, patients undergoing EUS-FNA of either adrenal gland from 1997-2011 in our tertiary care center were included. Medical records were reviewed and results of EUS, cytology, adrenal size change on follow-up imaging ≥6 mo after EUS and any repeat EUS or surgery were abstracted. A lesion was considered benign if: (1) EUS-FNA cytology was benign and the lesion remained <1 cm from its original size on follow-up computed tomography (CT), magnetic resonance imaging or repeat EUS ≥6 mo after EUS-FNA; or (2) subsequent adrenalectomy and surgical pathology was benign.

Results.—Ninety-four patients had left ($n = 90$) and/or right ($n = 5$) adrenal EUS-FNA without adverse events. EUS indications included: cancer staging or suspected recurrence ($n = 31$), pancreatic ($n = 20$), mediastinal ($n = 10$), adrenal ($n = 7$), lung ($n = 7$) mass or other indication ($n = 19$). Diagnoses after adrenal EUS-FNA included metastatic lung ($n = 10$), esophageal ($n = 5$), colon ($n = 2$), or other cancer ($n = 8$); benign primary adrenal mass or benign tissue ($n = 60$); or was non-diagnostic ($n = 9$). Available follow-up confirmed a benign lesion in 5/9 non-diagnostic aspirates and 32/60 benign aspirates. Four of the 60 benign aspirates were later confirmed as malignant by repeat biopsy, followup CT, or adrenalectomy. Adrenal EUS-FNA diagnosed metastatic cancer in 24, and ruled out metastasis in 10 patients. For the diagnosis of malignancy, EUS-FNA of either adrenal had sensitivity, specificity, positive predictive value and negative predictive value of 86%, 97%, 96% and 89%, respectively.

Conclusion.—Adrenal gland EUS-FNA is safe, minimally invasive and a sensitive technique with significant impact in the management of adrenal gland mass or enlargement.

▶ Endoscopic ultrasound-guided fine-needle aspiration (EUS-FNA) is a relatively new method to sample the adrenal glands. Martinez et al report that adrenal gland EUS-FNA is accurate, although false negatives and false positives do occur. Operator experience in performing EUS-FNA plays a large role in obtaining sufficient samples, and specimen quality plays a huge role in determining institutional sensitivity and specificity. For further reading, see reference list.[1,2]

S. Raab, MD

References

1. Kuruba R, Gallagher SF. Current management of adrenal tumors. *Curr Opin Oncol.* 2008;20:34-46.
2. Harisinghani MG, Maher MM, Hahn PF, et al. Predictive value of benign percutaneous adrenal biopsies in oncology patients. *Clin Radiol.* 2002;57:898-901.

Making Mock-FNA Smears from Fresh Surgical Pathology Specimens to Improve Smear Preparation Technique and to Create Cytohistological Correlation Series

Mezei T, Contac A, Iacob A, et al (Univ of Medicine and Pharmacy of Tirgu Mures, Romania)

PLoS One 9:e104983, 2014

Background.—Fine needle aspiration (FNA) cytology is a well-established diagnostic method based on the microscopic interpretation of often scant cytological material; therefore, experience, good technique and smear quality are equally important in obtaining satisfactory results.

Aims of Study.—We studied the use of fresh surgical pathology specimens for making so-called mock-FNA smears with the potential of cytohistological correlation. Additionally, we studied how this process aids the improvement of preparation technique and smear quality.

Methods.—Cytological aspirates from 32 fresh biopsy specimens from various sites: lung (20), lymph nodes (6), and breast (6) were obtained, all with a clinical diagnosis of tumor. Aspiration was performed from grossly palpable tumors. 25G needle and Cameco-type syringe holder was used with minimal or no suction.

Results.—Unfixed surgical specimens provided sufficient cytological material that resulted in good quality smears. After standard processing of specimens into microscopic sections from paraffin embedded tissues, cytohistological case-series were created. No significant alteration was reported in tissue architecture on hematoxylin-eosin stained sections after the aspiration procedure. A gradual, but steady improvement was observed in smear quality just after a few preparations.

Discussions and Conclusions.—Our study proved that surgical specimens may be used as a source of cytological material to create cytohistological correlation studies and also to improve FNA cytology skills. The use of very fine gauge needle (25G, 0,6 mm diameter) during the sampling process does not alter tissue architecture therefore the final histopathological diagnosis is not compromised. We conclude that by using fresh surgical specimens useful cytohistological collections can be created both as a teaching resource and as improving experience.

▶ The development of study sets based on the fine-needle aspiration of surgical pathology specimens, which Mezei et al propose as a method to improve smear technique, was practiced by those who introduced fine-needle aspiration into institutions that generally did not perform the procedure. It is a fantastic method for learning interpretation skills, the variability in lesion appearance based on sampling, and the effect of technique on sampling quality. Unfortunately, many individuals do not have the time or inclination to practice in this manner. Some residency and fellowship programs build study sets using this method and also use this practice as a training tool. For additional reading, see reference list below.[1,2]

S. Raab, MD

References

1. Das DK. Fine-needle aspiration cytology: its origin, development, and present status with special reference to a developing country, India. *Diagn Cytopathol.* 2003; 28:345-351.
2. Siddig E. Fine needle aspiration: past, current practice and recent developments. *Biotech Histochem.* 2014;89:241-244.

'Suspicious for Papillary Thyroid Carcinoma' before and after The Bethesda System for Reporting Thyroid Cytopathology: Impact of Standardized Terminology

Olson MT, Boonyaarunnate T, Atlinboga AA, et al (Johns Hopkins Hosp, Baltimore, MD; Ankara Univ School of Medicine, Turkey; et al)

Acta Cytol 58:15-22, 2014

Background.—The high-risk 'suspicious for papillary thyroid carcinoma' (SPTC) is a clinically relevant diagnosis in the cytological interpretation of thyroid aspirates. While The Bethesda System for Reporting Thyroid Cytopathology (TBSRTC) has provided invaluable terminology standardization, a performance comparison for this diagnostic category has not been performed. Therefore, this study evaluates the SPTC diagnosis before and after the introduction of TBSRTC in a large meta-analysis and at a single institution.

Materials and Methods.—The meta-analysis analyzed publications of SPTC or similar diagnoses before and after the introduction of TBSRTC. Similarly our own institutional experience was analyzed for the 8 years surrounding the introduction of TBSRTC. A correlation of the cytopathology and surgical pathology diagnoses was performed.

Results.—The introduction of TBSRTC coincided with a significant decrease in the fraction of cases called SPTC in the meta-analysis (4.5–3.1%, $p < 0.00001$) and in the institutional review (1.7–0.9%, $p = 0.005$). Meanwhile, the malignancy risk for those cases increased significantly in the meta-analysis from 62.5 to 80.5% ($p < 0.00001$) and trended upwards in the institutional review from 69 to 79% ($p = 0.4$). The follow-up rate was similar in both time periods in the meta-analysis and the institutional review.

Conclusions.—The introduction of TBSRTC coincided with a decrease in the fraction of cases called SPTC and an increase in the malignancy risk associated with that diagnosis.

▶ Although Olson et al showed that the probability of malignancy based on a diagnosis of suspicion for papillary thyroid carcinoma (PTC) increased after the introduction of the Bethesda System for Reporting Thyroid Cytopathology from 69% to 79% (based on institutional review), I am still surprised that the frequency of a non-PTC diagnosis is still 20%, which seems high. Olson et al report little data of the benign conditions, although of 17 patients with follow-up, 11 patients had an adenomatous nodule. A more detailed root cause analysis is necessary, but possible causes include diagnostic variability or the lack of precision, in both surgical pathology and cytopathology diagnosis. It would be interesting to determine if the cytopathologist who originally made the diagnosis of suspicion for PTC was consulted on the surgical pathology specimen or if the non-PTC surgical pathology case underwent consensus review. For additional reading, see reference list below.[1,2,3]

S. Raab, MD

References

1. Raparia K, Min SK, Mody DR, Anton R, Amrikachi M. Clinical outcomes for 'suspicious' category in thyroid fine-needle aspiration biopsy: patient's sex and nodule size are possible predictors of malignancy. *Arch Pathol Lab Med.* 2009; 133:787-790.
2. Cibas ES, Ali SZ. The bethesda system for reporting thyroid cytopathology. *Thyroid.* 2009;19:1159-1165.
3. Seningen JL, Nassar A, Henry MR. Correlation of thyroid nodule fine-needle aspiration cytology with corresponding histology at Mayo Clinic, 2001–2007: an institutional experience of 1,945 cases. *Diagn Cytopathol.* 2012;40:E27-E32.

Investigating MicroRNA Expression Profiles in Pancreatic Cystic Neoplasms

Lee LS, Szafranska-Schwarzbach AE, Wylie D, et al (Brigham and Women's Hosp, Boston, MA; Asuragen, Austin, TX; et al)

Clin Transl Gastroenterol 5:e47, 2014

Objectives.—Current diagnostic tools for pancreatic cysts fail to reliably differentiate mucinous from nonmucinous cysts. Reliable biomarkers are needed. MicroRNAs (miRNA) may offer insights into pancreatic cysts. Our aims were to (1) identify miRNAs that distinguish benign from both premalignant cysts and malignant pancreatic lesions using formalin-fixed, paraffin-embedded (FFPE) pathology specimens; (2) identify miRNAs that distinguish mucinous cystic neoplasm (MCN) from branch duct-intraductal papillary mucinous neoplasm (BD-IPMN).

Methods.—A total of 69 FFPE pancreatic specimens were identified: (1) benign (20 serous cystadenoma (SCA)), (2) premalignant (10 MCN, 10 BD-IPMN, 10 main duct IPMN (MD-IPMN)), and (3) malignant (19 pancreatic ductal adenocarcinoma (PDAC)). Total nucleic acid extraction was performed followed by miRNA expression profiling of 378 miRNAs interrogated using TaqMan MicroRNA Arrays Pool A and verification of candidate miRNAs. Bioinformatics was used to generate classifiers.

Results.—MiRNA profiling of 69 FFPE specimens yielded 35 differentially expressed miRNA candidates. Four different 4-miRNA panels differentiated among the lesions: one panel separated SCA from MCN, BD-IPMN, MD-IPMN, and PDAC with sensitivity 85% (62, 97), specificity 100% (93, 100), a second panel distinguished MCN from SCA, BD-IPMN, MD-IPMN, and PDAC with sensitivity and specificity 100% (100, 100), a third panel differentiated PDAC from IPMN with sensitivity 95% (76, 100) and specificity 85% (72, 96), and the final panel diagnosed MCN from BD-IPMN with sensitivity and specificity approaching 100%.

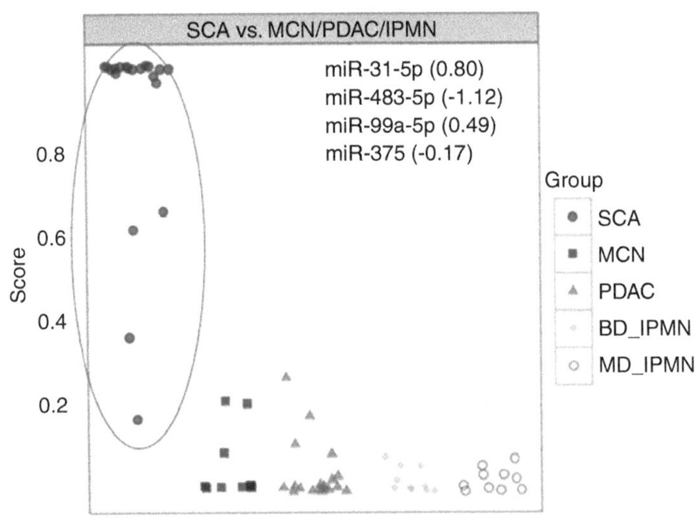

FIGURE 2.—Serous cystadenoma classifier. The "score" for each specimen is the probability that the specimen is a SCA and not a MCN, IPMN, or PDAC. The values next to the listed miRNAs represent the coefficients from the logistic regression model. IPMN, intraductal papillary mucinous neoplasm; MCN, mucinous cystic neoplasm; PDAC, pancreatic ductal adenocarcinoma; SCA, serous cystadenoma. (Reprinted from Lee LS, Szafranska-Schwarzbach AE, Wylie D, et al. Investigating MicroRNA expression profiles in pancreatic cystic neoplasms. *Clin Transl Gastroenterol.* 2014;5:e47, with permission from American College of Gastroenterology.)

Conclusions.—MiRNA profiling of surgical pathology specimens differentiates serous cystadenoma from both premalignant pancreatic cystic neoplasms and PDAC and MCN from BD-IPMN (Fig 2).

▶ The diagnosis of pancreatic cystic lesions is a challenge on endoscopic ultrasound-guided fine-needle aspiration. In many situations, even with experienced operators, the sample is limited and consists mostly of cyst fluid with rare cells. Lee et al[1] report that microRNA profiling of surgical pathology specimens differentiates serous cystadenomas from premalignant pancreatic cystic neoplasms and ductal adenocarcinomas (Fig 2) and mucinous cystic neoplasms from branch duct-intraductal papillary mucinous neoplasm. The challenge for many institutions will be developing methods to provide these tests to assist in differentiation.

S. Raab, MD

References

1. Lee LS, Clancy T, Kadiyala V, Suleiman S, Conwell DL. Interdisciplinary management of cystic neoplasms of the pancreas. *Gastroenterol Res Pract.* 2012;2012: 513163.

An Assessment of Gynecological Cytology Screening Practices Among Health Care Providers Nationwide

Darwish-Yassine M, Garvin AD, Johnston CM, et al (Michigan Public Health Inst, Okemos; Univ of Michigan Health System, Ann Arbor; et al)
Arch Pathol Lab Med 139:650-655, 2015

Context.—The Michigan Public Health Institute and the Michigan Cancer Consortium's Cervical Cancer Committee conducted a national survey of health care providers, thanks to funding from the Centers for Disease Control Cooperative Agreement 5U47CI000743-02. Papanicolaou test screening practices were examined, emphasizing the relationship between clinical and laboratory practices. This survey found differing screening practices among providers of women's health care.

Objectives.—To collect information from family medicine practitioners, women's nurse practitioners, obstetricians and gynecologists, and certified nurse-midwives on Papanicolaou and human papillomavirus testing; to discuss how those practices align with current cytology screening and follow-up recommendations from professional organizations (US Preventive Services Task Force, American Cancer Society, American College of Obstetricians and Gynecologists, and American Society for Colposcopy, and Cervical Pathology); and ultimately, to make recommendations aimed at standardizing practice performance.

Design.—This survey was conducted in part to examine clinicians' practices and their perceptions of laboratory performance, to evaluate items that are known to enhance quality of care, and to examine factors that

TABLE 7.—Type of Human Papillomavirus (HPV) Tests Ordered By Providers, n = 1550

HPV Testing	GM/FPs, No. (%)	OB/GYNs, No. (%)	WHNPs, No. (%)	CNMs, No. (%)
Test ordered?				
No	54 (18.5)	24 (4.1)	19 (7.0)	26 (6.5)
Yes	238 (81.5)	560 (95.9)	253 (93.0)	376 (93.5)
Which type?				
Low-risk HPV test	19 (6.5)	25 (4.3)	13 (4.8)	24 (6.0)
Low-risk and high-risk together	96 (32.9)	110 (18.8)	66 (24.3)	122 (30.3)
High-risk HPV test	138 (58.0)	449 (76.9)	195 (71.7)	253 (62.9)

Abbreviations: CNMs, certified nurse-midwives; GM/FPs, general medicine/family practice providers; OB/GYNs, obstetricians and gynecologists; WHNPs, women's health nurse practitioners.

may prohibit universal implementation of best standards of care. The survey used a self-administered questionnaire, distributed to 9366 clinicians, with 1601 (17.1%) completed surveys.

Results.—This assessment shows a clear lack of consensus among practitioners in performing Papanicolaou testing. It demonstrates how differently patients are tested, based on the providers' screening practices, and demonstrates specific cervical cancer screening practice disparities between and among the 4 provider groups, both in Papanicolaou testing and in the use of human papillomavirus testing.

Conclusion.—A unified mandate for screening is needed to standardize screening practices (Table 7).

▶ Darwish-Yassine and colleagues present national survey data on existing provider cytopathology practices for cervical cancer screening. Not surprisingly, cervical cancer screening practice differs among and within provider groups (eg, family medical practitioners, nurse practitioners). For example, providers follow different published guidelines, reflecting the different opinions of our medical societies and colleges rather than those of the providers themselves. Table 7 shows provider ordering patterns for human papillomavirus (HPV) testing, with greater than 20% of providers (in all provider groups) ordering low-risk HPV testing, even though most guidelines do not advocate its use. For additional reading, see reference list below.[1-3]

S. Raab, MD

References

1. Smith RA, Cokkinides V, Brooks D, Saslow D, Brawley OW. Cancer screening in the United States, 2010: a review of current American Cancer Society guidelines and issues in cancer screening. *CA Cancer J Clin.* 2010;60:99-119.21.
2. Wright TC Jr, Massad LS, Dunton CJ, Spitzer M, Wilkinson EJ, Solomon D, American Society for Colposcopy and Cervical Pathology-sponsored Consensus

Conference. 2006 consensus guidelines for the management of women with abnormal cervical cancer screening tests. *Am J Obstet Gynecol.* 2007;196:346-355.

3. Tworek JA, Henry MR, Blond B, Jones BA. College of American Pathologist Gynecologic cytopathology quality consensus conference on good laboratory practices in gynecologic cytology: background, rationale and organization. *Arch Pathol Lab Med.* 2013;137:158-163.

The Utility of Liquid-Based Cytology in Salivary Gland Fine-Needle Aspirates: Experience of an Academic Institution

Rarick JM, Wasman J, Michael CW (Univ Hosps Case Med Ctr/Case Western Reserve Univ, Cleveland, OH)

Acta Cytol 58:552-562, 2014

Objective.—To review the morphological features of salivary gland fine-needle aspirates (FNA) on ThinPrep® (TP) preparations. Emphasis is placed on the commonalities and specific differences between TP and conventional smear (CS) preparations.

Study Design.—The cytology and surgical pathology archives were searched for 'salivary' or 'parotid' at our institution from 2003 to 2013 for cases processed by TP and with a range of specified diagnoses and surgical followup. These cases were reviewed by the authors. A review of the known literature was also performed.

Results.—Morphological features and artifacts were noted for the most common salivary gland lesions. General features noted in the literature were identified, along with novel features identified on our review of cases. Emphasis was placed on cellular alterations, extracellular differences and architectural changes.

Conclusions.—The multitude of both benign and malignant lesions coupled with the unique artifacts encountered on TP makes salivary gland FNAs difficult for most practicing pathologists and cytopathologists. For this reason, many laboratories have been reluctant to implement TP preparations for these lesions. With knowledge of the specific artifacts and differences on TP compared to CS, TP can be used with confidence without a compromise in diagnostic accuracy for adequately cellular samples.

▶ A challenge in pathology that is often not directly addressed is the problem of specimen quality. One area that limits specimen quality is artifact, which, generally speaking, depends on technical issues within the laboratory or preanalytic issues related to specimen handling. Often, we learn about artifacts through experience (sometimes by making a mistake) or by reading the literature, in which specific artifacts are discussed as "limitations." A key learning from this article is the list of ThinPrep artifacts seen in fine-needle aspiration specimens of the salivary gland. An important follow-up would be seeing numerous examples of these artifacts in practice, which in our current environment generally depends on seeing lots of cases. For additional reading, see reference list.[1,2]

S. Raab, MD

References

1. Al-Khafaji BM, Afify AM. Salivary gland fine-needle aspiration using the ThinPrep® technique: diagnostic accuracy, cytologic artifacts and pitfalls. *Acta Cytol.* 2001;45:567-574.
2. Parfitt JR, McLachlin CM, Weir MM. Comparison of ThinPrep and conventional smears in salivary gland fine-needle aspiration biopsies. *Cancer.* 2007;111: 123-129.

4 Head and Neck

Epidemiological Trends in Head and Neck Cancer and Aids in Diagnosis

Vigneswaran N, Williams MD (The Univ of Texas School of Dentistry at Houston; UT MD Anderson Cancer Ctr, Houston, TX)

Oral Maxillofac Surg Clin North Am 26:123-141, 2014

Head and neck squamous cell carcinoma is the sixth most common cancer worldwide predominately associated with tobacco use. Changing cause and increased incidence in oropharyngeal carcinomas is associated with high-risk types of human papilloma virus and has an improved survival. Optical devices may augment visual oral examination; however, their lack of specificity still warrants tissue evaluation/biopsy. Histologic factors of oral carcinomas are critical for patient management and prognostic determination. Clinical biomarkers are still needed to improve early detection, predict malignant transformation, and optimize therapies.

▶ Vigneswaran and Williams provide this excellent review article, from the clinical and pathology perspective, of head and neck squamous cell carcinoma. Of note, human papillomavirus (HPV) testing is routinely performed as a prognostic biomarker for patients with a squamous cell carcinoma arising in the oropharynx. In situ hybridization is the most commonly used method to screen for high-risk HPV types (16, 18, 31, 33, 35, 39, 45, 51, 52, 56, 58, and 66). The immunohistochemical p16 study may be used as a surrogate marker for HPV. In some clinical trials, p16 expression in primary oropharyngeal squamous cell carcinomas strongly correlated with HPV status and improved survival.

S. Raab, MD

Lymphoepithelial-like carcinomas of the head and neck

Wenig BM (Mount Sinai Health System, NY)

Semin Diagn Pathol 32:74-86, 2015

Lymphoepithelial-like carcinomas (LELC) of the head and neck represent malignant neoplasms that are histologically similar to nasopharyngeal carcinoma (NPC), nonkeratinizing undifferentiated type but arise in locations other than the nasopharynx. The most common location for LELC in the head and neck is the salivary glands, in particular the parotid gland. However, LELC may arise in other sites including the oropharynx (tonsils, base of tongue), sinonasal tract, larynx, and middle ear/temporal bone. Unlike the nonkeratinizing undifferentiated type of NPC which is

A B C D E F

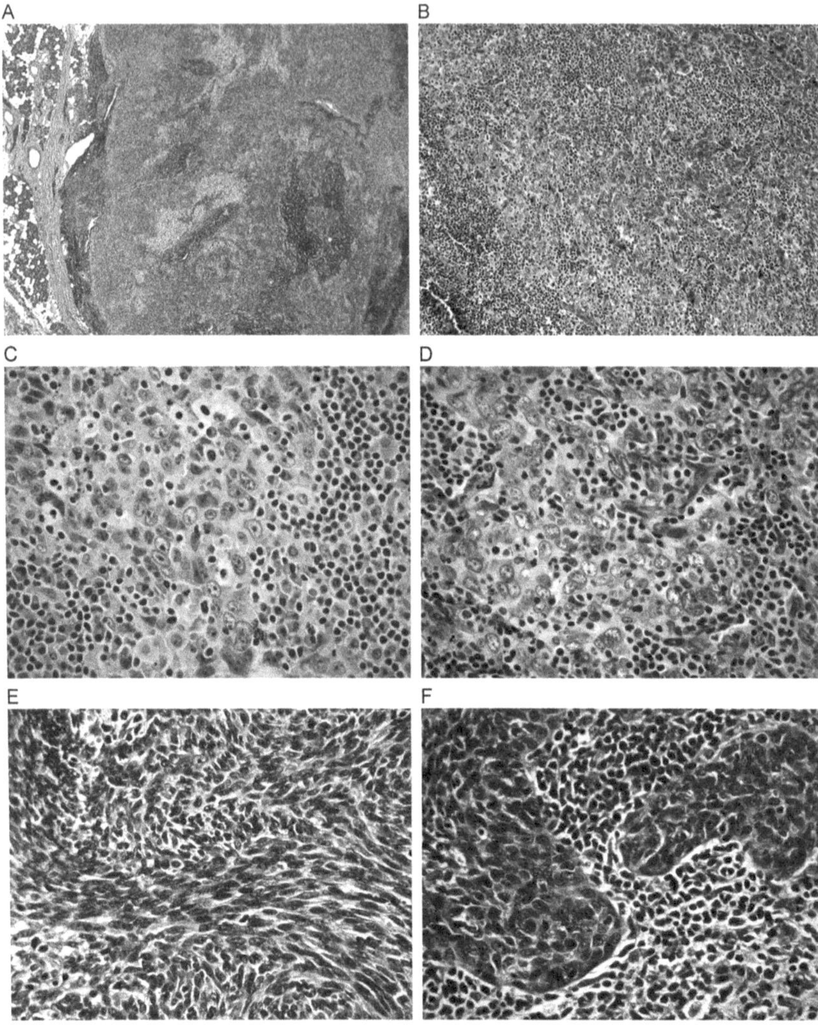

FIGURE 1.—Lymphoepithelial-like carcinoma of the parotid gland. (A and B) Infiltrative but circumscribed cellular proliferation separated from the adjacent parotid gland parenchyma (left); the proliferation includes cluster so flighter-staining neoplastic foci in a background of dense lymphocytic cell infiltrate including germinal centers. Note the absence of an associated desmoplastic reaction to the infiltrative neoplasm. (C and D) Cohesive cluster of neoplastic cells characterized by cells with enlarged vesicular nuclei, prominent eosinophilic nucleoli, and in distinct borders creating a syncytial growth. These histologic features are similar to nasopharyngeal carcinoma nonkeratinizing undifferentiated type. Variant histologic features may include (E) fascicular growth with spindle-shaped neoplastic cells and (F) basaloid cell features. (Reprinted from Wenig BM. Lymphoepithelial-like carcinomas of the head and neck. *Semin Diagn Pathol.* 2015;32:74-86, with permission from Elsevier.)

etiologically linked to Epstein-Barr virus (EBV), LELCs are not uniformly associated with EBV. The differential diagnosis for LELC varies per site and depending on the site of occurrence may include lymphoepithelial sialadenitis, sinonasal undifferentiated carcinoma (SNUC), and large cell neuroendocrine carcinoma. Treatment in general includes combined (multimodality) therapy including surgical resection, neck dissection, radiation therapy and/or chemotherapy. The prognosis may vary per site overall favorable owing to a good response to therapy (Figs 1, 4-6).

▶ This is a nice review on the uncommon entity of lymphoepithelial-like carcinomas (LELC) of the head and neck of nonnasopharyngeal origin (occurring in the salivary glands, oropharynx, sinonasal tract, larynx, and middle ear) but that show similar morphology and in some instances can be also associated with

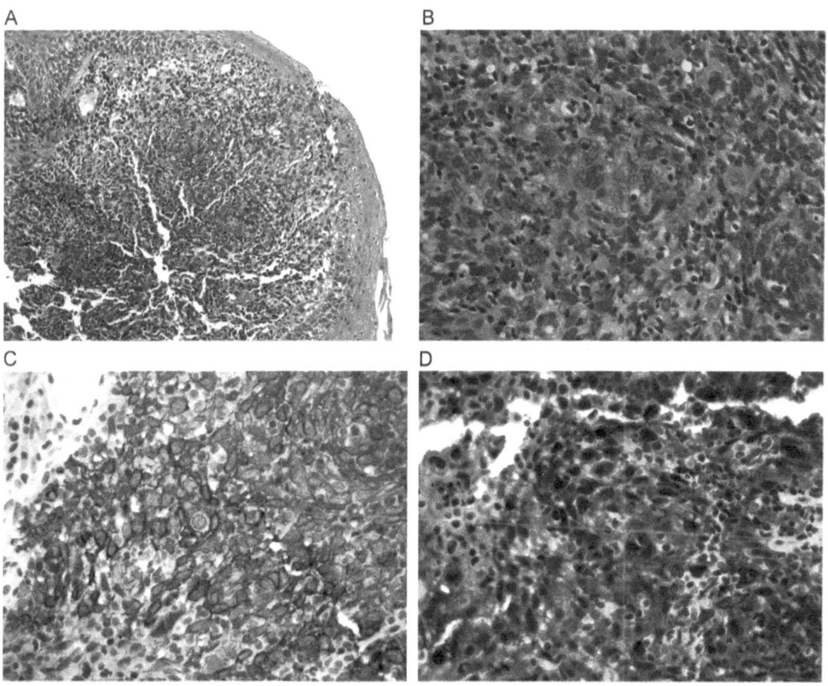

FIGURE 4.—Lymphoepithelial-like carcinoma of the oropharynx. (A) Submucosal clusters of lesional cells with associated dense lymphoplasmacytic cell infiltrate and absence of stromal desmoplastic reaction. (B) Histomorphologic features are similar to those of EBV-associated nasopharyngeal carcinoma nonkeratinizing undifferentiated type, including cells with enlarged pleomorphic and vesicular nuclei and prominent nucleoli. Lesional cells are (C) cytokeratin positive and (D) p16 positive. EBER staining was negative (not shown). Subsequent evaluation by polymerase chain reaction confirmed the presence of high-risk human papilloma virus (not shown). This carcinoma can metastasize to cervical neck lymph nodes as an occult primary carcinoma. In such a scenario, purely based on the light microscopic features, a primary (EBV-associated) nasopharyngeal carcinoma would be the most likely consideration. EBER staining would be negative and unless consideration was given for a possible oropharyngeal origin, p16 staining which would be diagnostic might not be ordered. (Reprinted from Wenig BM. Lymphoepithelial-like carcinomas of the head and neck. *Semin Diagn Pathol.* 2015;32:74-86, with permission from Elsevier.)

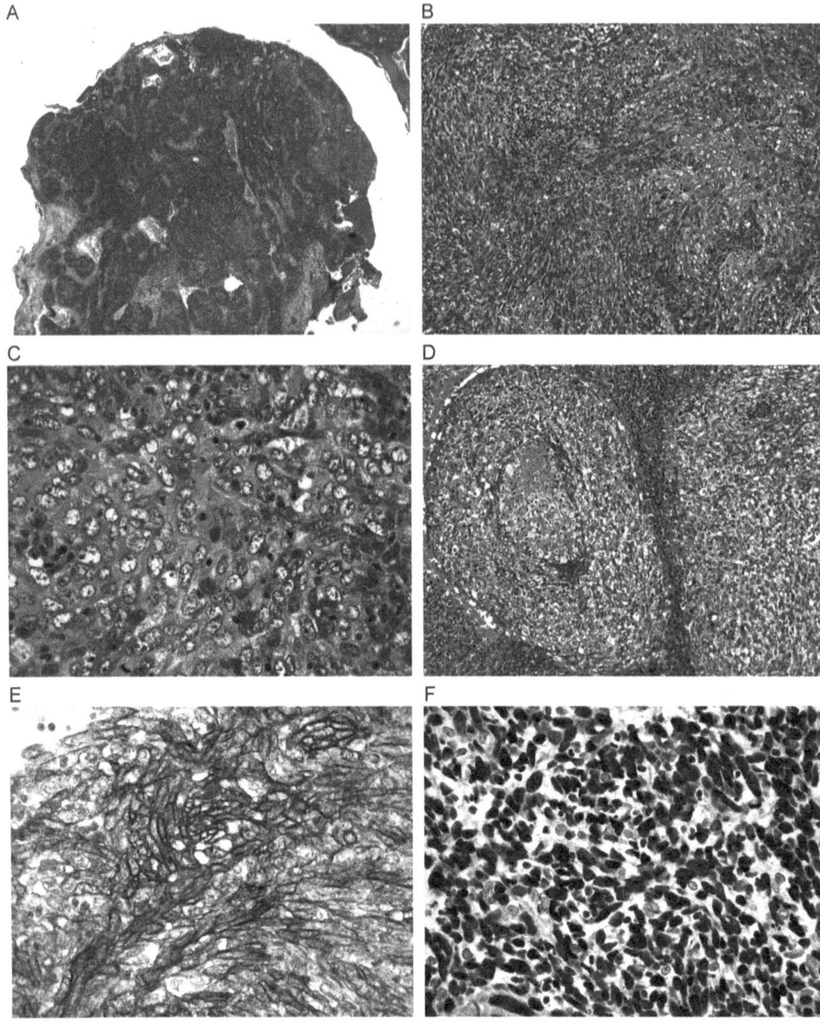

FIGURE 5.—Sinonasal lymphoepithelial-like carcinoma. (A) Polypoid invasive lesion with broad interconnecting cords of tumor similar to the growth pattern seen in sinonasal nonkeratinizing carcinoma. (B) The lesional cells are epithelioid and spindle-shaped. (C) Both cell types (epithelioid shown here) are comprised of enlarged vesicular nuclei and prominent eosinophilic nuclei. Increased mitotic activity is present. (D) A focus of central comedotype necrosisis present. Lesional cells are immunoreactive for (E) cytokeratin (AE1/AE3) and (F) in situ hybridization for Epstein–Barr encoded RNA (EBER). (Reprinted from Wenig BM. Lymphoepithelial-like carcinomas of the head and neck. *Semin Diagn Pathol.* 2015;32:74-86, with permission from Elsevier.)

Epstein-Barr virus (EBV). The article reviews the different morphologic (Figs 1, 4-6), immunohistochemical, and differential aspects of these tumors. It shows that many of these tumors can also be Epstein-Barr virus-encoded small RNA (EBER) positive like their naso-opharyngeal counterpart, although not always. The article discusses the oropharyngeal LELC, which is found to be linked more

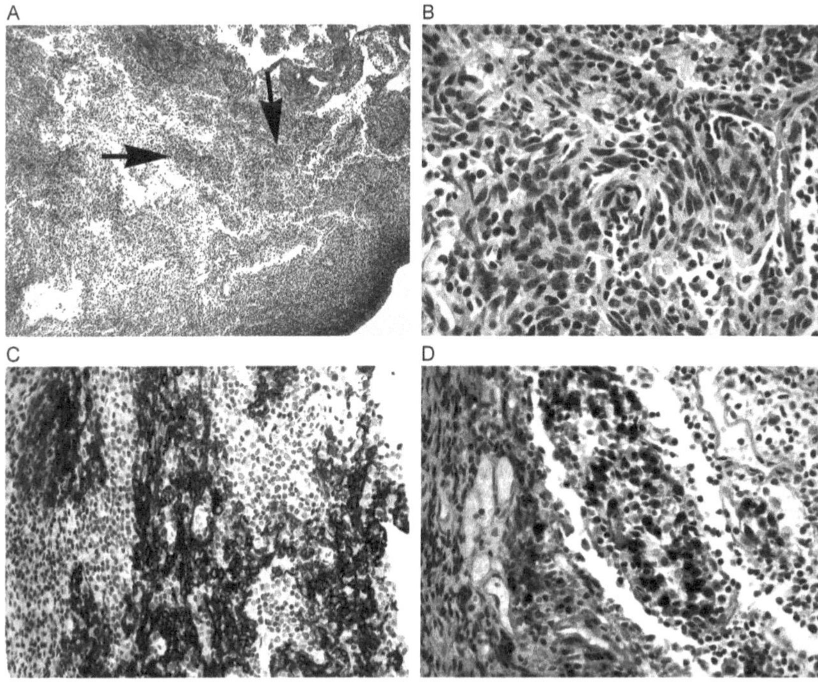

FIGURE 6.—Primary middle early mphoepithelial-like carcinoma. (A) Polypoid lesion that originated from the middle ear with dense submucosal lymphoid proliferation obscuringan infiltrative neoplasm (arrows). (B) At higher magnification epithelioid and spindle-shaped cells with enlarged vesicular nuclei and prominent eosinophilic nuclei are identified. (C) Lesional cells are immunoreactive for cytokeratin (AE1/AE3). (D) In situ hybridization for Epstein–Barr encoded RNA (EBER). (Reprinted from Wenig BM. Lymphoepithelial-like carcinomas of the head and neck. *Semin Diagn Pathol.* 2015;32:74-86, with permission from Elsevier.)

to human papilloma virus than to EBER in spite of the identical morphologic features to primary EBV nasopharyngeal lymphoepithelial carcinoma. The article also describes the more rare sites of these tumors, such as those seen in the middle ear or temporal bone (only 6 cases reported in the literature). One of the important aspects of this article is the areas of differential diagnosis of these tumors in these variable head and neck sites, as reaching the correct diagnosis will influence the modalities of treatment and prognosis of these patients. A good example of this is the differentiation between sinonasal undifferentiated carcinoma (SNUC) and sinonasal LELC, for although the mortality rate of adequately treated LELC appears to be low, SNUC generally speaking, has a worse prognosis.

M. S. Said, MD, PhD

Papillary Thyroid Carcinoma in a Branchial Cleft Cyst without a Thyroid Primary: Navigating a Diagnostic Dilemma

Ruhl DS, Sheridan MF, Sniezek JC (Tripler Army Med Ctr (TAMC), honolulu, HI; Tri-State Otolaryngology-Head & Neck Surgery, Huntington, WV)

Case Rep Otolaryngol 2013:405342, 2013

We report a rare case of papillary thyroid carcinoma incidentally found within a branchial cleft cyst. Only four other cases have been described in the literature. A total thyroidectomy and selective neck dissection was performed, and no evidence of occult primary disease was found after review of fine sections. Branchial cleft cysts are the most common lateral neck masses. Ectopic thyroid tissue within a branchial cleft cyst is an unusual phenomenon, and papillary thyroid carcinoma arising from this tissue is extremely rare. Clinicians are left with a diagnostic dilemma when presented with thyroid tissue neoplasm within a neck cyst in the absence of a thyroid primary—is this a case of metastatic disease with a missed primary or rather carcinoma arising in ectopic thyroid tissue? A thorough discussion of the etiologies of these lateral neck masses is reviewed including the embryogenesis of thyroid tissue in a branchial cleft cyst. The prognosis of patients with papillary thyroid carcinoma in lateral neck cysts without a primary site identified appears to be good following excision of the cyst and total thyroidectomy. Other management recommendations regarding these unique lateral neck malignancies are also presented (Figs 2 and 3).

► Reports of papillary carcinoma in neck sites other than the thyroid gland indicate that it is usually seen in the central neck thyroglossal duct cyst, which contains thyroid follicle tissue in its wall and is considered the site of origin of these cancers. Reports in laterally located branchial cleft neck cysts without a thyroid

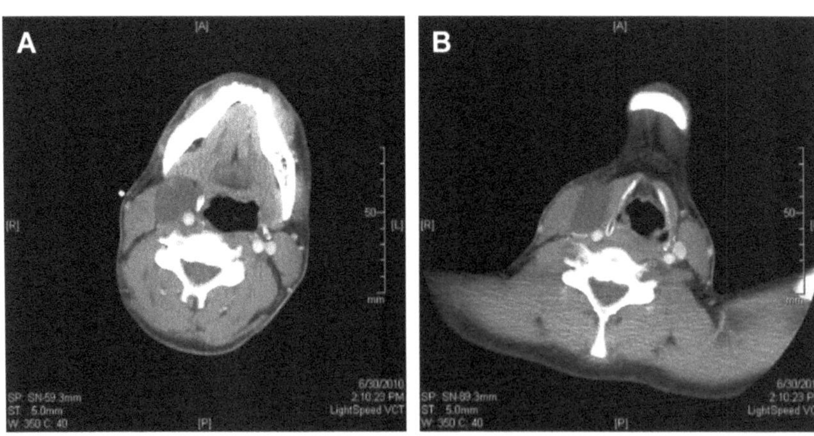

FIGURE 2.—Axial CT Scan with contrast showing the cystic neck mass lateral to the great vessels. (Reprinted from Ruhl DS, Sheridan MF, Sniezek JC. Papillary thyroid carcinoma in a branchial cleft cyst without a thyroid primary: navigating a diagnostic dilemma. *Case Rep Otolaryngol.* 2013;2013:405342, with permission from Douglas S. Ruhl et al.)

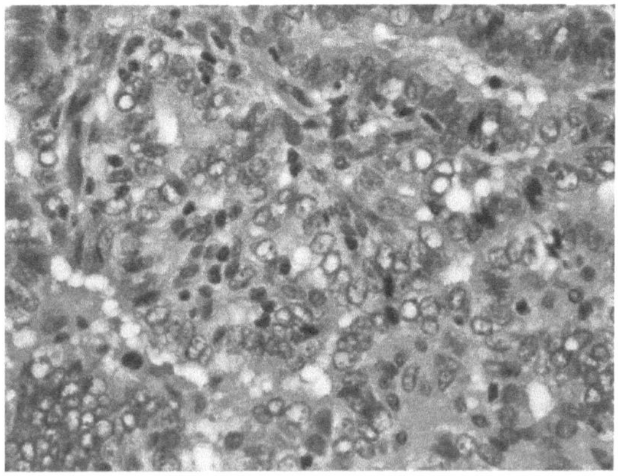

FIGURE 3.—High power (40×) microscopy of the lateral neck mass showing cells with enlarged nuclei, intranuclear cytoplasmic inclusions, nuclear grooves and powdery chromatin which is diagnostic for papillary thyroid carcinoma. (Reprinted from Ruhl DS, Sheridan MF, Sniezek JC. Papillary thyroid carcinoma in a branchial cleft cyst without a thyroid primary: navigating a diagnostic dilemma. *Case Rep Otolaryngol.* 2013;2013:405342, with permission from Douglas S. Ruhl et al.)

primary are extremely rare, with only 4 cases reported in the existing literature.[1] This case report highlights an additional case in a 20-year-old man (Figs 2 and 3). Theories on the mechanism of these incidents remain unclear and poorly defined, but some suggest an inclusion or an entrapped thyroid tissue during branchial pouch developments. Similar to events in which papillary carcinoma is found in a thyroglossal duct cyst or even those occurring in the ovary as struma ovarii, total thyroidectomy is recommended because experience has taught us that papillary microcarcinoma can be seen in the thyroid gland when thyroid cancer is seen in these extrathyroidal sites. Despite the rarity of these cases, awareness of their existence in important in trying to explain the origin of papillary thyroid cancer in which no obvious thyroid primary can be detected.

M. Sherif Said, MD, PhD

Reference

1. Mehmood RK, Basha SI, Ghareeb E. A case of papillary carcinoma arising in ectopic thyroid tissue within a branchial cyst with neck node metastasis. *Ear Nose Throat J.* 2006;85:675-676.

Polymorphous Low Grade Adenocarcinoma has a Consistent p63+/p40− Immunophenotype that Helps Distinguish it from Adenoid Cystic Carcinoma and Cellular Pleomorphic Adenoma

Rooper L, Sharma R, Bishop JA (The Johns Hopkins Med Institutions, Baltimore, MD)

Head Neck Pathol 2014 [Epub ahead of print]

Polymorphous low grade adenocarcinoma (PLGA) is a tumor of minor salivary glands that exhibits considerable morphologic overlap with adenoid cystic carcinoma and cellular pleomorphic adenoma, especially in small biopsy specimens. Unlike these other tumor types. PLGAs do not harbor a myoepithelial component, yet their frequent positivity for p63 diminishes the usefulness of this particular myoepithelial marker as a discriminating immunostain. p40 is an antibody that recognizes ΔNp63, a p63 isoformthat is more specific for true myoepithelial differentiation. As such, p40 immunostaining could help distinguish PLGAs from adenoid cystic carcinomas and pleomorphic adenomas. In this study, p63 and p40 immunohistochemistry was performed on paraffin embedded, formalin fixed tissue from 11 PLGAs, 101 adenoid cystic carcinomas, and 31 pleomorphic adenomas. All 11 PLGAs (100 %) were positive for p63 but completely negative for p40. Among adenoid cystic carcinomas, 91 of 101 (90 %) were positive for p63 and 90/101 (89 %) were positive for p40. The single discordant p63+/p40– adenoid cystic carcinoma exhibited solid architecture and high grade features not typically seen in PLGA. Among pleomorphic adenomas, 21/31 (68 %) were positive for p63 and 13/31 (42 %) were positive for p40. For the pleomorphic adenomas, the discordant p63+/p40– staining pattern was seen only in the overtly mesenchymal chondromyxoid stroma. The cellular epithelial component of the pleomorphic adenomas demonstrated concordant p63+/p40+ or p63–/p40– immunophenotypes. PLGA consistently exhibits a p63+/p40– immunophenotype that can help distinguish it from adenoid cystic carcinoma and cellular pleomorphic adenoma, tumors that characteristically demonstrate concordant p63 and p40 immunostaining patterns. A p63/p40 immunohistochemical panel can provide a valuable tool for making the distinction between these morphologically similar but clinically divergent entities (Fig 1, Table 1).

▶ Differentiating among polymorphous low-grade adenocarcinoma (PLGA), adenoid cystic carcinoma, and cellular pleomorphic adenoma can sometimes be difficult, particularly when dealing with a small biopsy. Differentiation has depended mostly on morphologic evaluation of the specimen with little support from ancillary studies, and although molecular testing can be somewhat helpful in certain instances, the practicality and speed of immunohistochemistry, if applicable, can be quite useful. This article highlights the usefulness of P40 as a more specific marker for myoepithelial differentiation than P63, thus making it more useful in identifying PLGA based on the fact that PLGA does not show evidence of myoepithelial differentiation yet can be diffusely and strongly positive for P63 (Fig 1, Table 1). Previous attempts to use C-kit, Ki-67, CD43, BCL2, and S100 immunohistochemistry have not been successful in definitively differentiating among the 3 entities. The uniform negativity of PLGA to P40 shown in this article certainly helps in that differentiation, although some reservations remain, as the authors show that in some cases of high-grade adenoid cystic carcinoma, P40 negativity can also be seen. I believe that their finding is a

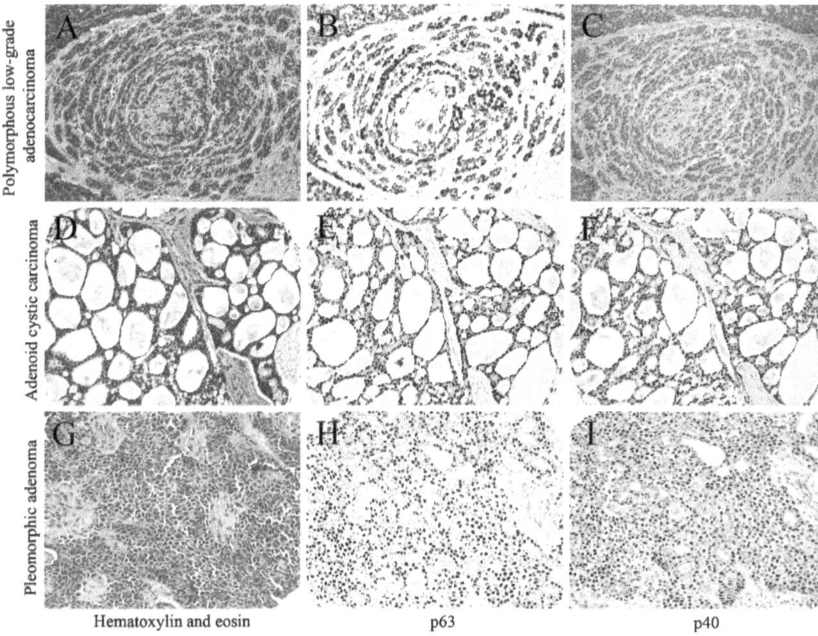

FIGURE 1.—All polymorphous low grade adenocarcinomas (H&E, **a**) showed diffuse, strong, positivity for p63 (**b**) but complete negativity for p40 (**c**). In contrast, most of the adenoid cystic carcinomas (H&E, **d**) and pleomorphic adenomas (H&E, **g**) demonstrated positivity for both p63 (**e**, **h**) and p40 (**f**, **i**) in a peripheral (myoepithelial cell) pattern. (Reprinted from Rooper L, Sharma R, Bishop JA. Polymorphous low grade adenocarcinoma has a consistent p63+/p4o- immunophenotype that helps distinguish it from adenoid cystic carcinoma and cellular pleomorphic adenoma. *Head Neck Pathol.* 2014, with permission from Springer Science+Business Media.)

TABLE 1.—p63/p40 Immunophenotypes in Polymorphous Low-Grade Adenocarcinoma, Adenoid Cystic Carcinoma, and Pleomorphic Adenoma

	p63+/p40+	p63+/p40−	p63−/p40−
Polymorphous low-grade adenocarcinoma	0/11 (0 %)	11/11 (100 %)	0/11 (0 %)
Adenoid cystic carcinoma	90/101 (89 %)	1/101 (1 %)	10/101 (10 %)
Pleomorphic adenoma	13/31 (42 %)	8/31 (26 %)	10/31 (32 %)

Reprinted from Rooper L, Sharma R, Bishop JA. Polymorphous low grade adenocarcinoma has a consistent p63+/p4o- immunophenotype that helps distinguish it from adenoid cystic carcinoma and cellular pleomorphic adenoma. *Head Neck Pathol.* 2014, with permission from Springer Science+Business Media.

useful tool that can be used in concert with the morphologic findings or other previously attempted immunohistochemical methods to reach a diagnosis.

M. Sherif Said, MD, PhD

Multifocal Fibrosing Thyroiditis and Its Association with Papillary Thyroid Carcinoma Using BRAF Pyrosequencing

Frank R, Baloch ZW, Gentile C, et al (Univ of Pennsylvania, Philadelphia)

Endocr Pathol 25:236-240, 2014

Multifocal fibrosing thyroiditis (MFT) is characterized by numerous foci of fibrosis in a stellate configuration with fibroelastotic and fibroblastic centers entrapping epithelial structures. MFT has been proposed as a risk factor for papillary thyroid carcinoma (PTC) development. We attempted to identify whether MFT showed such molecular changes and could possibly be related to PTC. We identified seven cases of PTC with MFT in our institutional pathology database and personal consult service of one of the authors (VAL) for the years 1999 to 2012. Areas of PTC, MFT, and normal tissue were selected for *BRAF* analysis. Macrodissection, DNA extraction and PCR amplification, and pyrosequencing were performed to detect *BRAF* mutations in codon 600. All of the MFT lesions and normal thyroid tissue were negative for *BRAF* mutations. Of the seven PTCs analyzed, five (71 %) were negative for *BRAF* mutations, while two cases were positive. In our study, none of the MFT lesions harbored *BRAF* mutations, whereas 29 % (two of seven) PTCs in the same gland were positive. Hence, in this small study, we found no evidence that the MFT lesion is a direct precursor to PTC. It is likely an incidental bystander in the process and a reflection of the background thyroiditis (Figs. 1 and 3).

▶ Certain factors have been identified as, or at least believed by some to be, risk factors for papillary carcinoma, including radiation exposure and Hashimoto thyroiditis. This article explored the role of multifocal fibrosing thyroiditis (MFT) as a risk factor for papillary carcinoma. Foci of MFT can be seen in some papillary carcinoma cases and in cases that do not show cancer; its etiology remains ill

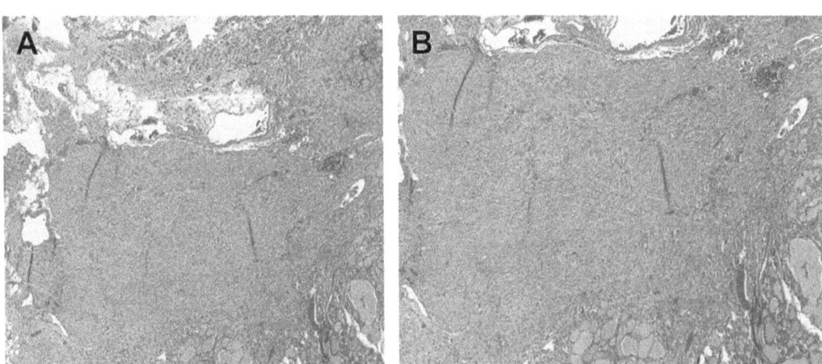

FIGURE 1.—Representative focus of multifocal fibrosing thyroiditis scar showing stellate-shaped area of fibrosis located separate from the areas of PTC with intervening benign thyroid tissue: a H&E ×2, b H&E ×4. (With kind permission from Springer Science+Business Media. Frank R, Baloch ZW, Gentile C, et al. Multifocal fibrosing thyroiditis and its association with papillary thyroid carcinoma using BRAF pyrosequencing. *Endocr Pathol.* 2014;25:236-240, with permission from Springer Science+Business Media New York.)

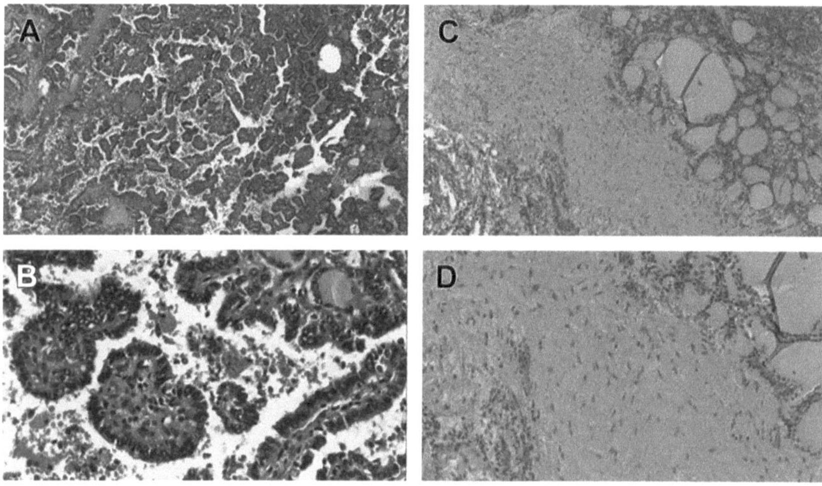

FIGURE 3.—Representative case of PTC with MFT with *BRAF* mutation: **a** PTC H&E ×10, **b** PTC H&E ×20, **c** multifocal fibrosing scar H&E ×10, **d** multifocal fibrosing scar H&E ×20. (With kind permission from Springer Science+Business Media. Frank R, Baloch ZW, Gentile C, et al. Multifocal fibrosing thyroiditis and its association with papillary thyroid carcinoma using BRAF pyrosequencing. *Endocr Pathol.* 2014;25:236-240, with permission from Springer Science+Business Media New York.)

defined, although it is usually seen accompanying lymphocytic thyroiditis. The authors discussed the current suggestion that MFT is analogous to radial scar in breast tissue that is related to progression to breast cancer. However, as the abstract indicates, none of the cases of MFT showed *BRAF* mutation, and thus a direct relationship of progression to cancer was not found (Figs 1 and 3); however, the theory the authors advanced is interesting, citing that MFT, like other thyroid injuries, can lead to epithelial hyperplasia, atypia, and stromal response, each of which may be an early stage in the pathogenesis of papillary thyroid carcinoma.

M. Sherif Said, MD, PhD

SMARCB1 (INI-1)-deficient Carcinomas of the Sinonasal Tract

Bishop JA, Antonescu CR, Westra WH (The Johns Hopkins Med Institutions, Baltimore, MD; Memorial Sloan Kettering Cancer Ctr, NY)

Am J Surg Pathol 38:1282-1289, 2014

SMARCB1 (*INI-1*) is a tumor-suppressor gene located on chromosome 22q11.2. Its gene product is ubiquitously expressed in nuclei of all normal tissues. *SMARCB1* gene inactivation has been implicated in the pathogenesis of a diverse group of malignant neoplasms that tend to share "rhabdoid" cytomorphology. This group of SMARCB1-deficient tumors is now further expanded by a subset of carcinomas arising in the sinonasal tract. *SMARCB1* immunostaining was performed on 142 sinonasal carcinomas. Tumors that showed loss of expression were further characterized for SMARCB1 deletions by fluorescence in situ hybridization. Nine of 142

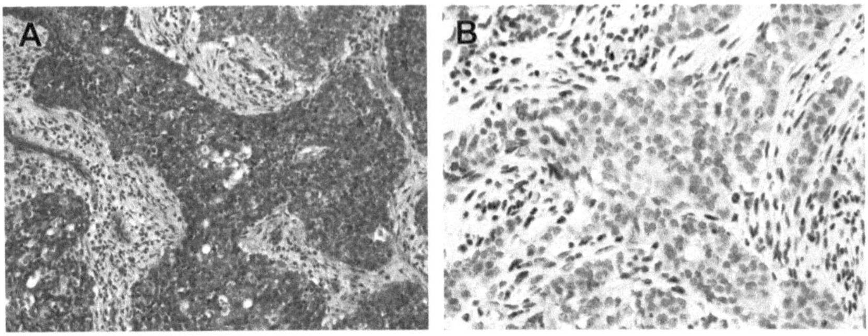

FIGURE 1.—A, Most of the carcinomas were composed of basaloid nests and lobules with intervening desmoplastic stroma (case 3). B, All tumors exhibited complete loss of SMARCB1 immunostaining, with stromal and inflammatory cells serving as an internal positive control (case 3). (Reprinted from Bishop JA, Antonescu CR, Westra WH. SMARCB1 (INI-1)-deficient carcinomas of the sinonasal tract. *Am J Surg Pathol.* 2014;38:1282-1289, with permission from Lippincott Williams & Wilkins.)

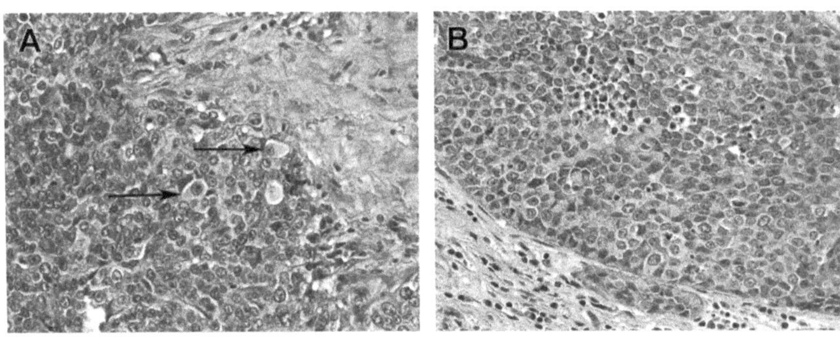

FIGURE 2.—. Each SMARCB1-deficient sinonasal carcinoma exhibited a component of rhabdoid cells, but their distribution was variable. In some cases, the rhabdoid cells (arrows) were individually dispersed among the basaloid tumor cells (A, case 2), whereas in others the rhabdoid cells predominated (B, case 6). (Reprinted from Bishop JA, Antonescu CR, Westra WH. SMARCB1 (INI-1)-deficient carcinomas of the sinonasal tract. *Am J Surg Pathol.* 2014;38:1282-1289, with permission from Lippincott Williams & Wilkins.)

(6%) primary sinonasal carcinomas showed loss of SMARCB1 expression by immunohistochemistry. Five patients were women, and patients ranged in age from 33 to 78 years (mean 59 y). The SMARCB1-deficient tumors were characterized by nests, sheets, and cords of cells without any histologic evidence of specific (eg, squamous or glandular) differentiation. The tumors comprised varying proportions of basaloid and rhabdoid cells. The SMARCB1-deficient carcinomas had been diagnosed as nonkeratinizing squamous cell carcinomas (n = 3), sinonasal undifferentiated carcinomas (n = 2), myoepithelial carcinoma (n = 2), nonintestinal adenocarcinoma (n = 1), and carcinoma, not otherwise specified (n = 1). Fluorescence in situ hybridization analysis revealed *SMARCB1* deletions in 6 of 8 (75%) carcinomas. The SMARCB1-deficient carcinomas did not harbor human papillomavirus or NUT-1 alterations. Six patients presented

TABLE 1.—SMARCB1-Deficient Sinonasal Carcinomas

Case	Original Diagnosis	Mucicarmine	INI-1	AE1/AE3	p63/p40	S100	SMA	SYN	CHR	NUT-1	p16/HR HPV ISH	INI-1 FISH
1	Nonintestinal adenocarcinoma	Focal	–	+	Focal	Focal	–	Focal	–	–	–/–	Homozygous deletion
2	NKSCC	–	–	+	+	–	–	Focal	–	–	+/–	Homozygous deletion
3	SNUC	–	–	+	–	–	–	–	–	–	+/–	Homozygous deletion
4	NKSCC	–	–	+	+	–	–	–	–	–	–/–	Homozygous deletion
5	SNUC	–	–	+	–	–	–	Focal	–	–	–/–	Homozygous deletion
6	NKSCC	–	–	+	+	–	–	–	–	–	–/–	Heterozygous deletion
7	Myoepithelial carcinoma	–	–	+	–	–	–	Focal	–	–	–/–	Normal
8	Myoepithelial carcinoma	–	–	+	–	–	–	Focal	–	–	–/–	Normal
9	Carcinoma NOS	Focal	–	+	–	–	–	NA	–	–	–/–	NA

CHR indicates chromogranin; HR HPV ISH, high-risk HPV in situ hybridization; NA, not available due to inadequate tissue; NKSCC, nonkeratinizing squamous cell carcinoma; NOS, not otherwise specified; SMA, smooth muscle actin; SYN, synaptophysin; SNUC, sinonasal undifferentiated carcinoma.

Reprinted from Bishop JA, Antonescu CR, Westra WH. SMARCB1 (INI-1)-deficient carcinomas of the sinonasal tract. *Am J Surg Pathol.* 2014;38:1282-1289, with permission from Lippincott Williams & Wilkins.

TABLE 2.—Clinical Characteristics of the Patients with SMARCB1-deficient Sinonasal Carcinomas

Case	Age	Sex	Presentation	Site	Stage	Primary Treatment	Clinical Course	Current Status (Follow-up) (mo)
1	71	F	Sinus pain	Maxillary	T3 N0 M0	Surgery+XRT initially	Local recurrence	DWD (15)
2	46	F	Headaches	Frontal, ethmoid	T4 N0 M0	Surgery+XRT	NED	NED (57)
3	33	M	Proptosis, vision defects	Nasal, ethmoid, frontal	T4 N0 M0	Surgery+XRT	Local recurrence, distant metastases	DWD (30)
4	60	M	Nasal obstruction	Ethmoid	T4 N0 M0	Surgery+XRT	NED	Died of unclear reasons (10)
5	54	F	Headache, nasal discharge	Nasal, ethmoid, maxillary	T4 N0 M0	Surgery+CT+XRT	Local recurrence	DWD (15)
6	44	M	Eye swelling, tearing	Ethmoid	T4 N0 M0	Surgery+planned XRT	NA	NA (0)
7	78	F	Nasal obstruction	Nasal, ethmoid	T3 N0 M0	Surgery	NED	NED (26)
8	77	M	Headache, eye pain	Ethmoid	T4 N0 M0	Surgery+CT+XRT	Distant metastases	DWD (17)
9	67	F	Headache, ear ache	Ethmoid	T4 N0 M0	Surgery+CT+XRT	Locoregional recurrence	NED (16)

CT indicates chemotherapy; DM, distant metastases; DWD, died with disease; F, female; LR, local recurrence; M, male; NA, not applicable; NED, no evidence of disease; RM, regional metastases; RT, radiation therapy.

Reprinted from Bishop JA, Antonescu CR, Westra WH. SMARCB1 (INI-1)-deficient carcinomas of the sinonasal tract. *Am J Surg Pathol.* 2014;38:1282-1289, with permission from Lippincott Williams & Wilkins.

with T4 disease, 5 patients developed local recurrences and/or distant metastases, and 4 died of their disease. Inactivation of the *SMARCB1* tumor-suppressor gene appears to be involved in the pathogenesis of a subset of sinonasal carcinomas, further expanding the family of SMARCB1-deficient neoplasms and further delineating a bewildering group of poorly/undifferentiated, aggressive carcinomas arising at this site. The ability to detect SMARCB1 loss by immunohistochemistry, particularly when dealing with poorly differentiated carcinomas with basaloid or rhabdoid features, should facilitate a more comprehensive understanding of these sinonasal carcinomas including clinical behavior and response to targeted therapies (Figs. 1 and 2, Tables 1 and 2).

▶ Sinonasal carcinomas are difficult cancers with significant management and psychologic implications; proper classification and characterization of the cancer type carries important implications on their treatment strategies. This article, as noted in the abstract, identified a subset of carcinomas exhibiting INI-1 deficiency (Fig 1, Table 1). The authors emphasized that all these tumors focally exhibited rhabdoid features (Fig 2). They also emphasized that these INI-1-positive tumors had a tendency for aggressive course, as evidenced by advanced stage at presentation, potential for metastasis, and a 50% mortality rate. Identifying this subset of INI-1-deficient carcinomas can help design a more efficient and targeted therapy to combat these aggressive tumors, and it would be beneficial to see additional studies from variable institutions to compare their findings with those of this study.

M. Sherif Said, MD, PhD

Prognostic features in mucoepidermoid carcinoma of major salivary glands with emphasis on tumour histologic grading

Katabi N, Ghossein R, Ali S, et al (Memorial Sloan-Kettering Cancer Ctr, NY)

Histopathology 2014 [Epub ahead of print]

Aims.—To compare the different grading systems of mucoepidermoid carcinoma (MEC) and identify the most reliable and objective histopathologic features predictive of outcome.

Methods and Results.—Seventy-two cases diagnosed as MEC were subjected to a meticulous histopathologic re-review. 20 of 72 (28%) cases were originally misdiagnosed as MEC including 16 as high grade (HG). Among the 52 confirmed MEC, median follow up (FU) was 59 months. Mitosis ($\geq$4/10 High Power Fields), necrosis, pleomorphism, focal keratinization, desmoplasia, and lymph node metastasis were associated with adverse disease specific survival (DSS) and recurrence free survival (RFS) ($P < 0.002$). In all grading systems, low and intermediate grade had similar DSS and RFS but much better outcome than HG ($P < 0.007$). All patients with tumour harboring low mitotic rate and no necrosis did not recur except for one patient with a positive margin. All cases with high mitotic rate and necrosis died or recurred.

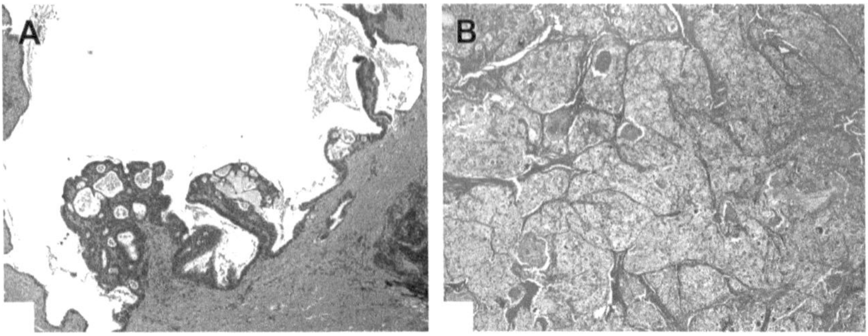

FIGURE 1.—(A–B) **A**, Low grade mucoepidermoid carcinoma: predominantly cystic; **B**, Intermediate grade mucoepidermoid carcinoma: solid growth pattern with bland cytology. (Reprinted from Katabi N, Ghossein R, Ali S, et al. Prognostic features in mucoepidermoid carcinoma of major salivary glands with emphasis on tumour histologic grading. *Histopathology*. 2014 [Epub ahead of print], with permission from Blackwell Publishing Lmt.)

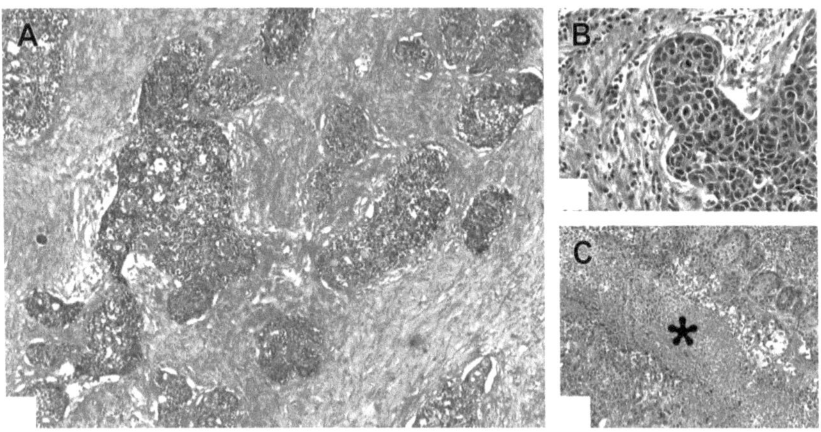

FIGURE 2.—(A–C) High grade mucoepidermoid carcinoma: **A**, Infiltration and solid growth pattern; **B**, increased mitotic activity; **C**, tumour necrosis (star). (Reprinted from Katabi N, Ghossein R, Ali S, et al. Prognostic features in mucoepidermoid carcinoma of major salivary glands with emphasis on tumour histologic grading. *Histopathology*. 2014 [Epub ahead of print], with permission from Blackwell Publishing Lmt.)

Conclusions.—The majority of previously diagnosed HG MEC cases are misclassified. There is no difference in outcome between low and intermediate grade in all grading schemes. Consideration should be given to stratify MEC based on relatively objective criteria such as mitosis and necrosis (Figs 1 and 2, Tables 1, 2 and 5).

▶ Mucoepidermoid carcinoma is the most common salivary gland malignancy in children and adults alike and hence has been the subject of interest of many pathologists over the years, with a number of histologic classification schemes, most famously among the Armed Forces Institute of Pathology, Brandwein, and modified Healy systems (Table 1). The authors aimed at defining more objective

TABLE 1.—AFIP, Brandwein, and Modified Healy Grading Systems (Modified From Seethala)[5]

AFIP		Brandwein		Modified Healy
Intracystic component <20%	+2	Intracystic component <25%	+2	Low grade:
				• Macrocysts and microcysts
Neural invasion	+2	Neural invasion	+2	• Differentiated mucin with 1/1 mucin/ epidermoid with minimal to moderate intermediate cells
		Tumour invades in small nests	+2	
Mitosis (≥4/10HPFs)	+3	Mitosis (≥4/10HPFs)	+3	• Absent to minimal pleomorphism and rare mitoses
				• Broad front or circumscribed borders
				• Pools of extravasated mucin
Necrosis	+3	Necrosis	+3	Intermediate grade:
		Vascular invasion	+3	• Solid nests, few microcysts, no macrocysts
Anaplasia	+4	Nuclear atypia	+3	
		Bone invasion	+3	• Mild to moderate pleomorphism, few mitoses, prominent nuclei and nucleoli
				• Invasive, well defined and uncircumscribed with fibrosis separating tumour nests Peripheral chronic inflammation
Grade	Score	Grade	Score	High grade:
Low grade	0–4	Low grade	0	• Predominately solid with no macrocysts
Intermediate grade	5–6	Intermediate grade	2–3	
High grade	≥7	High grade	≥4	• Tumour cells range from poorly differentiated to epidermoid and intermediate cells to ductal cells adenocarcinoma
				• Marked pleomorphism and easily found mitoses
				• Perineural and vascular invasions, soft tissue invasion, and desmoplasia
				• Less common peripheral chronic inflammation

Editor's Note: Please refer to original journal article for full references.

Reprinted from Katabi N, Ghossein R, Ali S, et al. Prognostic features in mucoepidermoid carcinoma of major salivary glands with emphasis on tumour histologic grading. *Histopathology.* 2014 [Epub ahead of print], with permission from Blackwell Publishing Lmt.

TABLE 2.— Our own (Memorial Sloan-Kettering Cancer Center) Grading System

	Low Grade	Intermediate Grade	High Grade
Predominant growth pattern	Cystic	Predominantly solid	Any (usually solid)
Infiltration	Well circumscribed borders	Well circumscribed or infiltrative borders	Any (usually infiltrative borders)
Mitosis	0–1/10 HPF	<4/10 HPFs	≥4/10 HPFs
Tumour necrosis	Absent	Absent	Present

HPF: high power fields. Mitotic rate was determined by counting mitoses in 10 contiguous HPF (400×) in the areas of greatest concentrations of mitoses, these 10 HPF correspond to 2.4 mm^2.

Reprinted from Katabi N, Ghossein R, Ali S, et al. Prognostic features in mucoepidermoid carcinoma of major salivary glands with emphasis on tumour histologic grading. *Histopathology.* 2014 [Epub ahead of print], with permission from Blackwell Publishing Lmt.

TABLE 5.—Pathological Predictors of Disease Specific Survival and Recurrence Free Survival

	Number	5-Years DSS %	*P* Value	5-Years RFS %	*P* Value
Tumour size					
<2 cm	34	100	0.06	100	0.006
≥2 cm	18	86		72	
Tumour border					
Circumscribed	30	100	0.23	100	0.002
Partial circumscribed	15	93		93	
Infiltration	7	80		50	
Lymphoid stroma					
Absent	9	89	0.3	76	0.14
Present	43	96		94	
% Cystic component					
<80	22	89	0.12	83	0.21
≥80	30	100		95	
% Intermediate cells					
<60	25	95	0.97	83	0.27
≥60	27	94		95	
% Mucous cells					
<20	32	92	0.29	88	0.66
≥20	20	100		92	
% Epidermoid cells					
<10	32	100	0.1	95	0.17
≥10	20	88		82	
Vascular invasion					
Absent	49	100	<0.0001	97	<0.0001
Present	3	33		0	
Perineural invasion					
Absent	42	97	0.37	94	0.16
Present	10	88		75	
Pleomorphism					
Absent	49	100	<0.0001	97	<0.0001
Present	3	50		0	
Mitoses					
<4	48	100	<0.0001	97	<0.0001
≥4	4	33		0	
Keratin					
Absent	47	100	<0.001	97	<0.0001
Present	5	60		40	
Desmoplasia					
Absent	44	100	0.002	97	0.0005
Present	8	70		55	
Necrosis					
Absent	49	100	<0.0001	97	<0.001
Present	3	33		0	
Own Grade					
LG	30	100	<0.0001	95	<0.0001
IG	19	100		100	
HG	3	33		0	
AFIP Grade					
LG	47	100	<0.0001	97	<0.0001
IG	2	100		100	
HG	3	33		0	
Brandwein Grade					
LG	28	100	0.007	95	0.004
IG	17	100		100	
HG	7	71		57	
Healy Grade					
LG	30	100	<0.0001	95	<0.0001
IG	19	100		100	
HG	3	33		0	

(*Continued*)

TABLE 5. (*continued*)

	Number	5-Years DSS %	*P* Value	5-Years RFS %	*P* Value
EPE					
Absent	42	100	0.004	100	<0.0001
Present	8	73		55	
Margin					
Negative	32	100	0.09	100	0.01
Positive/close	19	87		74	
LN Metastasis					
Absent	41	100	<0.0001	100	<0.0001
Present	4	54		25	

DSS, Disease specific survival; RFS, Recurrence free survival; LG, low grade; IG, intermediate grade; HG, high grade; EPE, extraparenchymal extension; LN, lymph node.

Reprinted from Katabi N, Ghossein R, Ali S, et al. Prognostic features in mucoepidermoid carcinoma of major salivary glands with emphasis on tumour histologic grading. *Histopathology.* 2014 [Epub ahead of print], with permission from Blackwell Publishing Lmt.

criteria, citing that there is a lack of consensus among the current grading systems, a fact many practicing pathologists appreciate. Table 5 highlights and summarizes the study's objective of correlating pathologic predictors to specific survival and recurrence-free survival. Accordingly, the authors concluded with the suggestion of a new classification scheme (Memorial Sloan Kettering grading system; Table 2, Figs 1 and 2). The authors also concluded that high mucoepidermoid carcinoma is less frequent than it is believed to be in the existing literature; they considered the high grade form a rarity among types of mucoepidermoid carcinoma and thought that mitosis and necrosis are the 2 most important parameters in judging whether the tumor is a high grade.

M. Sherif Said, MD, PhD

Pediatric sinonasal tumors in the United States: incidence and outcomes

Gerth DJ, Tashiro J, Thaller SR (Univ of Miami, FL)
J Surg Res 190:214-220, 2014

Background.—Sinonasal tumors in the pediatric population are exceedingly rare.

Materials and Methods.—Surveillance, Epidemiology, and End Results database was used to identify 250 cases of sinonasal malignancy in patients aged <20 y (1973–2010). Malignant histology codes were based on the International Classification of Disease for Oncology, third edition coding scheme. Incidence rates were adjusted to the 2000 U.S. population. Survival outcomes were plotted using the Kaplan–Meier method and compared with the log-rank test. All other analyses were performed using standard statistical methods.

Results.—Overall incidence was 0.052 per 100,000. Rhabdomyosarcoma had the highest incidence among histologic groups. Regional stage was the most common at diagnosis (59%). Overall survival at 5-y

TABLE 1.—Incidence Rates of Pediatric Sinonasal Malignancies

Overall	0.0515
Gender	
Female	0.0543
Male	0.0488
Race	
White	0.0487
Black	0.0676
Other	0.0410
Age (y)	
<1	0.0147
1–4	0.0452
5–9	0.0422
10–14	0.0395
15–19	0.0849
Type	
Rhabdomyosarcomas	0.0214
Sarcomas	0.0052
Germ cell tumors	
Neuroectoderm tumors/ Neuroblastomas	0.0099
Lymphomas	0.0085
Other	0.0062
Stage	
In situ	0.0000
Localized	0.0063
Regional	0.0217
Distant	0.0063

Reprinted from Gerth DJ, Tashiro J, Thaller SR. Pediatric sinonasal tumors in the United States: incidence and outcomes. *J Surg Res*. 2014;190:214-220, with permission from Elsevier.

follow-up was 62.5%. Patients in age groups 1–4 and 15–19 y had the worst survival rates, as median survival was 205 and 104 mo, respectively. Distant metastases at the time of diagnosis signified a poor prognosis. These were associated with a 39-mo median survival. Survival improved during the study period, $P = 0.003$. Gender, race, site of lesion, or histology did not appear to affect mortality.

Conclusions.—Sinonasal tumors are rare in children and adolescents. Long-term survival is dependent on age and clinical stage at the time of diagnosis. Cancer-related surgery confers a survival advantage. Gender, race, and histologic type are not associated with mortality (Tables 1, 2 and 4).

▶ This is an interesting review and analysis on the Surveillance, Epidemiology, and End Results database analysis of pediatric sinonasal malignancies. The literature on this topic is rather limited in children.[1] Sinonasal malignancies in children are rare and in some instances are not diagnosed early in the course of the cancer because of the nonspecificity of symptoms; however, it is important to be aware of the possibility, although remote, in our pediatric population, particularly when symptoms are not resolved reasonably quickly or if the symptoms are thought to be due to more benign common childhood conditions.

TABLE 2.—Demographics and Clinical Characteristics

Category	*n* (% of total)
Gender	
Female	116 (46)
Male	134 (54)
Race	
White	182 (74)
Black	45 (18)
Other	19 (8)
Age (y)	
<1	6 (2)
1–4	42 (17)
5–9	42 (17)
10–14	57 (23)
15–19	103 (41)
Type	
Rhabdomyosarcoma	104 (47)
Sarcomas	23 (10)
Neuroectoderm tumors/ neuroblastomas	44 (20)
Lymphoma	40 (18)
Other	12 (5)
Site	
Nasal cavity	95 (38)
Maxillary sinus	76 (30)
Ethmoid sinus	40 (16)
Sphenoid sinus	10 (4)
Overlapping lesion of accessory sinuses	10 (4)
Accessory Sinus, numbers	19 (8)
Surgery	
Surgery	122 (49)
No surgery	127 (51)
Radiation	
Radiation	157 (63)
No radiation	91 (37)
Staging	
In situ	0 (0)
Localized	31 (18)
Regional	102 (59)
Distant	39 (23)
Diagnosis (y)	
1973–1978	9 (4)
1979–1984	14 (6)
1985–1991	25 (10)
1992–1997	33 (13)
1998–2003	66 (26)
2004–2010	103 (41)

Reprinted from Gerth DJ, Tashiro J, Thaller SR. Pediatric sinonasal tumors in the United States: incidence and outcomes. *J Surg Res.* 2014;190:214-220, with permission from Elsevier.

Tables 1, 2, and 4 give the reader a general comprehensive idea about the incidence and demographics of these cancers. Rhabdomyosarcoma remains the most common head and neck sarcoma, including the sinonasal tract with neuroectodermal tumors and lymphomas following. In contrast, squamous cell carcinoma is the most common type in adults. The nasal cavity in the pediatric

TABLE 4.—Survival by Demographic and Clinical Characteristics. Log-Rank Tests were Performed on Each Category to Evaluate for Statistical Significance

Category	Median Survival (mo)	5-y Survival (%)	15-y Survival (%)	30-y Survival (%)	P
Overall	NR	63	59	57	
Gender					NS
Female	NR	64	64	60	
Male	NR	61	54	—	
Race					NS
White	NR	64	60	60	
Black	205	55	51	—	
Other	NR	62	62	—	
Age (y)					0.018
<1	NR	100	100	—	
1–4	205	55	55	—	
5–9	NR	78	78	78	
10–14	NR	71	60	—	
15–19	104	52	49	—	
Histologic type					NS
Rhabdomyosarcoma	NR	54	54	54	
Sarcomas	NR	86	64	64	
Neuroectoderm tumors/ neuroblastomas	NR	65	57	—	
Lymphoma	NR	68	64	—	
Other	NR	65	65	—	
Site					NS
Nasal cavity	NR	70	67	67	
Maxillary sinus	NR	58	53	—	
Ethmoid sinus	NR	57	57	57	
Sphenoid sinus	NR	72	72	—	
Overlapping lesion of accessory sinuses	NR	72	54	—	
Accessory Sinus, numbers	52	47	47	—	
Surgery					0.042
Surgery	—	69	64	64	
No surgery	205	55	53	50	
Radiation					NS
Radiation	NR	59	58	55	
No radiation	NR	70	62	62	
Staging					0.001
In situ	NR	—	—	—	
Localized	NR	89	89	—	
Regional	NR	67	64	—	
Distant	39	43	32	—	
Diagnosis (y)					
1973–1978	14	22	22	22	0.003
1979–1984	27	36	36	36	
1985–1991	NR	50	50	—	
1992–1997	NR	71	68	—	
1998–2003	NR	66	—	—	
2004–2010	NR	69	—	—	

Reprinted from Gerth DJ, Tashiro J, Thaller SR. Pediatric sinonasal tumors in the United States: incidence and outcomes. *J Surg Res*. 2014;190:214-220, with permission from Elsevier.

population is the most common sinonasal site, and that, as the authors mention, could be because sinuses are not fully developed until adulthood.

M. Sherif Said, MD, PhD

Reference

1. Shapiro NL, Bhattacharyya N. Staging and survival for sinus cancer in the pediatric population. *Int J Pediatr Otorhinolaryngol.* 2009;73:1568-1571.

Basal Cell Adenocarcinoma and Basal Cell Adenoma of the Salivary Glands: A Clinicopathological Review of Seventy Tumors with Comparison of Morphologic Features and Growth Control Indices

Wilson TC, Robinson RA (Univ of Iowa)

Head Neck Pathol 2014 [Epub ahead of print]

Basal cell adenoma and basal cell adenocarcinoma represent uncommon basaloid salivary gland neoplasms that show marked morphologic similarity. We wished to compare clinical outcome and morphologic features as well as growth and proliferation associated markers for both neoplasms.

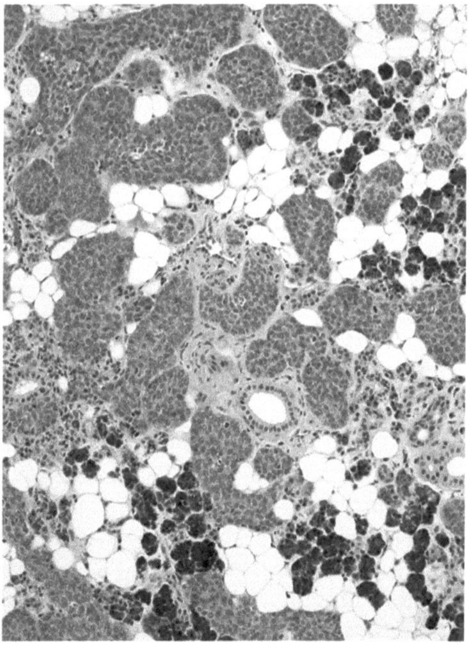

FIGURE 3.—Basal cell adenocarcinoma. Nests of basaloid cells with minimal atypia invade into the adjacent salivary gland tissue. (Reprinted from Wilson TC, Robinson RA. Basal cell adenocarcinoma and basal cell adenoma of the salivary glands: a clinicopathological review of seventy tumors with comparison of morphologic features and growth control indices. *Head Neck Pathol.* 2014 [Epub ahead of print], with permission from Springer Science+Business Media New York.)

TABLE 1.—Patient Demographics

	Basal Cell Adenoma	Basal Cell Adenocarcinoma
Tumors (N)*	41	29
Men	17	12
Women	24	17
Age (years)	14–86 (mean 58)	40–90 (mean 67)
Cases with follow-up (months)	30 (1–342 months; mean 75, median 48)	18 (1–170 months; mean 59, median 70)
Site		
Parotid	33	22
Submandibular	1	1
Sublingual	0	1
Oral cavity**	6	3
Parapharyngeal***	1	2

*70 Tumors in 69 patients; one man with basal cell adenoma and subsequent contralateral basal cell adenocarcinoma.

**Sites of oral cavity basal cell adenomas included lip (3), buccal mucosa (1), maxillary mucosa (1), and palate (1). Sites of oral cavity basal cell adenocarcinomas included lip (2) and buccal mucosa (1).

***The authors have maintained the parapharyngeal sites as the primary site although it is possible that these sites actually represented extensions from a parotid gland primary. No additional clinical or pathology data could lend support to a parotid origin.

Reprinted from Wilson TC, Robinson RA. Basal cell adenocarcinoma and basal cell adenoma of the salivary glands: a clinicopathological review of seventy tumors with comparison of morphologic features and growth control indices. *Head Neck Pathol.* 2014 [Epub ahead of print], with permission from Springer Science+Business Media New York.

TABLE 3.—Comparison of Growth and Proliferation-Related Markers of Basal Cell Adenoma and Basal Cell Adenocarcinoma

	Basal Cell Adenoma	Basal Cell Adenocarcinoma	*p* Value
Available tissue (N)	36	18	
Maximum mitotic rate (per 10 HPF)	0–5 (mean 0.7)	1–43 (mean 8.6)	<.001****
Ki-67 index*	0.1–10.5 % (mean 3.3)	0.4–53.3 % (mean 15.5)	<.001****
Apoptotic index**	0–9 (mean 1.0)	0–37 (mean 10.1)	<.001****
p53 overexpression	3 (8.3 %)	8 (44.4 %)	.004***
Loss of bcl-2 Expression	4 (11.1 %)	3 (16.7 %)	.429***

*Proliferation index calculated by number of cells with Ki-67 expression per at least 1,000 cells. Areas of greatest Ki-67 (hot spots) were selected for counting.

**Apoptotic Index calculated by counting maximum number of cells positive for caspase 3 per 10 high power fields.

***$\chi 2$, Fisher exact.

*****t* test, unpaired.

Reprinted from Wilson TC, Robinson RA. Basal cell adenocarcinoma and basal cell adenoma of the salivary glands: a clinicopathological review of seventy tumors with comparison of morphologic features and growth control indices. *Head Neck Pathol.* 2014 [Epub ahead of print], with permission from Springer Science+Business Media New York.

We reviewed the pathologic features of 70 neoplasms diagnosed as basal cell adenoma or basal cell adenocarcinoma. Observations included maximum mitotic activity and presence or absence of invasion into surrounding normal tissues as well as immunohistochemical studies for Ki-67, caspase 3, p53, and bcl-2. Establishing malignancy on the basis of invasion into surrounding benign tissues, 41 basal cell adenomas and 29 basal cell adenocarcinomas were identified. For tumors with follow-up, recurrence rates were 6.7 % for basal cell adenoma and 16.7 % for basal cell adenocarcinoma. One patient with basal cell adenocarcinoma had distant metastases and died of disease. Overall basal cell adenocarcinomas showed significantly higher values for growth and proliferation markers compared to basal cell adenomas. Salivary gland basal cell adenoma and basal cell adenocarcinoma show morphologic similarity. Basal cell adenocarcinoma can exhibit a locally aggressive behavior and has potential metastatic behavior. The overall mitotic rate and Ki-67 expression were higher in basal cell adenocarcinoma compared to basal cell adenoma, but overlap between the results of these observations in each tumor did not allow for accurate diagnosis or prediction of outcome in individual cases. We conclude that morphologic observation of local tissue invasion is the best marker for separating basal cell adenoma from basal cell adenocarcinoma (Fig 3, Tables 1 and 3).

► Many pathologists appreciate that differentiating basal cell adenocarcinoma from basal cell adenoma in small biopsies or fine-needle aspirates is a difficult if not impossible task. The subtlety of appreciating malignancy in differentiating these cases requires demonstration of invasive features such as tissue infiltration and perineural or angiolymphatic invasion; hence, an adequate sample and/or total resection with the margins well sampled is necessary. Usually, although not in all cases, necrosis alerts many pathologists to the possibility of malignant change in salivary glands (for example, in pleomorphic adenoma or myoepithelioma), but this change is not seen in basal cell adenocarcinomas. This study, comprising 70 patients with basal cell adenoma and carcinoma (Table 1), is interesting in that it sought to identify additional markers that may help in this task, including mitotic rate, Ki-67 index, apoptotic index, P53 expression, and BCL2 expression (Table 3). The authors' findings indicate only limited value for increased Ki-67 and mitotic activity and confirm that the observation of invasion (Fig 3) is the most valid parameter. This study is a good example of the fact that largely negative results in an investigation can be useful to focus the pathologists and investigators on what works best in evaluating these kinds of tumors.

M. Sherif Said, MD, PhD

A Prospective Assessment Defining the Limitations of Thyroid Nodule Pathologic Evaluation

Cibas ES, Baloch ZW, Fellegara G, et al (Brigham and Women's Hosp and Harvard Med School, Boston, MA; Univ of Pennsylvania, Philadelphia; Centro Diagnostico Italiano, Milan, Italy; et al)

Ann Intern Med 159:325-332, 2013

Background.—Clinical management of thyroid neoplasms is based on light microscopic diagnosis, but its accuracy and precision are poorly defined.

Objective.—To assess inter- and intraobserver variability of preoperative cytopathologic and postoperative histopathologic thyroid diagnoses.

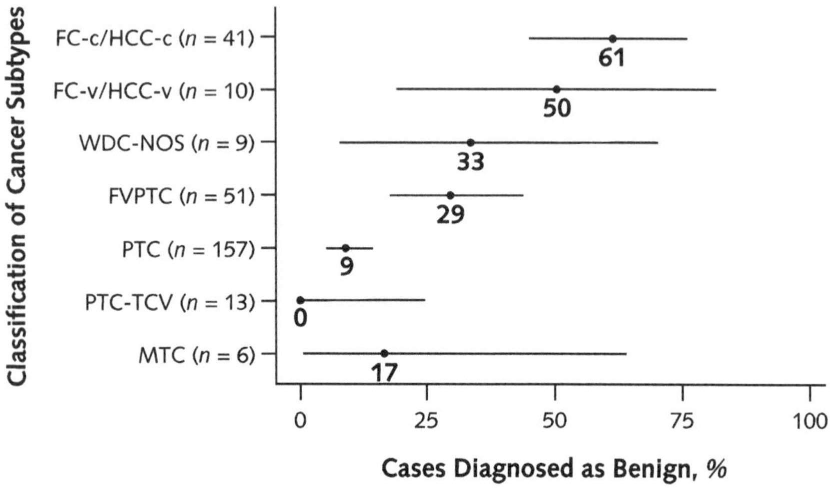

FIGURE 1.—Analysis of disagreements in categorical benign versus malignant diagnoses made by expert histopathologists, as a function of specific cancer subtypes. The y-axis represents all patients where at least 1 of the experts diagnosed the patient as having cancer. The x-axis represents the proportion of nodules diagnosed as benign by at least 1 expert for each cancer subtype (*y*-axis). Categorization in both axes was done while the expert was unaware of the other expert's diagnosis and the local pathologist's diagnosis. The averages of the 2 experts and 95% CIs are shown. Follicular and Hürthle cell carcinomas with capsular invasion resulted in the highest percentage of disagreement before the next step of conferral between the central histopathologists. FC-c/HCC-c = follicular/Hürthle cell carcinoma with capsular invasion; FC-v/HCC-v = follicular/Hürthle cell carcinoma with vascular invasion; FVPTC = follicular variant of papillary thyroid carcinoma; MTC = medullary thyroid carcinoma; PTC = papillary thyroid carcinoma; PTC-TCV = papillary thyroid carcinoma, tall cell variant; WDC-NOS = well-differentiated carcinoma, not otherwise specified. (Reprinted from Cibas ES, Baloch ZW, Fellegara G, et al. A prospective assessment defining the limitations of thyroid nodule pathologic evaluation. *Ann Intern Med.* 2013;159:325-332, with permission from American College of Physicians.)

Design.—Samples were collected in a prospective, multicenter trial validating a gene expression classifier between June 2009 and December 2010.

Setting.—14 academic and 35 community clinical sites.

Patients.—653 patients with 776 surgically resected thyroid nodules of 1 cm or greater.

Measurements.—Intraobserver concordance among 2 or more central histopathologists who independently read histopathology slides was calculated. Interobserver concordance between the diagnoses made by the central histopathologists and those made by local pathologists were calculated. Intra- and interobserver concordance for cytopathology was similarly calculated by comparing diagnoses made by local pathologists with those made by a central panel of 3 cytopathologists.

Results.—Concordance on the histopathologic distinction between benign and malignant diagnoses was 91% comparing local with central histopathologists and 90% comparing 2 central histopathologists. Using the 6-category Bethesda System, 64.0% of diagnoses made by local and central cytopathologists and 74.7% of intraobserver diagnoses were

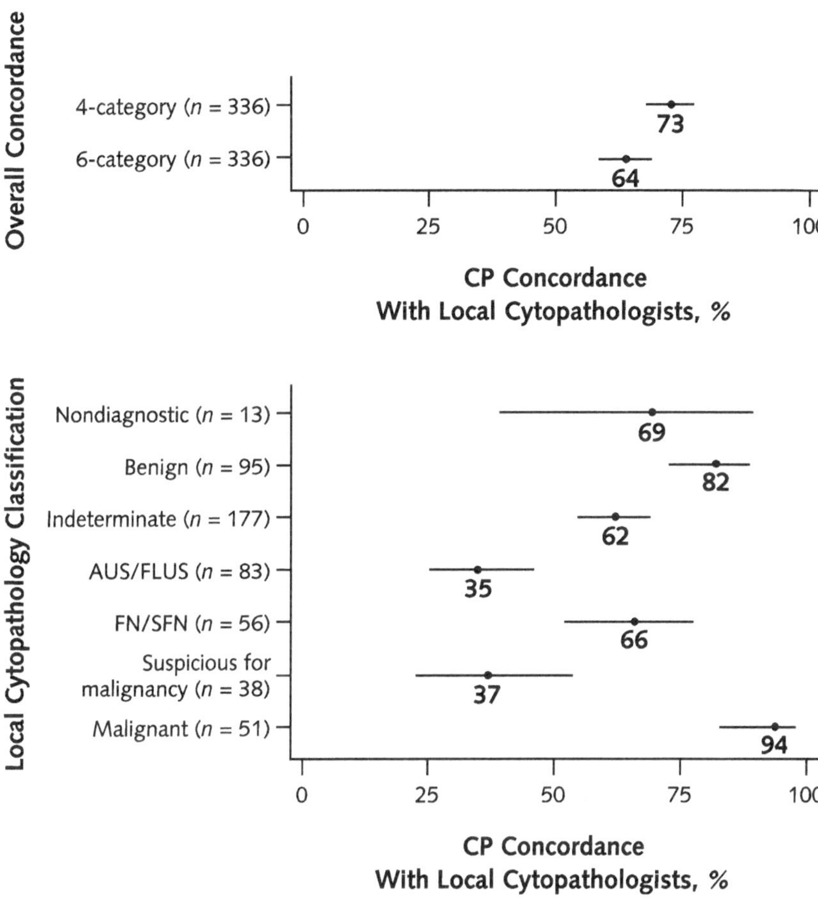

FIGURE 2.—Interobserver concordance of thyroid FNA cytopathologic diagnoses. Concordance (95% CI) of diagnoses between local pathologists and central CP members (interobserver) are shown. AUS/FLUS = atypia of undetermined significance/follicular lesion of undetermined significance; CP = cytopathology panel; FN/SFN = follicular neoplasm/suspicious for follicular neoplasm; FNA = fine-needle aspiration. **Top.** Overall concordance for the 6-category system is lower than that for the 4-category system. **Bottom.** CP vs. local cytopathology diagnostic concordance is highest for benign nodules and cancer diagnoses and lowest for AUS/FLUS diagnoses and nodules suspicious for malignancy. (Reprinted from Cibas ES, Baloch ZW, Fellegara G, et al. A prospective assessment defining the limitations of thyroid nodule pathologic evaluation. *Ann Intern Med.* 2013;159:325-332, with permission from American College of Physicians.)

concordant. Central cytopathologists made fewer indeterminate diagnoses than local pathologists (41.2% vs. 55.0%).

Limitations.—Many local pathologists did not use the Bethesda System, so their reports were translated to allow comparison. The study required histopathology, and the study population and specimens did not encompass all newly evaluated patients with a thyroid nodule.

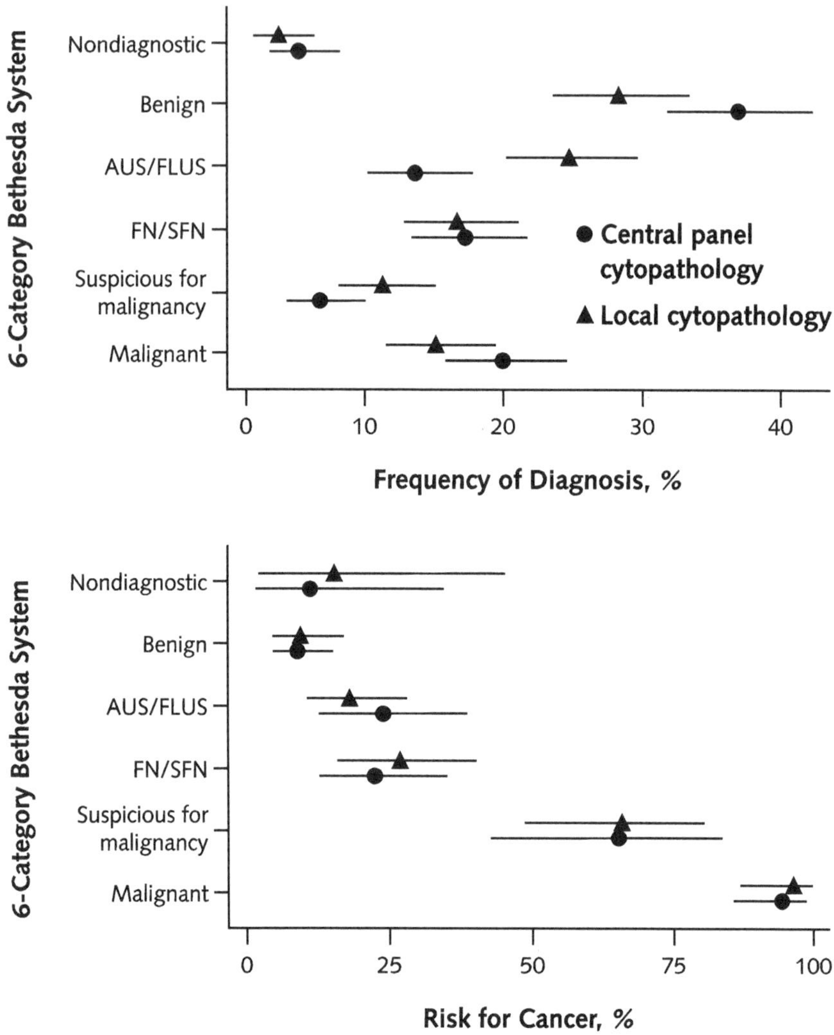

FIGURE 3.—Frequency distribution of central panel versus local cytopathologic diagnoses and risk for malignant thyroid nodule by cytology category, stratified by CP versus local pathologist. This figure and Table 3 depict results for local cytopathology and CP. AUS/FLUS = atypia of undetermined significance/ follicular lesion of undetermined significance; CP = cytopathology panel; FN/SFN = follicular neoplasm/ suspicious for follicular neoplasm. **Top.** Point estimates and 95% CIs are shown for the frequency of each cytopathologic diagnosis. **Bottom.** Risk for cancer was determined postoperatively for each cytopathologic diagnosis. For findings, see Table 3. Definitive cytopathologic diagnoses of benign nodules or cancer are made more often by the CP members, but those of AUS/FLUS and nodules suspicious for malignancy are made less often. Fewer cytologically indeterminate calls are made by the CP without a change in the risk for cancer for any given diagnostic category (e.g., the CP made more benign diagnoses, but the risk for cancer was not changed significantly from the local pathologists' benign diagnoses). (Reprinted from Cibas ES, Baloch ZW, Fellegara G, et al. A prospective assessment defining the limitations of thyroid nodule pathologic evaluation. *Ann Intern Med.* 2013;159:325-332, with permission from American College of Physicians.)

Conclusion.—Substantial inter- and intraobserver variability exists in the cytopathologic and histopathologic evaluation of thyroid nodules, confirming an inherent limitation of visual microscopic diagnosis (Figs 1-3).

▶ It is well known to pathologists reviewing thyroid specimens either in cytology or in a surgical pathology setting that variations in the interpretations of thyroid nodules exist among pathologists. Historically, this has sometimes created controversies and strong opinions among pathologists and even called into question in the confidence level some patients have in the cytological/histological interpretation of their specimens; hence, it is not infrequent that patients ask for second opinion or even multiple opinions. This interesting study, encompassing multiple institutions, aimed to assess this interobserver variability (Figs 1–3), only to confirm the substantial variability and indicate that the future of more concordant or decreasing interpretation differences rests, although not completely, on adding additional parameters in the methods used for diagnosis. For the time being, this seems to point toward molecular studies. I also want to add that this study was conducted by a number of eminent and experienced cytopathologists, pathologists, and clinicians, which adds a great deal of credibility to the findings. I think this work can add to our patients' understanding of the inherent problems in interpreting thyroid nodules.

M. Sherif Said, MD, PhD

Malignant triton tumour of the sinonasal tract: Case report and literature review

Zakzouk A, Hammad F, Langlois O, et al (Univ Hosp of Rouen, France)
Int J Surg Case Rep 5:608-612, 2014

Introduction.—The objective is to report a rare tumour of the sinonasal tract and conduct a literature review.

Malignant triton tumour is a subtype of malignant schwannoma with rhabdomyoblastic differentiation. It is a very rare tumour, with only 15 reported cases involving the sinonasal region.

Presentation of Case.—Forty-seven years old female presented with a right-sided epistaxis, progressive right sided nasal obstruction and anosmia and a visible mass in the right nasal cavity. Imaging studies showed a mass extending from the piriform aperture to the nasopharynx in contact with the dura and the orbital content. The mass was biopsied and the result was consistent with malignant triton tumour. The patient refused the surgery at first so chemotherapy with MAID protocol was started. After the fourth course of chemotherapy the treatment was stopped due to patient intolerance and a thrombosis of the jugular vein. Patient then underwent surgery with frontal craniotomy and dural excision, endoscopic control was done at the end to ensure a complete removal. The patient received radiotherapy in the postoperative period (56 Greys). At

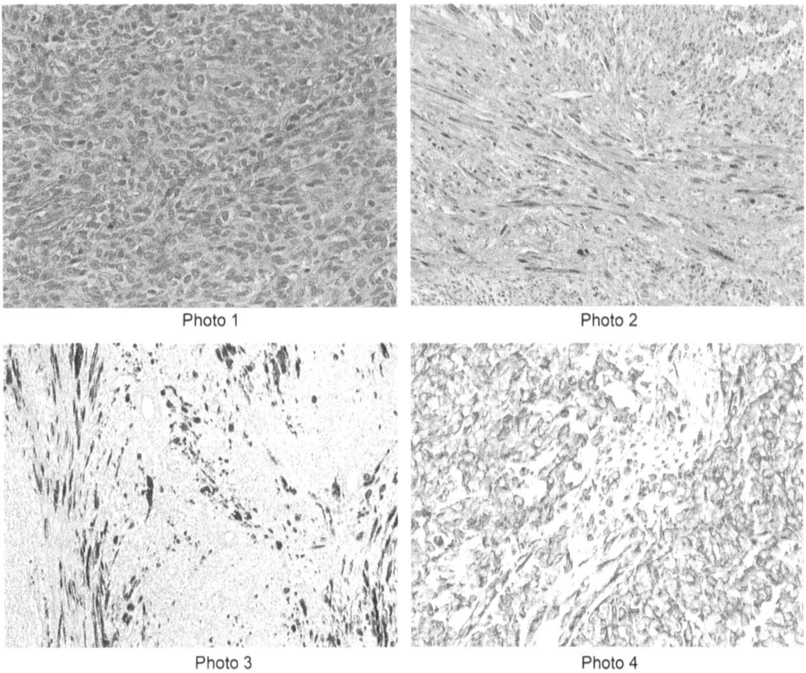

FIGURE 2.—Photo 1: immunohistochemical analysis showing focal positive Ps 100 staining (indicating a nerve sheet origin) with scattered spindle cells (IHC ×40). Photo 2: immunohistochemical analysis showing strong focal positive myogenin staining (indicating a striated muscle cells IHC ×25). Photo 3: immunohistochemical analysis showingstrong positive desmine staining (indicating a striated muscle cells IHC ×10). Photo 4: immunohistochemical analysis showing strong positive vimentin staining (indicatinga mesenchymal cells IHC ×40). (Reprinted from Zakzouk A, Hammad F, Langlois O, et al. Malignant triton tumour of the sinonasal tract: Case report and literature review. *Int J Surg Case Rep.* 2014;5:608-612, with permission from The Authors.)

5 years of follow-up the patient is doing fine with no signs of recurrence and normal ophthalmological findings.

Discussion.—Sixteen cases, including our case, have been reported to date in the literature. The mean age at presentation is 61 years. None of the cases were associated with neurofibromatosis type 1. Eight patients were reported to be alive 5 years post-treatment, and 2 patients were reported to have died of the disease. The prognosis for triton tumours in the sinonasal tract is better than that for triton tumours in other locations.

Conclusion.—Malignant triton tumour is a rare malignancy of the sinonasal tract. Otolaryngologists should be aware of this disease. The optimal treatment should include radical resection of the tumour (Fig 2, Table 1).

▶ Malignant triton tumor is a rare tumor in the head and neck, with only 53 cases reported in this location.[1] Some of these are recorded in the sinonasal tract (16 cases; Table 1), as mentioned in the review of this case report. Woodruff proposed the diagnostic criteria for this tumor in 1973.[2] Understandably, it

TABLE 1.—Review of the Literature on Malignant Triton Tumours of the Sinonasal Tract

Patients	Age/sex	NF 1	Localisation	Treatment	Radio-or Chemotherapy	Retreatment	Outcome
Shajrawi et al. [14]	75/M	No	Left paranasal sinuses	Debulking	RT	Surgical removal of recurrence at 36 months	Alive NED at 6 months
Bhatt et al. [11]	66/F	No	Left nasal cavity	Extended external ethmoidectomy			Alive with tumour at 27 months
Heffner and Gnepp [13]	64/M	No	Left nasal cavity	Incomplete excision			Died of tumour at 27 months, pulmonary metastasis and cranial extension
	58/M	No	Nasal cavity	Surgery	RT		Alive NED at 48 months
	56/F	No	Left nasal cavity	Local excision		Removal of recurrence at 11 and 15 years	Alive NED at 7 years
	59/M	No	Right nasal cavity	Transpalatal excision	RT		Alive NED at 7 years
	43/M	No	Right nasal cavity	N/A		Recurrence at 15 years, treatment N/A	Alive NED at 7 years
Nicolai et al. [5]	81/F	No	Right nasal cavity	Endoscopic excision			Alive NED at 36 months
Kim et al. [4]	38/F	No	Right nasal cavity	Medial maxilectomy	RT		Alive NED at 5 years
Tringali et al. [6]	80/F	N/A	Right nasal cavity	Extended midfacial resection		Recurrence at 8 months with cerebral involvement, midfacial and sub frontal excision and RT. 3 endoscopic partial resections in 5 years	Alive with disease at 5 years
Xue et al. [7]	47/F	N/A	Right paranasal sinuses	Lateral rhinotomy	RT		Alive NED at 5 years
Terzic et al. [2]	35/F	no	Right nasal cavity	Craniotomy with sub-cranial resection			Alive NED at 30 months
	77/M	No	Left nasal cavity	Partial endoscopic resection		RT for lymph node metastasis at 6 months	Alive with tumour at 7.5 months
	73/F	No	Right maxillary sinus	Partial endoscopic resection		Endoscopic resection with RT for recurrence at 18 months	Died of other causes at 5.5 years
	76/M	no	Left sinonasal CAVITY	Refused treatment			Died of tumour at 1.5 months
Present case	49/F	N/A	Right nasal cavity	Craniotomy with sub-cranial resection	RT		Alive NED at 5 years

N/A: not available or not specified, NED: no evidence of disease, RT: radiotherapy.
Editor's Note: Please refer to original journal article for full references.

is not a familiar entity among pathologists because of its scarcity. The differential diagnosis of this tumor can include entities more familiar in this region, including rhabdomyosarcoma, Ewing sarcoma, olfactory neuroblastoma, and neuroendocrine tumors. Fig 2 describes its major histological features. Although sometimes NF-1-associated cases occur, none seen in the sinonasal tract have shown this association, as mentioned in the accompanying abstract.

It is important to be familiar with malignant triton tumor and include it in the differential diagnosis of sinonasal tract malignancies. As the author mentioned, although it is usually of low grade, histologic malignancy, metastasis, and intracranial extension can occur, and from the report, it appears that 3 of the reported sinonasal tract patients died from the tumor. It is also important to note from this review that most of these tumors are of low histologic grade in the head and neck region, and patients with tumors in this region have better survival than those with tumors in other body sites.[2]

M. Sherif Said, MD, PhD

References

1. Terzic A, Bode B, Gratz KW, Stoeckli SJ. Prognostic factors for the malignant triton tumor of the head and neck. *Head Neck.* 2009;31:679-688.
2. Woodruff JM, Chernik NL, Smith MC, Millett WB, Foote FW Jr. Peripheral nerve tumors with rhabdomyosarcomatous differentiation (malignant "triton tumors"). *Cancer.* 1973;32:426-439.

Cerebellopontine Angle and Intracanalicular Masses Mimicking Vestibular Schwannomas

Calzada AP, Go JL, Tschirhart DL, et al (Univ of Southern California, Los Angeles, CA; St. Vincent Med Ctr, Los Angeles, CA)
Otol Neurotol 2014 [Epub ahead of print]

Objective.—To describe the clinical and radiographic characteristics in a series of patients with non-vestibular schwannoma cerebellopontine angle (CPA) and intracanalicular (IAC) masses, who underwent microsurgery for presumed vestibular schwannoma (VS).

Study Design.—Retrospective case series.

Setting.—Tertiary neurotologic referral center.

Patients.—One thousand five hundred ninety-three patients underwent microsurgery for apparent VS from 2002 to 2013. Of these, 53 patients (3%) were discovered to have a diagnosis other than VS.

Interventions.—Middle fossa, translabyrinthine, and retrosigmoid craniotomy.

Main Outcome Measures.—Clinical presentation, radiologic analysis, and histopathology examination.

Results.—There were 17 facial schwannomas, 15 meningiomas, 9 hemangiomas, 6 lipochoristomas, 3 inflammatory reactions, and one each of lymphoma, glial heterotopia, solitary fibrous tumor, ependymoma, and a non-diagnostic mass. Excluding facial schwannomas, 23 cases were

TABLE 3.—Histopathology of CPA Tumors in 53 Subjects with Non-Vestibular Schwannoma

Tumor Type	Total (n = 55)[a]
Facial nerve schwannoma	17 (30.9%)
Meningioma	15 (27.3%)
Hemangioma	9 (16.4%)
Lipochoristoma	6 (10.9%)
Inflammation	3 (5.5%)
Lymphoma	1 (1.8%)
Glial heterotopia	1 (1.8%)
Solitary fibrous tumor	1 (1.8%)
Ependymoma	1 (1.8%)
Non-diagnostic	1 (1.8%)

[a]*Note*: 2 patients had two non-vestibular schwannoma tumor types on pathologic examination, for a total of 55 tumors in 53 patients.

Reprinted from Calzada AP, Go JL, Tschirhart DL, et al. Cerebellopontine Angle and Intracanalicular Masses Mimicking Vestibular Schwannomas. *Otol Neurotol*. 2014 [Epub ahead of print], with permission from otology & Neurotology, Inc.

misdiagnosed as VS in the first half of the study period, compared to only 15 cases in the latter half ($p = 0.09$). Ninety-six percent of patients presented with some combination of sensorineural hearing loss, balance disturbance, and tinnitus. In the subset of patients with available preoperative MRI scans for retrospective review, only 4 of 28 patients had radiologic findings suggestive of pathology other than VS. The most common missed radiologic diagnoses were facial schwannoma, lipochoristoma, and meningioma.

Conclusion.—A subgroup of patients with CPA and IAC masses who present with radiologic findings diagnostic of VS will have an alternative histopathologic diagnosis. Optimal radiologic imaging and experienced interpretation can improve diagnostic accuracy. The most common tumors that mimic VS despite ideal radiologic imaging are facial schwannomas, meningiomas, and hemangiomas (Table 3).

▶ This is a combined radiologic and histopathologic study of 1593 patients on the evaluation cerebellopontine and intracanalicular masses that highlights the types of pathologies seen in this region, in addition to the classic finding of schwannomas (Table 3). From this article, it seems clear that although improved radiologic methodology may improve the preoperative diagnostic impressions of these tumors, histologic evaluation remains the ultimate method for classifying them, and pathologists should be aware of these nonvestibular schwannomas types in their evaluation of tumors from that site, particularly when the tumor fragments are small or only small biopsies are available. It is also interesting to note that meningiomas and hemangiomas are at the top of the list of these tumors, which are also seen in nearby anatomic sites intracranially or extracranially.

M. Sherif Said, MD, PhD

Recent advances in the diagnostic pathology of salivary carcinomas

Simpson RHW, Skálová A, Di Palma S, et al (Univ of Calgary, Alberta, Canada; Charles Univ in Prague, Czech Republic; Royal Surrey County Hosp, Guildford, UK; et al)

Virchows Arch 465:371-384, 2014

This review concentrates on the most important developments since the WHO classification of 2005. In particular, the identification of specific translocations is revolutionising the way salivary tumours are considered and will have a major impact on future diagnostic practice. This is true so far in four malignancies: mammary analogue secretory, mucoepidermoid, adenoid cystic and hyalinising clear cell carcinomas. In each, the gene rearrangement is found in 80% or more of cases. Two 2014 publications have added further possible candidates with molecular abnormalities to the list (cribriform adenocarcinoma of the tongue and minor salivary glands and epithelial-myoepithelial carcinoma), but these findings have yet to be confirmed by other investigators. The advances in molecular pathology have also allowed reevaluation of the morphology; for example, it is now realised that the histological spectrum of hyalinising clear cell

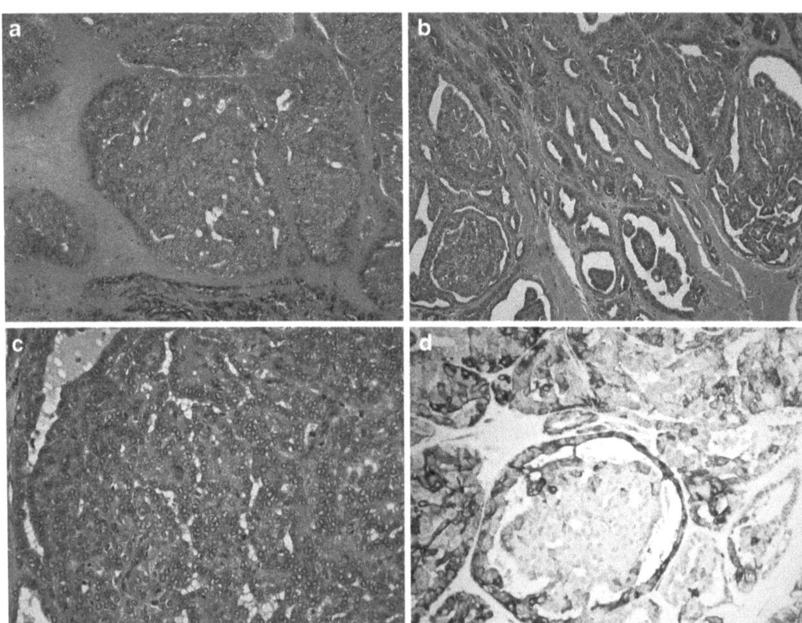

FIGURE 2.—**a** CATS: areas of cribriform growth. **b** CATS: tubules with characteristic glomeruloid structures. **c** CATS: clear nuclei resembling those of papillary thyroid carcinoma. **d** CATS: patchy reaction with basal/myoepithelial markers, highlighting particularly the peripheral cells of the glomeruloid structures (smooth muscle myosin). (With kind permission from Springer Science+Business Media. Simpson RHW, Skálová A, Di Palma S, et al. Recent advances in the diagnostic pathology of salivary carcinomas. *Virchows Arch*. 2014;465:371-384, with permission from Springer-Verlag Berlin Heidelberg.)

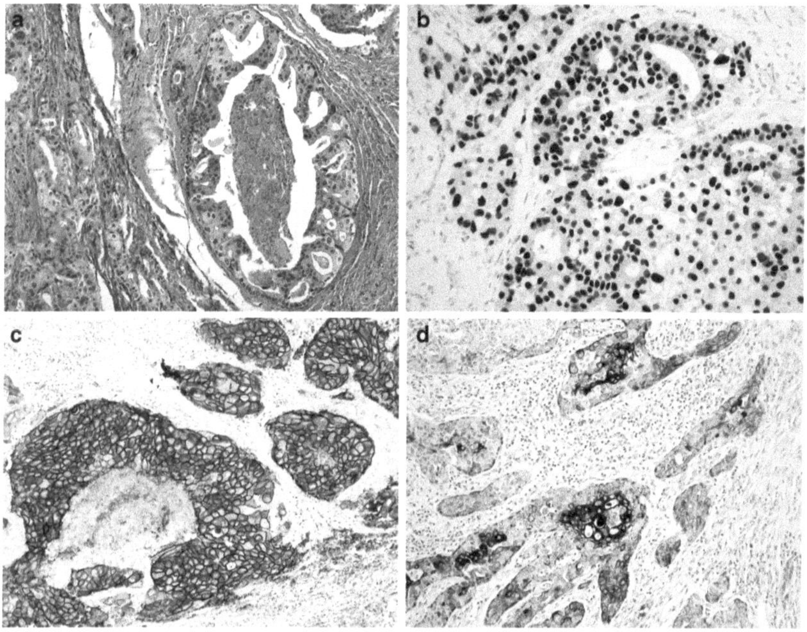

FIGURE 6.—**a** SDC: in situ and infiltrating patterns. **b** SDC: luminal subtype with strong nuclear staining for androgen receptors in almost all nuclei. **c** SDC: HER2 subtype with strong staining for HER2 protein, graded as 3+. **d** SDC: basal phenotype showing positivity for cytokeratin 5/6. (With kind permission from Springer Science+Business Media. Simpson RHW, Skálová A, Di Palma S, et al. Recent advances in the diagnostic pathology of salivary carcinomas. *Virchows Arch.* 2014;465:371-384, with permission from Springer-Verlag Berlin Heidelberg.)

TABLE 1.—Salivary Carcinomas and Molecular Abnormalities

	Tumour	Translocation	Genes Involved	Approx %
Well-established abnormalities in relatively common carcinomas	MASC	t(12;15) (p13;q25)	*ETV6-NTRK3*	Translocation 80 % ETV6 break 99 %
	MEC	t(11;19) (q21; p13) t(11;15)(q21;q26)	*CRTC1-MAML2* *CRTC3-MAML2*	60-80 % 6 % or less
	AdCC	t(6;9)(q22-23;p23-24)	*MYB-NFIB*	80-90 %
	HCCC	t(12;22)(q13;q12)	*EWSR1-ATF1*	80 %
Rare salivary malignancies	DSRCT	t(11;22)(p13;q12)	*EWS-WT1*	Up to 97 %
	NUT carcinoma	t(15;19)(q14, p13.1) t(9;15)(q34.2;q14) t(15;?)(q14;unknown)	*BRD4-NUT* *BRD3-NUT* *NUT-variant*	approx. 67 % remaining third of cases
Few studies, so not yet well-established	CATS	t(1;14)(p36.11;q12) t(X;14)(p11.4;q12)	*ARID1A-PRKD1* DDX3X-PRKD1 Other abnormalities of *PRKD2* and *PRKD3*	possibly as many as 80 %.
	EMC	No translocations, but a mutation	*HRAS* exon 3, codon 61	27 % in one small series

Reprinted from Simpson RHW, Skálová A, Di Palma S, et al. Recent advances in the diagnostic pathology of salivary carcinomas. *Virchows Arch.* 2014;465:371-384.

carcinoma includes intracellular mucin in over half of cases, as well as tumours with only scanty clear cells. In a separate development, it is now proposed that salivary duct carcinoma can be subdivided along molecular lines, in ways analogous to breast cancer, suggesting new therapeutic prospects in an otherwise highly aggressive malignancy (Figs 2 and 6, Table 1).

▶ This is a useful article updating the reader on salivary gland tumors, which as we know is a rich field with a wealth of new information added to it almost yearly. The article reviews the significant molecular abnormalities reported in salivary gland tumors as seen in Table 1, and contain reviews of 2 more recently identified salivary tumors: one that received wide interest and is more frequently diagnosed and previously highlighted in the YEAR BOOK head and neck review, mammary analogue secretory carcinoma; the other, the less frequently encountered cribriform adenocarcinoma of the tongue and minor salivary glands (CATS; Fig 2), which was classified by the World Health Organization in 2005 as a possible subtype of polymorphous low-grade adenocarcinoma (PLGA), the nuclei of which bear a surprising resemblance to the cells of papillary thyroid carcinoma. This type is now believed to be a distinct subtype rather than a subtype of PLGA. The tumor cells are negative immunohistochemically for TTF and thyroglobulin; *BRAF*, *KRAS*, and *PDGFRa* genes are negative as well. Few cases showed *Ret* and *H-RAS* mutations. CATS shows gene rearrangement for *PRKD1-3*.

The article also reviews recent molecular studies in other salivary gland carcinomas mentioned in the abstract. Perhaps most interestingly, it points out a study[1] that classified salivary duct carcinoma into 3 molecular subtypes (Fig 6): luminal subtype, *HER2* subtype, and basal phenotype. Overall, it is a useful article for pathologist reviewing various salivary gland tumors in their practices.

M. Sherif Said, MD, PhD

Reference

1. Di Palma S, Simpson RHW, Marchio C, et al. Salivary duct carcinomas can be classified into luminal androgen receptor-positive, HER2 and basal-like phenotypes. *Histopathology*. 2012;61:629-643.

5 Kidney

Defining the spectrum of immunoglobulin A–dominant/codominant glomerular deposition in diabetic nephropathy

Cossey LN, Messias N, Messias E, et al (Nephropath, Little Rock, AR; Univ of Arkansas for Med Sciences, Little Rock)
Hum Pathol 45:2294-2301, 2014

In patients with diabetic nephropathy (DN), the spectrum of immunoglobulin A (IgA)–dominant/codominant glomerular deposition (IgAGD) has not been addressed in the literature. The aim of our study is to detail the clinicopathological and outcome findings in patients with DN and IgAGD. Our database was retrospectively searched over a 10-year period for patients with DN and IgAGD. A total of 132 patients were included in the study, 55 with outcome data. All cases were reviewed by light microscopy, immunofluorescence, and electron microscopy. Mean age was 59 ± 13 years, with a 2:1 male-to-female ratio. Indications for biopsy were often multiple, with proteinuria/nephrotic syndrome and acute renal failure being the most common. All patients showed IgAGD and mesangial deposits by electron microscopy. Seventy-three (55.3%) patients had no proliferative glomerular changes and no clinical history of infection and were most consistent with IgA nephropathy on DN, whereas 19 (14.4%) showed proliferative glomerular changes, had a history of infection, and were most consistent with IgA-dominant infection-associated glomerulonephritis. Forty (30.3%) patients showed a mixture of these findings and did not fit into either category. Patients with a mean of 42 (2-120 range) months of follow-up showed an overall poor prognosis, with 59% of all respondents proceeding to renal replacement therapy or death (RRT/D) over an average of 23 (range, 4-54) months. Progression to RRT/D was most frequent in those most consistent with IgA-dominant infection-associated glomerulonephritis (71%), and by multivariate analysis, only advanced Tervaert morphologic classification (classes III and IV) was associated with progression to RRT/D.

► Most patients with diabetic nephropathy are followed closely, and a renal biopsy is rarely performed, as the diagnosis is presumptive. However, when there is a permanent change in renal function or in the degree of proteinuria, clinicians may consider a renal biopsy to evaluate for the possibility of superimposed glomerular diseases. One of the more common and recently described glomerular diseases, which may complicate diabetic nephropathy, is that of immunoglobulin A (IgA)-dominant/codominant glomerular deposition. This report describes the clinical presentation and progression of disease in this cohort of patients. All the patients were selected because of the presence of both diabetic nephropathy and IgA-dominant/codominant deposition within the mesangial regions of the glomeruli. This was confirmed by immunofluorescence and electromicroscopy. However, 3 distinct patient groups were defined by the report. It is not surprising that the patient group with a history of infection and proliferative changes by light microscopy on the kidney biopsy showed the most frequent progression to renal replacement therapy/death. One of the important take-home messages from this report is that not all patients with diabetes and mesangial IgA deposition are associated with a superimposed idiopathic IgA nephropathy. Instead, most diabetic patients likely have a component of postinfectious glomerular nephritis, which is IgA dominant/codominant. This distinction may have important treatment repercussions.

For additional review of IgA dominant/codominant postinfectious glomerular nephritis in the setting of diabetic nephropathy, I refer the readers to Nasr et al.[1,2]

M. L. Smith, MD

References

1. Nasr SH, Share DS, Vargas MT, D'Agati VD, Markowitz GS. Acute poststaphylococcal glomerulonephritis superimposed on diabetic glomerulosclerosis. *Kidney Int.* 2007;71:1317-1321.
2. Nasr SH, Markowitz GS, Whelan JD, et al. IgA-dominant acute poststaphylococcal glomerulonephritis complicating diabetic nephropathy. *Hum Pathol.* 2003;34: 1235-1241.

Focal and segmental glomerulosclerosis: clinical and kidney biopsy correlations

Sethi S, Zand L, Nasr SH, et al (Mayo Clinic College of Medicine, Rochester, MN)

Clin Kidney J 7:531-537, 2014

Background.—Primary focal segmental glomerulosclerosis (FSGS) is a common glomerular disease in adults and ranks among the top causes of a primary glomerular disease causing end-stage renal disease (ESRD). Primary FSGS is, however, a diagnosis of exclusion and distinction between primary versus secondary FSGS is not always obvious, resulting in a number of patients with secondary FSGS undergoing unnecessary immunosuppressive therapy.

Methods.—We reviewed the Mayo Clinic Renal Pathology Database for patients with a diagnosis of FSGS on native renal biopsy and divided the patients into nephrotic syndrome-associated (NS-associated) and non-nephrotic syndrome-associated (NNS-associated) FSGS as a first approximation followed by dividing the lesion according to the degree of foot process effacement (FPE) on electron microscopy (EM) examination.

Results.—A total of 41 patients with FSGS with complete evaluation were identified. Of these, 18 were classified as having NS and 23 were classified as having NNS. Baseline characteristics (age, gender, body mass index, serum creatinine and hematuria) were not different between the groups. All of the patients with NS showed diffuse FPE ranging from 80 to 100% (mean 96%). On the other hand, of the 23 patients in the NNS group, 22 had segmental FPE and showed patchy effacement, with all cases showing 20–60% FPE (mean of 48%).

Conclusion.—Adult patients presenting with NS, an FSGS lesion on LM, extensive FPE (≥80%) on EM examination and no risk factors associated with secondary FSGS are likely to have primary FSGS. Conversely, the absence of NS in a patient with segmental FPE on EM strongly suggests a secondary FSGS. Dividing FSGS into the presence or absence of NS together with the degree of FPE on EM examination is more helpful as it provides a more practical way to separate patients into cases of primary versus secondary FSGS.

▶ The distinction between primary and secondary focal segmental glomerulosclerosis (FSGS) has important clinical implications. Primary FSGS is typically treated with robust immunosuppressive therapy, whereas secondary focal segmental glomerulosclerosis is not treated with aggressive immunosuppression. Instead, treatment of secondary FSGS focuses on identifying the driving lesion (malignancy, connective tissue disease, drug reaction, etc). However, the distinction between primary and secondary FSGS is not always clear based on the biopsy specimen. In general, patients with primary FSGS show tip lesions as opposed to the perihilar scars of secondary FSGS. In addition, by electron microscopy, primary FSGS shows diffuse foot process effacement involving more than 90% of the glomerular basement membranes, whereas secondary FSGS shows more patchy foot process effacement. However, these changes are not seen universally, and better ways to easily and accurately classify patients as primary or secondary FSGS are needed. This article suggests that involving the clinical information as to the presence of nephrotic syndrome, which is defined by nephronic-range proteinuria (> 3.5 g of protein/24 h) as well as low serum albumin levels (defined as < 3.5 g/dL). When separating cases of FSGS by the Columbia criteria into the different subtypes, this study showed no correlation with the degree of proteinuria; however, this may be related to the relatively small number of patients studied (n = 481). These new proposed criteria may improve the ease of identification of patients most likely to have primary focal segmental glomerulosclerosis.

For additional review of the topic, I refer readers to D'Agati et al.[1]

M. L. Smith, MD

Reference

1. D'Agati VD, Fogo AB, Bruijn JA, Jennette JC. Pathologic classification of focal segmental glomerulosclerosis: a working proposal. *Am J Kidney Dis.* 2004;43: 368-382.

Tuberous Sclerosis–associated Renal Cell Carcinoma: A Clinicopathologic Study of 57 Separate Carcinomas in 18 Patients

Guo J, Tretiakova MS, Troxell ML, et al (Cleveland Clinic, OH; Univ of Washington, Seattle; Oregon Health & Science Univ, Portland; et al)
Am J Surg Pathol 38:1457-1467, 2014

Tuberous sclerosis complex (TSC) is an autosomal dominant disorder with characteristic tumors involving multiple organ systems. Whereas renal angiomyolipoma (AML) is common in TSC, renal cell carcinoma (RCC) is rarely reported. Fifty-seven RCCs from 13 female and 5 male TSC patients were reviewed. Age at surgery ranged from 7 to 65 years (mean: 42 y). Nine patients (50%) had multiple synchronous and/or metachronous RCCs (range of 2 to 20 RCCs) and 5 had bilateral RCCs (28%). Seventeen patients (94%) had histologically confirmed concurrent renal AMLs, including 15 with multiple AMLs (88%) and 9 (50%) with AMLs with epithelial cysts. None of the 15 patients with available clinical follow-up information had evidence of distant metastatic disease from 6 to 198 months after their initial surgery (mean: 52 mo). The 57 RCCs exhibited 3 major distinct morphologies: (1) 17 RCCs (30%) had features similar to tumors previously described as "renal angiomyoadenomatous tumor" or "RCC with smooth muscle stroma"; (2) 34 RCCs (59%) showed features similar to chromophobe RCC; and (3) 6 RCCs (11%) showed a granular eosinophilic-macrocystic morphology. Distinct histologic changes were also commonly present in the background kidney parenchyma and included cysts or renal tubules lined by epithelial cells with prominent eosinophilic cytoplasm, nucleomegaly, and nucleoli. Immunohistochemically, all RCCs tested showed strong nuclear reactivity for PAX8 and HMB45 negativity. Compared with sporadic RCCs, TSC-associated RCCs have unique clinicopathologic features including female predominance, younger age at diagnosis, multiplicity, association with AMLs, 3 recurring histologic patterns, and an indolent clinical course. Awareness of the morphologic and clinicopathologic spectrum of RCC in this setting will allow surgical pathologists to better recognize clinically unsuspected TSC patients.

▶ This article serves as a good reminder to general surgical pathologists that not all renal cell carcinomas encountered in clinical practice are sporadic renal cell carcinomas. Specifically, female patients who present at a younger age and with multiple lesions should raise suspicion for the possibility of a genetically associated condition. Most pathologists are well familiar with the association between tuberous sclerosis complex and renal angiomyolipoma. However, in younger female patients with renal angiomyolipoma and features suggestive of renal cell carcinoma, a particularly high suspicion for tuberous sclerosis complex should be entertained. Unfortunately, the histopathology of renal cell carcinomas in this setting is not specific for tuberous sclerosis complex and overlaps significantly with sporadic renal cell carcinomas of chromophobe type and of eosinophilic/clear cell renal cell carcinoma type. The one exception is the renal angiomyoadenomatous tumor for renal angiomyoadenomatous tumor-like renal cell carcinoma in which the stroma contains abundant smooth muscle. Fortunately, from an immunohistochemical perspective, the renal cell carcinomas show typical staining of PAX8 positivity and HMB-45 negativity supporting an epithelial origin. The recognition of this clinical pathologic entity may have prognostic significance as well because patients developing renal cell carcinoma in the setting of tubular sclerosis complex may show an improved survival and an indolent course.

For a nice review of the tuberous sclerosis complex, clinical presentation, and diagnostic features, I refer the readers to Crino et al.[1]

M. L. Smith, MD

Reference

1. Crino PB, Nathanson KL, Henske EP. The tuberous sclerosis complex. *N Engl J Med.* 2006;355:1345-1356.

Validation of a histopathologic classification scheme for antineutrophil cytoplasmic antibody–associated glomerulonephritis

Nohr E, Girard L, James M, et al (Foothills Medical Center, Calgary, Alberta, Canada)

Hum Pathol 45:1423-1429, 2014

Antineutrophil cytoplasmic antibody–associated small-vessel vasculitides cause multiple organ system disease including rapidly progressive glomerulonephritis. Recently, Berden et al (*J Am Soc Nephrol.* 2010; 21:1628-1636) proposed a new histopathologic classification scheme separating renal biopsies into 4 classes: focal, crescentic, mixed, and sclerotic. We validated the prognostic implications of this classification scheme in a retrospective cohort study of 67 individuals with antineutrophil cytoplasmic antibody glomerulonephritis who underwent kidney biopsy in Calgary, Alberta, between 2005 and 2010. Their biopsies were rescored according to the classification scheme of Berden et al. Additional tubulointerstitial parameters were also scored. Clinical information including demographics and creatinine values at presentation and 1-year follow-up was retrieved. The mean age was 60 years. Forty-one percent were female. Biopsies were classified as follows: 35% crescentic, 32% mixed, 21% focal, and 11% sclerotic. Ten patients (14%) died within 1 year. Among surviving patients, the overall mean (95% confidence interval) change in estimated glomerular filtration rate (eGFR) at 1 year was 11 (7-15) mL/min per 1.73 m^2, and this change significantly differed ($P = .02$) between the classes: 19 (11-27) mL/min per 1.73 m^2 with crescentic histology, 11 (1-21) mL/min per 1.73 m^2 with focal, 8 (3-13) mL/min per 1.73 m^2 with mixed, and −4 (−7 to −1) mL/min per 1.73 m^2 with sclerotic. Tubulointerstitial pathology parameters did not predict outcomes. Patients with crescentic class biopsies showed significantly more improvement in eGFR at 1 year compared with the mixed ($P = .04$) and sclerotic ($P = .005$) classes. The

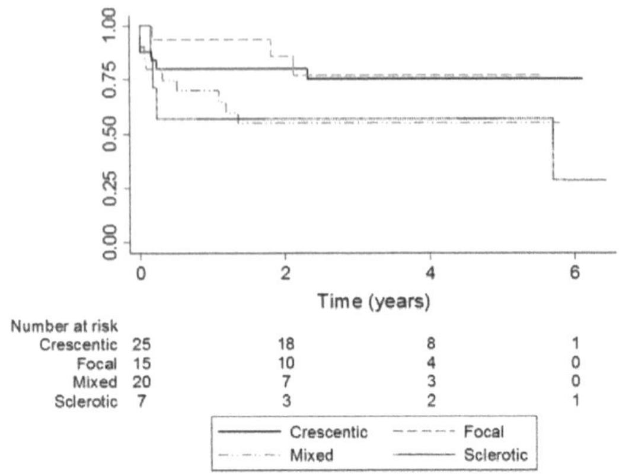

FIGURE 2.—Kaplan-Meier plot of time to chronic dialysis, kidney transplant, or death according to histologic class, censoring for loss to follow-up. (Reprinted from Human Pathology. Nohr E, Girard L, James M, et al. Validation of a histopathologic classification scheme for antineutrophil cytoplasmic antibody—associated glomerulonephritis. *Hum Pathol.* 2014;45:1423-1429, with permission from Elsevier.)

focal class was associated with the highest eGFR values at presentation and 1 year. These findings validate the prognostic utility of the Berden classification scheme and suggest that it may be generalizable (Fig 2).

▶ All proliferative glomerulonephritides have the potential to develop nephron loss, elevated creatinine levels, and loss of glomerular filtration rate. Any classification scheme should have clinical or prognostic significance to support its use. Otherwise, it is classification for the simple means of classification. Until a few years ago, the classification of antineutrophil cytoplasmic antibody (ANCA)-associated glomerulonephritis did not have a well-described and used classification system. This article validates a recently proposed classification system with regard to patient prognosis. Fig 2 shows nicely the different survival curves of the 4 different classes of ANCA-associated glomerulonephritis: crescentic, focal, mixed, and sclerotic. It is not surprising that the focal diseases are associated with the best prognosis, and the sclerotic diseases are associated with the worst prognosis. The differences in organ survival are most notable at 1 year, likely attributable to the treatable nature of ANCA-associated glomerulonephritis and the lack of significant relapse. I find it surprising in this article that the degree of tubulointerstitial fibrosis and atrophy was not independently associated with prognosis. Strengths of this article include the large number of ANCA-associated glomerulonephritis from this single institution (123).

For additional reading regarding the classification system, I refer the readers to Berden et al.[1]

M. L. Smith, MD

Reference

1. Berden AE, Ferrario F, Hagen EC, et al. Histopathologic classification of ANCA-associated glomerulonephritis. *J Am Soc Nephrol.* 2010;21:1628-1636.

Granulomatosis With Polyangiitis Presenting as a Renal Tumor

Ward A, Konya C, Mark EJ, et al (Harvard Med School, Boston, MA; Harvard Med School Massachusetts General Hosp, Boston)

Am J Surg Pathol 38:1444-1448, 2014

Inflammatory tumors of the kidney are uncommon and include primary inflammatory processes and systemic diseases such as sarcoidosis, IgG4 disease, and granulomatosis with polyangiitis (GPA). There are approximately 15 cases of the latter in the literature. Tumors in GPA are well described and have been reported in several organs including breast, orbit, mediastinum, central nervous system, and especially the lung. We report the case of a 48-year-old woman who presented with diffuse frontal headaches. Imaging showed both a cranial/sinus and renal mass. The pathology of the dura and nasal sinus biopsies were unrevealing. A nephrectomy was performed that demonstrated a discrete lesion with extensive necrosis, granulomatous inflammation, and crescentic pauci-immune glomerulonephritis, findings consistent with GPA (Fig 3).

► The authors present a most unusual case of mass forming granulomatosis with polyangiitis masquerading as a primary renal neoplasm. Fig 3 highlights the main resection specimen and the low-power histopathology showing typical geographic zones of necrosis of granulomatosis with polyangiitis. Although granulomatosis with polyangiitis has been reported as a mass lesion in several different organs in the past, this case report serves as good reminder for the general surgical pathologist that granulomatosis polyangiitis can mimic both infectious etiologies and neoplastic etiologies and should remain on any differential diagnosis. It is interesting in this case that an initial needle core biopsy showed extensive necrosis with lymphoplasmacytic inflammation, and a diagnosis of granulomatosis with polyangiitis was not able to be made. In our institution, we recently had a patient present with bilateral lung masses and was found to have pulmonary granulomatosis with polyangiitis on transbronchial biopsy. The patient had typical serologic studies in keeping with this diagnosis. Patients with this diagnosis subsequently present with multiple mass lesions within the liver. A needle core biopsy showed extensive necrosis with neutrophilic inflammation and occasional multinucleated giant cells. Without knowledge of the prior diagnosis of granulomatosis with polyangiitis, the liver biopsy was signed out descriptively, and an infectious etiology was favored. However, upon review, it seems the biopsy result was entirely in keeping with granulomatosis with polyangiitis involving the hepatic parenchyma in mimicking mass forming neoplasms by radiographic imaging and infectious etiologies by histopathology.

M. L. Smith, MD

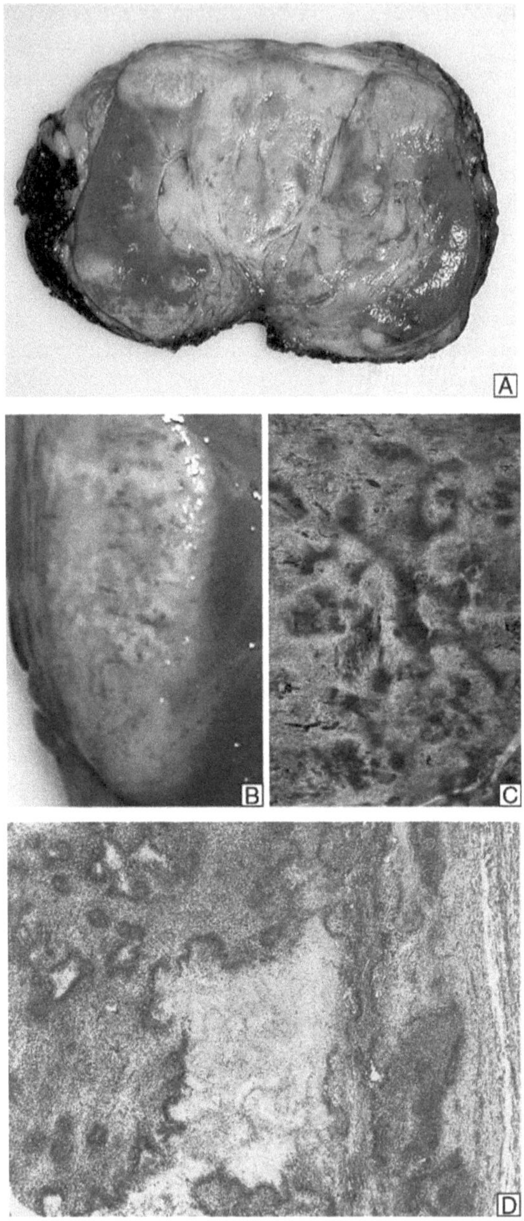

FIGURE 3.—A, The tumor measures 11 cm, is tan-yellow, firm, and well circumscribed. It is centrally located, leaving the polar regions largely uninvolved. B, High-power gross image of tumor showing a focal white reticulated pattern. C, Immunofluorescence stain for fibrin demonstrates that the reticular pattern seen likely relates to fibrin deposition. D, Low-power image of vimentin strain highlights the edge of a large geographic zone of necrosis. The absence of staining within the zonal area suggests complete mesenchymal destruction. (Reprinted from Ward A, Konya C, Mark EJ, et al. Granulomatosis with polyangiitis presenting as a renal tumor. *Am J Surg Pathol*. 2014;38:1444-1448.)

Rhabdoid Differentiation is Associated With Aggressive Behavior in Renal Cell Carcinoma: A Clinicopathologic Analysis of 76 Cases With Clinical Follow-up

Przybycin CG, McKenney JK, Reynolds JP, et al (Robert J. Tomsich Pathology and Laboratory Medicine Inst, Cleveland, OH; et al)

Am J Surg Pathol 38:1260-1265, 2014

Rhabdoid differentiation has been associated with aggressive behavior in carcinomas from different organ systems. A recent consensus statement of the International Society of Urological Pathology (ISUP), in addition to proposing a nucleolar grading system (ISUP grade) for renal cell carcinoma (RCC) to replace the Fuhrman system, recommended reporting the presence of rhabdoid differentiation in RCC and considering tumors with rhabdoid differentiation to be ISUP grade 4. Although it has been shown that rhabdoid differentiation is associated with increased grade and stage of RCC, it has not been fully demonstrated whether it has an adverse effect independent of this association with increased grade and stage. We provide the largest clinicopathologic analysis of RCC with rhabdoid differentiation to date (76 cases), including characterization of metastatic disease. In addition, by constructing a multivariable model including tumor grade, stage, necrosis, and distant metastasis to compare a series of 49 clear cell RCC with rhabdoid differentiation with a cohort of 41 clear cell RCCs without rhabdoid differentiation, we demonstrate that the presence of rhabdoid differentiation in clear cell RCC confers an increased risk of death (hazard ratio = 5.25; 95% confidence interval, 2.1-14.3) independent of these other adverse prognostic factors. These findings underscore the significance of rhabdoid differentiation in RCC as an adverse prognostic factor and support the recent reporting and grading recommendations of the ISUP (Table 3).

▶ This is the largest study looking at the clinical outcome of renal cell carcinoma showing rhabdoid differentiation to date. Important aspects of this report include the precise definition used for rhabdoid differentiation, which was sheets and clusters of variably cohesive, large epithelioid cells with vesicular nuclei, prominent nucleoli, and large paranuclear intracytoplasmic inclusions.

TABLE 3.—Factors Associated With Death—Multivariable Analysis

Factor	Hazard Ratio	95% CI	*P*
Rhabdoid differentiation	5.25	2.1-14.3	< 0.001
Tumor stage ≥ T3a	4.1	1.8-9.3	< 0.001
Tumor grade 4*	2.42	1.2-5.1	0.016

*Grade of the nonrhabdoid component in tumors with rhabdoid differentiation.

The second important aspect is the mean clinical follow-up time, which was 86 months with a range of 13 to 179 months. The main findings, on multivariate analysis, are given in Table 3. It is interesting that only 3 pathologic features on multivariate analysis show clinical significance, and rhabdoid differentiation seems to show the most clinical significance with a hazard ratio associated with death of 5.25. These findings underscore the importance to the general surgical pathologist of looking for areas of rhabdoid differentiation and reporting them within the sinapic surgical pathology report. These patients likely should be treated more aggressively and surveilled more closely. The results of this study also emphasize the importance of rhabdoid differentiation being associated with a high nuclear grade as recommended by the International Society of Urological Pathology.[1]

For additional reading regarding nuclear grading of renal cell carcinoma, I refer the readers to Delahunt et al.[1]

M. L. Smith, MD

Reference

1. Delahunt B, Cheville JC, Martignoni G, et al. The International Society of Urological Pathology (ISUP) grading system for renal cell carcinoma and other prognostic parameters. *Am J Surg Pathol.* 2013;37:1490-1504.

Diagnostic Approach to Eosinophilic Renal Neoplasms

Kryvenko ON, Jorda M, Argani P, et al (Univ of Miami Miller School of Medicine, FL; The Johns Hopkins Med Institutions, Baltimore, MD)
Arch Pathol Lab Med 138:1531-1541, 2014

Context.—Eosinophilic renal neoplasms include a spectrum of solid and papillary tumors ranging from indolent benign oncocytoma to highly aggressive malignancies. Recognition of the correct nature of the tumor, especially in biopsy specimens, is paramount for patient management.

Objective.—To review the diagnostic approach to eosinophilic renal neoplasms with light microscopy and ancillary techniques.

Data Sources.—Review of the published literature and personal experience.

Conclusions.—The following tumors are in the differential diagnosis of oncocytic renal cell neoplasm: oncocytoma, chromophobe renal cell carcinoma (RCC), hybrid tumor, tubulocystic carcinoma, papillary RCC, clear cell RCC with predominant eosinophilic cell morphology, follicular thyroid-like RCC, hereditary leiomyomatosis–associated RCC, acquired cystic disease–associated RCC, rhabdoid RCC, microphthalmia transcription factor translocation RCC, epithelioid angiomyolipoma, and unclassified RCC. In low-grade nonpapillary eosinophilic neoplasms, distinction between oncocytoma and lowgrade RCC mostly rests on histomorphology; however, cytokeratin 7 immunostain may be helpful. In high-grade nonpapillary lesions, there is more of a role for ancillary techniques, including immunohistochemistry for cytokeratin 7, CA9, CD10, racemase, HMB45,

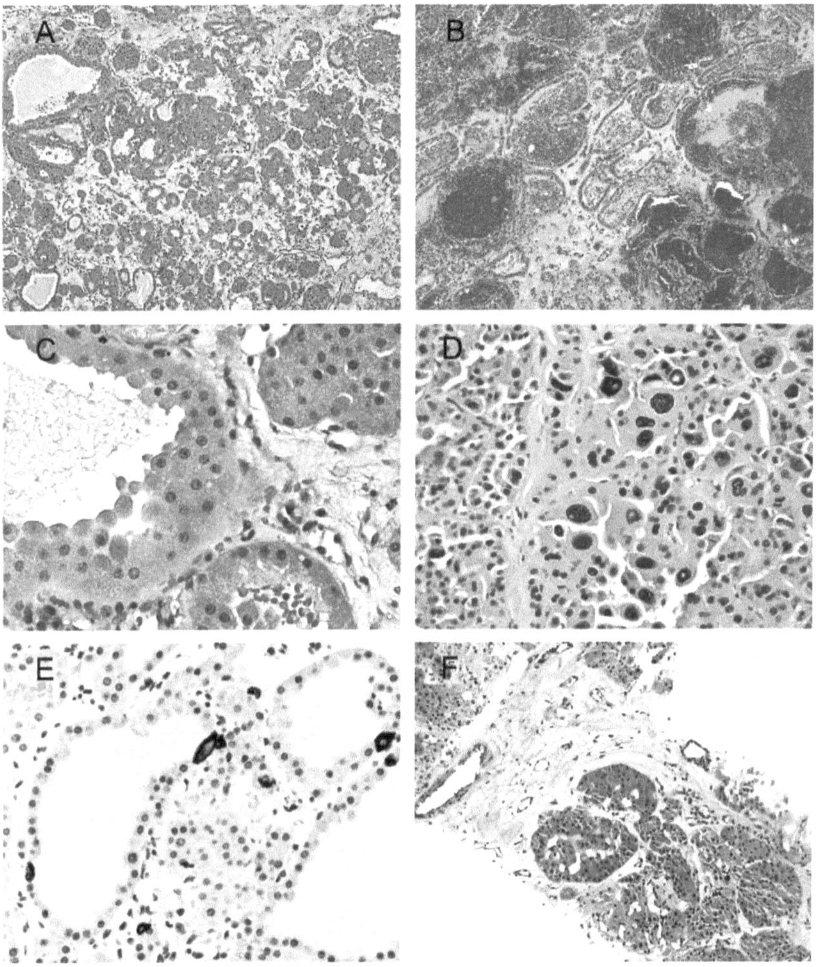

FIGURE 1.—A, Classic appearance of oncocytoma with small solid nests with myxoid or hyalinized background. B, Tubular architecture of oncocytoma with hemorrhage. C, Classic cytology of oncocytoma with abundant eosinophilic cytoplasm; indistinct cell borders; small, uniform nuclei; and prominent nucleoli. D, A cluster of degenerative-type atypia seen in oncocytoma. E, Scattered cytokeratin 7 immunoreactivity in oncocytoma. F, Biopsy of an oncocytic renal neoplasm consistent with oncocytoma (hematoxylin-eosin, original magnifications ×100 [A, B, and F], ×600 [C], and ×400 [D]; original magnification ×400 [E]). (Reproduced with permission of College of American Pathologists from Kryvenko ON, Jorda M, Argani P, et al. Diagnostic approach to eosinophilic renal neoplasms. *Arch Pathol Lab Med.* 2014;138:1531-1541; permission conveyed through Copyright Clearance Center, Inc.)

and Melan-A. In papillary eosinophilic neoplasms, it is important to distinguish sporadic type 2 papillary RCC from microphthalmia transcription factor translocation and hereditary leiomyomatosis–associated RCC. Histologic and cytologic features along with immunohistochemistry and fluorescence in situ hybridization tests for *TFE3* (Xp11.2) and *TFEB* [t(6;11)] are reliable confirmatory tests. Eosinophilic epithelial neoplasms with architecture, cytology, and/or immunoprofile not qualifying for either of the established types of RCC should be classified as unclassified eosinophilic RCC and arbitrarily assigned a grade (low or high) (Fig 1).

▶ There has been considerable change in progress in the classification and immunohistochemical workup of renal neoplasms over the past decade. In the past, there were a relatively limited number of distinct entities such as oncocytoma, papillary renal cell carcinoma, clear cell renal cell carcinoma, and chromophobe renal cell carcinoma. However, numerous distinct clinical pathologic entities have been identified, and their distinction from one another remains problematic in the general surgical pathology practice. This article highlights a comprehensive approach to the differential diagnosis of eosinophilic renal neoplasms. Fig 1 highlights the fairly broad differential diagnosis for renal tumors with eosinophilic cytoplasm. In the approach presented within this article, the primary 2 questions to ask to assist in classification include whether the tumor is a low-grade or high-grade tumor and also whether the tumor shows papillary or nonpapillary architecture. The answers to these 2 questions direct the additional workup. This provides a simple dichotomous approach to this challenging differential diagnosis. Fortunately, the immunohistochemical studies required in this workup are relatively common and should be available in many laboratories. However, the fluorescence in situ hybridization testing for hereditary renal cell carcinoma is less commonly available and may require send out testing.

For additional reading on the immunohistochemical distinction between renal neoplasms, I suggest Liu et al.[1]

M. L. Smith, MD

Reference

1. Liu L, Qian J, Singh H, Meiers I, Zhou X, Bostwick DG. Immunohistochemical analysis of chromophobe renal cell carcinoma, renal oncocytoma, and clear cell carcinoma: an optimal and practical panel for differential diagnosis. *Arch Pathol Lab Med.* 2007;131:1290-1297.

Biopsy-Proven Acute Interstitial Nephritis, 1993-2011: A Case Series

Muriithi AK, Leung N, Valeri AM, et al (Mayo Clinic, Rochester, MN; Columbia Univ, NY)

Am J Kidney Dis 64:558-566, 2014

Background.—Acute interstitial nephritis (AIN) is an important cause of acute kidney injury, especially in hospitalized patients. The cause and outcome of AIN, particularly that due to drugs, is changing with prevalent medication use. The effectiveness of steroids for treatment of AIN is debated.

Study Design.—Case series.

Setting & Participants.—133 patients with biopsy-proven AIN from 1993 through 2011 at a single center.

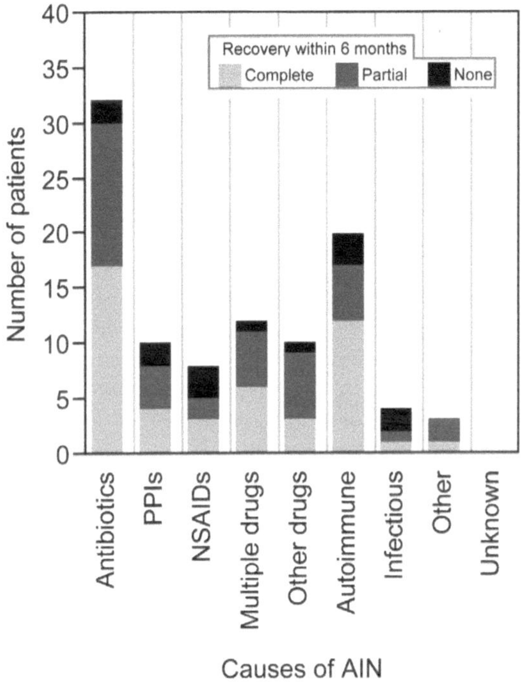

FIGURE 1.—All causes of acute interstitial nephritis (AIN) by recovery at 6 months. Abbreviations: NSAID, nonsteroidal antiinflammatory drug; PPI, proton pump inhibitor. (Reprinted from American Journal of Kidney Diseases. Muriithi AK, Leung N, Valeri AM, et al. Biopsy-proven acute interstitial nephritis, 1993-2011: a case series. *Am J Kidney Dis.* 2014;64:558-566, Copyright 2014, with permission from the National Kidney Foundation.)

Outcomes.—Recovery of kidney function by 6 months, either complete, partial, or none. Complete recovery was defined as improvement in serum creatinine level to within 25% of baseline (or <1.4 mg/dL), and partial recovery, as a ≥50% decrease in serum creatinine level from its peak value but not reaching within 25% of its baseline value.

Results.—Causes of AIN included drugs (70%), autoimmune diseases (20%), and infections (4%). Drug-induced AIN was due to antibiotics in 49%, proton pump inhibitors (PPIs) in 14%, and nonsteroidal anti-inflammatory drugs (NSAIDs) in 11%. Overall, the top 3 drug causes were omeprazole (12%), amoxicillin (8%), and ciprofloxacin (8%). Patients with drug-induced compared to non-drug-induced AIN were older and had higher baseline kidney function, but more severe acute kidney injury. Patients with PPI-induced AIN were older, were less symptomatic, and had longer durations of drug exposure and longer delays in getting kidney biopsy and steroids than for antibiotic-induced or NSAID-induced AIN. At 6 months postbiopsy, 49% of patients with drug-induced AIN treated with steroids achieved complete recovery; 39%, partial recovery; and 12%, no recovery. Correlates of poor recovery included a longer duration of drug exposure (15 vs 30 vs 130 days for complete, partial, and no recovery, respectively; $P = 0.04$) and longer delay in starting steroid therapy (8 vs 11 vs 35 days, respectively; $P = 0.05$).

Limitations.—Retrospective study, selection bias in patients who had kidney biopsy, single-center experience.

Conclusions.—The cause of AIN may be shifting; PPIs are emerging as an important contributor to this disease. Delays in discontinuation of the culprit drug and in initiating steroid treatment adversely affect recovery of kidney function (Fig 1).

▶ The authors retrospectively review one of the largest single-center case study series of acute interstitial nephritis. Their definition for a pathologic biopsy-proven diagnosis of acute interstitial nephritis includes the presence of prominent interstitial inflammation in the nonfibrotic cortex and tubulitis. Patients with an associated glomerular nephritis, young patients, and patients with primary vascular disease were excluded from the case series. In addition, this was based on native kidney biopsies alone as opposed to transplant kidney biopsies. Fig 1 highlights the main findings within this article and shows the distribution of etiologies associated with the acute interstitial nephritis. It is easy to see that adverse drug reactions led the etiology for interstitial nephritis followed closely by autoimmune diseases. Antibiotics are most often the offending agents, but surprisingly, in this study, proton pump inhibitors made up several cases as well. Surprisingly, the acute interstitial nephritis seemed to cause permanent renal failure in many patients. One of the important take-home messages from this study is that when an acute interstitial nephritis is found on the biopsy, a detailed review of the patient's medication list should be undertaken to exclude any possibilities of a drug-induced disease. If there are any possible drugs contributing to the interstitial nephritis, cessation of that drug should be done as soon as possible, and steroids should be initiated. There seemed to be improved recovery of kidney function in patients who have the drug stopped quickly and steroids started.

For additional review, I refer the readers to Raza et al.[1]

M. L. Smith, MD

Reference

1. Raza MN, Hadid M, Keen CE, Bingham C, Salmon AH. Acute tubular interstitial nephritis, treatment with steroid and impact on renal outcomes. *Nephrology.* 2012;17:748-753.

Membranous-like glomerulopathy with masked IgG kappa deposits

Larsen CP, Ambuzs JM, Bonsib SM, et al (Nephropath, Little Rock, AK; et al)
Kidney Int 86:154-161, 2014

The diagnostic classification of glomerulonephritis is determined by the interplay of changes seen using light, immunofluorescence, and electron microscopy of the renal biopsy. Routine direct immunofluorescence on

TABLE 2.—Morphologic Features on Initial Biopsy

Patient	LM Pattern	Fresh IgG	Fresh κ	Fresh λ	Pron IgG	Pron κ	Pron λ	Fresh C3	Deposit Location	Hump-Like Deposits	Hinge-Region Deposits
1	Normal	0	0	0	3	3	0	3	m, sp	Yes	Yes
2	Normal	0	0	0	3	3	0	2	m, sp	No	Yes
3	Normal	1	0	0	3	3	0	3	m, sp	Yes	Yes
4	Focal crescentic	0	0	0	3	3	0	3	m, sp	Yes	Yes
5	Normal	0	0	0	2	2	0	2	m, sp	No	Yes
6	Normal	0	0	0	3	2	0	1	m, sp	No	No
7	Normal	0	0	0	2	2	0	1	m, sp	No	Yes
8	Normal	0	0	0	3	3	0	3	m, sp	Yes	No
9	Normal	0	0	0	3	3	0	0	sp	No	No
10	Normal	1	0	0	3	3	0	1	sp	No	No
11	Normal	0	0	0	3	3	0	2	m, sp	Yes	No
12	Normal	0	0	0	3	3	0	1	m, sp	Yes	Yes
13	Focal crescentic	Tr	Tr	0	2	2	0	2	m, sp	No	No
14	Focal crescentic	Tr	0	0	3	3	0	2	m, sp	Yes	Yes

Abbreviations: LM, glomeruli on light microscopy; m, mesangial; Pron, pronase; sp, subepithelial; Tr, trace.

Reprinted with permission from Macmillan Publishers Ltd: Kidney International. Larsen CP, Ambuzs JM, Bonsib SM, et al. Membranous-like glomerulopathy with masked IgG kappa deposits. *Kidney Int*. 2014;86:154-161, with permission from International Society of Nephrology.

fresh tissue is currently considered the gold standard for the detection and characterization of immune deposits. We recently found a peculiar form of glomerular immune complex deposition in which masked deposits required an antigen-retrieval step to be visualized. Over a 2-year period, 14 cases were characterized by numerous, large subepithelial deposits visualized by electron microscopy and C3-predominant staining by routine immunofluorescence on fresh tissue with weak to negative immunoglobulin staining. Repeat immunofluorescence after digestion of the formalin-fixed paraffin-embedded tissue with pronase elicited strong IgG-κ staining restricted within the deposits. The patients were often young with a mean age of 26 years and commonly had clinical evidence of vague autoimmune phenomenon. The clinicopathologic findings in this unusual form of glomerulopathy do not fit neatly into any currently existing diagnostic category. We have termed this unique form of glomerulopathy membranous-like glomerulopathy with masked IgG-κ deposits (Table 2).

▶ The authors describe a small series of patients with peculiar light microscopy, immunofluorescence, and electron microscopy findings and suggest the term *membranouslike glomerulopathy with masked immunoglobulin G (IgG)* κ for this entity. The importance of this entity is that one might miss the diagnosis of an immune complex media process, particularly if only immunofluorescence is performed and electron microscopy is not done. All cases were negative for phospholipase A2 receptor performed on tissue that had undergone pronase digestion. This represents a peculiar example of a secondary-type membranous nephropathy. Table 2 highlights the morphologic features on the initial biopsy from this series of patients. One can see the marked difference between fresh IgG staining and pronase-digested IgG staining in each of the cases. Another take-home message from this case is the idea that pronase digestion may be of value in patients with confusing or negative initial immunofluorescence studies performed on fresh-frozen tissue. Interestingly, in this small series, most of the patients showed κ light chain restriction. However, no other evidence of a plasma cell dyscrasia or monoclonal process was identified in this series of patients, which may represent a sampling phenomenon. One of the major pitfalls in not recognizing these deposits by pronase immunofluorescence would be to classify these patients as having a C3 glomerulonephritis, a currently popular diagnosis. Further studies from other institutions are required to fully elucidate the clinical pathologic correlation to these histologic findings.

For further review of the pronase-digested immunofluorescence, I refer the readers to the Nasr et al.[1]

M. L. Smith, MD

Reference

1. Nasr SH, Galgano SJ, Markowitz GS, Stokes MB, D'Agati VD. Immunofluorescence on pronase digested paraffin sections: a valuable salvage technique for renal biopsies. *Kidney Int.* 2006;70:2148-2151.

The reproducibility and predictive value on outcome of renal biopsies from expanded criteria donors

Azancot MA, Moreso F, Salcedo M, et al (Universitat Autònoma Barcelona, Spain)

Kidney Int 85:1161-1168, 2014

Reproducibility and predictive value on outcome are the main criteria to evaluate the utility of histological scores. Here we analyze the reproducibility of donor biopsy assessment by different on-call pathologists and the retrospective evaluation by a single renal pathologist blinded to clinical outcomes. We also evaluate the predictive value on graft outcome of both evaluations. A biopsy was performed in donors with any of the following: age ≥55 years, hypertension, diabetes, creatinine >1.5 mg/dl, or stroke. Glomerulosclerosis, interstitial fibrosis, tubular atrophy, intimal thickening, and arteriolar hyalinosis evaluated according to the Banff criteria were added to obtain a chronic score. Biopsies were classified as mild (≥3), intermediate (4–5), or advanced (6–7) damage, and unacceptable (≥8) for transplantation of 127 kidneys biopsied. Weighted k value between both readings was 0.41 (95% CI: 0.28–0.54). Evaluation of biopsies by the renal pathologist was significantly and independently associated with estimated 12-month glomerular filtration rate and a significant composite outcome variable, including death-censored graft survival and time to reach an estimated glomerular filtration rate <30 ml/min per 1.73 m^2. Thus, there was no association between readings of on-call pathologists and outcome. The lack of association between histological scores obtained by the on-call pathologists and graft outcome suggests that a specific training on renal pathology is recommended to optimize the use of kidneys retrieved from expanded criteria donors (Fig 2).

▶ The decision to use a potential kidney allograft from an expanded criteria donor incorporates clinical information of the donor, laboratory data from the donor, histologic data from the donor kidney biopsy analysis, and considerations of the potential recipient. Surgeons will also take into account the gross examination of the organ as well as any anatomic variations. It has been suggested that the use of expanded criteria donors has the potential to markedly increase the donor pool and thus decrease various transplantation wait times. With the introduction of this practice, there has been an increase in pathology evaluations for potential kidney donor allograft biopsies. In addition to the increase in volume, an increase in frequency of disease has been identified as well due to the investigation of expanded criteria donors. In my opinion, there are 2 fundamental findings from this article, both present in Fig 2. In Fig 2b, there is a strong association between the evaluation of the biopsy before transplantation and the overall graft survival. This is encouraging and provides support to the use of pathologists in this critical decision as to whether to use an expanded criteria donor (ECD) kidney. However, panel b of Fig 2, does show some concerning data. When nontransplant pathologists evaluate potential kidney biopsies, there does not appear to be any correlation between the

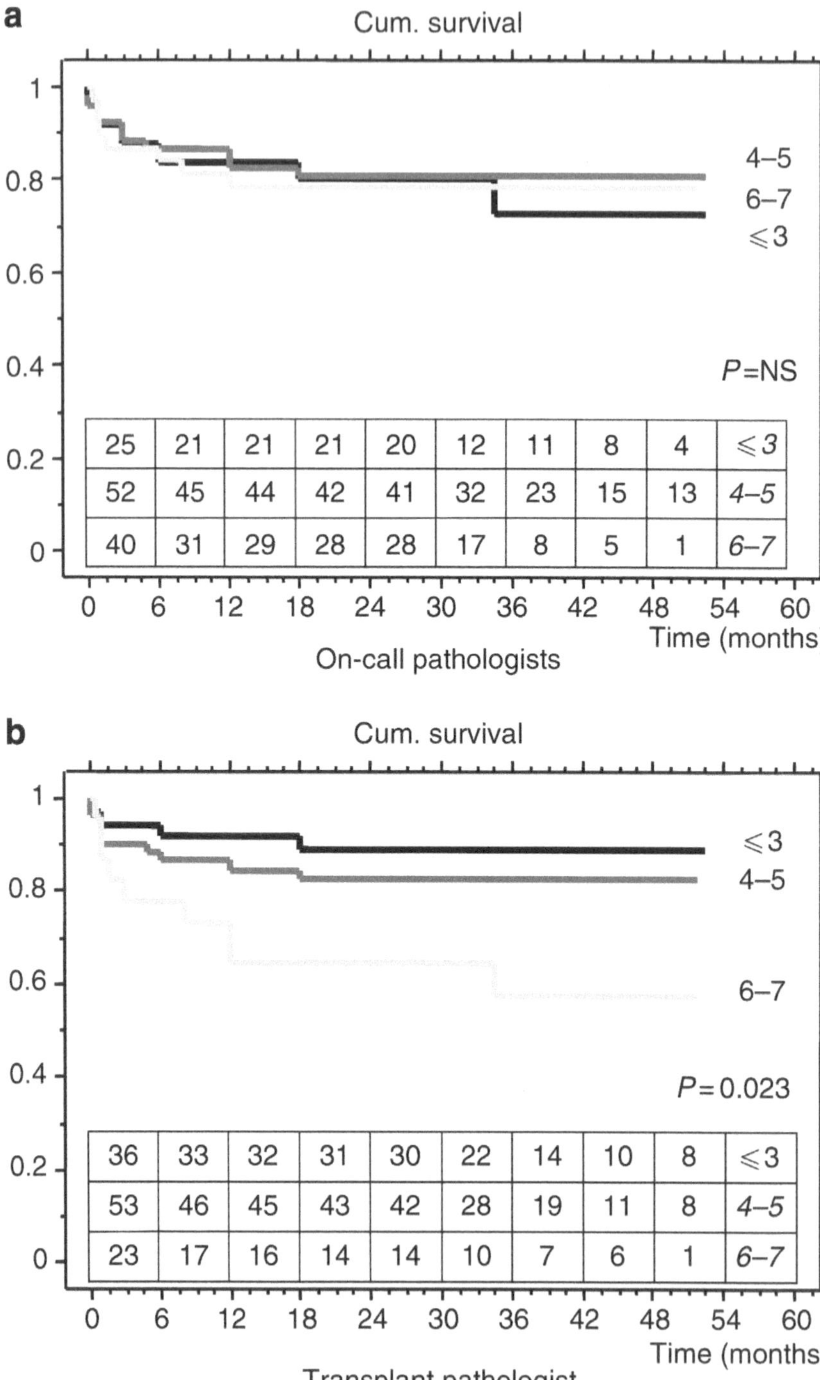

FIGURE 2.—Kaplan–Meier survival curves for the composite outcome variable. Kaplan–Meier survival curves for the composite outcome variable according to donor damage score evaluated by (**a**) on-call pathologists and (**b**) renal pathologist. The number of patients at risk at each time period is shown in the table. (Reprinted with permission from Macmillan Publishers Ltd: Kidney International. Azancot MA, Moreso F, Salcedo M, et al. The reproducibility and predictive value on outcome of renal biopsies from expanded criteria donors. *Kidney Int*. 2014;85:1161-1168, Copyright 2014.)

overall score and the graft cumulative survival. In contrast to the transplant pathologist, this suggests that the involvement of nonspecialist on-call pathologists does not contribute significant data to the decision to use ECD kidneys. This is a major challenge with regard to using expanded criteria donors because it is difficult for individual centers to have transplant pathologists on call 24 hours a day, 7 days a week. The article suggests additional training for on-call pathologists may be a solution to improve their recognition of the histologic features associated with poor graft survival. This is certainly 1 approach that deserves further study. An alternative approach may be to centralize the pathologic reading of transplant biopsies at the Organ Procurement and Transplant Network/United Network for Organ Sharing level, taking advantage of the increasing availability of whole-slide imaging.

For additional review of this topic, I refer the readers to Navarro et al.[1]

M. L. Smith, MD

Reference

1. Navarro MD, López-Andréu M, Rodríguez-Benot A, et al. Significance of pre-implantation analysis of kidney biopsies from expanded criteria donors and long-term outcome. *Transplantation.* 2011;91:432-439.

Best Practices Recommendations in the Application of Immunohistochemistry in the Kidney Tumors: Report From the International Society of Urologic Pathology Consensus Conference

Reuter VE, Members of the ISUP Immunohistochemistry in Diagnostic Urologic Pathology Group (Memorial Sloan-Kettering Cancer Ctr, NY; et al)

Am J Surg Pathol 38:e35-e49, 2014

Primary renal neoplasms comprise multiple distinct entities, some of which are well understood and others that are not. It is not uncommon for some of these entities to have overlapping morphologic features. Their clinical behavior is varied, ranging from highly malignant to benign, and metastatic renal cell carcinoma oftentimes enters into the differential diagnosis of tumors of unknown primary. In this age of personalized medicine, identifying biomarkers that can better predict clinical outcome and response to therapy is a pressing need. In 2013 the International Society of Urological Pathology held a meeting in which best practices recommendations on the use of immunohistochemical markers in urologic malignancies were discussed. In this review we make recommendations regarding immunohistochemical markers that are best suited to aid in establishing a diagnosis of renal primary, panels of antibodies that are most useful in classifying renal tumors, and the current status of prognostic and predictive biomarkers. Although no prognostic or predictive marker and set of

TABLE 2.—Tumors Composed Predominantly of "Clear" Cells

Tumor Type	CA IX	CK7	CD117	Cathepsin-K	HMB-45
Clear cell RCC	Positive, diffuse membranous	Negative	Negative	Negative	Negative
Clear cell PRCC	Positive, cup-like	Positive	Negative	Negative	Negative
Chromophobe RCC, classic	Negative	Positive, cytoplasmic	Positive, membranous	Negative	Negative
Epithelioid-AML	Negative	Negative	Negative	Positive,cytoplasmic	Positive, cytoplasmic
MiTF-TFE tumors					
Xp11 family	Variable but focal	Negative	Variable	Positive (50%), cytoplasmic	Negative
t(6;11)	Variable but focal	Negative	Negative	Positive, cytoplasmic	Positive (always focal)

Reprinted from Reuter VE, Members of the ISUP Immunohistochemistry in Diagnostic Urologic Pathology Group. Best practices recommendations in the application of immunohistochemistry in the kidney tumors. report from the international society of urologic pathology consensus conference. *Am J Surg Pathol.* 2014;38:e35-e49, with permission from Lippincott Williams & Wilkins.

TABLE 3.—Tumors With a Significant Papillary Component

	CAIX	CK7	AMACR	Cathepsin-K	34βE12	TFE3/ TFEB
ccRCC with papillary growth	Positive, membranous	Negative	Negative	Negative	Negative	Negative
PRCC "type I"	Negative	Positive	Positive	Negative	Negative	Negative
PRCC "type II"	Negative	± Positive	Positive	Negative	Negative	Negative
Clear cell PRCC	Positive, cup-like	Positive, diffuse	Negative	Negative	Negative	Negative
MiTF-TFE trans-assoc	Variable but focal	Negative	Positive	Positive (50%)	Negative	Positive*

*Antibodies are difficult to standardize on automated platforms. FISH assays are more reliable.

Reprinted from Reuter VE, Members of the ISUP Immunohistochemistry in Diagnostic Urologic Pathology Group. Best practices recommendations in the application of immunohistochemistry in the kidney tumors. report from the international society of urologic pathology consensus conference. *Am J Surg Pathol.* 2014;38:e35-e49, with permission from Lippincott Williams & Wilkins.

TABLE 4.—Solid PRCC Versus Metanephric Adenoma Versus Wilms Tumor

	CK7	AMACR	WT-1	CD57
Solid papillary	Positive	Positive	Negative	Negative
Metanephric adenoma	Negative or isolated cells	Negative	Positive, nuclear	Positive
Wilms	Negative or isolated cells	Negative	Positive, nuclear	Negative

Reprinted from Reuter VE, Members of the ISUP Immunohistochemistry in Diagnostic Urologic Pathology Group. Best practices recommendations in the application of immunohistochemistry in the kidney tumors. report from the international society of urologic pathology consensus conference. *Am J Surg Pathol.* 2014;38:e35-e49, with permission from Lippincott Williams & Wilkins.

TABLE 5.—Tumors With Oncocytic Features*

	CD117	CK7	Ksp-cadherin	HMB-45	Cathepsin-K
Oncocytoma	Positive, membranous	Negative	Positive	Negative	Negative
Chromophobe RCC, eosinophilic	Positive, membranous	Positive but variable	+/−Positive	Negative	Negative
Oncocytic PRCC	Negative	Positive but focal	Not known	Negative	Unknown
Oncocytic AML	Negative	Negative	Negative	Positive, focal	Negative

Other Abs said to be differentially expressed on oncocytomas and chromophobe RCC.

Positive in oncocytoma, negative in chromophobe: S100A1.

*Hale colloidal iron: Although a histochemical rather than an IHC stain, it can be useful in differentiating chromophobe carcinoma (cytoplasmic granular staining) from oncocytoma (negative or luminal staining). However, this is a technically demanding stain and reliability is laboratory-dependent.

Reprinted from Reuter VE, Members of the ISUP Immunohistochemistry in Diagnostic Urologic Pathology Group. Best practices recommendations in the application of immunohistochemistry in the kidney tumors. report from the international society of urologic pathology consensus conference. *Am J Surg Pathol.* 2014;38:e35-e49, with permission from Lippincott Williams & Wilkins.

TABLE 6.—Tumors With a Predominant Sarcomatoid Pattern of Growth*

	Vimentin†	CAIX‡	PAX8	CK7	34βE12	GATA3	P63
ccRCC	Positive	Positive, membranous	Positive	Negative	Negative	Negative	Negative
PRCC	Positive	Negative	Positive	Focal or negative	Negative	Negative	Negative
Chromophobe RCC	Positive	Negative	Positive	Positive	Negative	Negative	Negative
MTSC	Positive	Negative	Positive	Positive	Variable	Negative	Negative
Urothelial CA	Positive	+/−Negative	Negative§	Positive	Positive	Positive	Positive
Sarcoma	Positive	Negative	Negative	Negative	Negative	Negative	Negative

*Stains should be performed in the better differentiated or most epithelioid areas.
†In sarcomatoid component.
‡Positive adjacent to necrosis or focal cytoplasmic in high-grade areas of various tumors.
§Positive in up to 20% of upper tract UC.
Reprinted from Reuter VE, Members of the ISUP Immunohistochemistry in Diagnostic Urologic Pathology Group. Best practices recommendations in the application of immunohistochemistry in the kidney tumors. report from the international society of urologic pathology consensus conference. *Am J Surg Pathol.* 2014;38:e35-e49, with permission from Lippincott Williams & Wilkins.

TABLE 7.—"Distal Nephron-like" Carcinomas

	Collecting Duct Ca	Medullary Ca	Urothelial Ca
IN-1/BAF47	Retained*	Lost	Retained
OCT4	Negative	Positive†	Negative
GATA3	Negative	Negative	Positive
PAX8	Positive	Positive	Negative‡

*One study reports 15% of CDC with *INI-1* loss.
†Unpublished data.
‡20% positive.
Reprinted from Reuter VE, Members of the ISUP Immunohistochemistry in Diagnostic Urologic Pathology Group. Best practices recommendations in the application of immunohistochemistry in the kidney tumors. report from the international society of urologic pathology consensus conference. *Am J Surg Pathol.* 2014;38:e35-e49, with permission from Lippincott Williams & Wilkins.

markers have yet to be validated, ongoing research suggests that this fact is likely to change in the near future (Tables 2-7).

▶ Over the past decade, there have been considerable advances in the diagnosis and subclassification of primary neoplasms of the renal parenchyma. In the past, it was a relatively limited difference of diagnosis including oncocytoma, clear cell renal cell carcinoma, chromophobe renal cell carcinoma, and papillary renal cell carcinoma. Several new entities have been described and their immunohistochemical distinction has been slowly elucidated over time. This review article highlights several immunohistochemical panels to order depending on the initial histologic features of a biopsy and is an essential guide for surgical pathologists. Particularly, those surgical pathologists who are evaluating renal neoplasms on needle core biopsies, a practice that has increased in frequency as well. The article highlights that not all renal cell neoplasms require immunohistochemical evaluation and that only neoplasms with complex morphology, neoplasms suggestive of distal nephron origin, oncocytic lesions, and cases in which the architecture or its cytologic features are unusual deserve an additional immunohistochemical workup. Tables 2-7 highlight the different immunohistochemical panels suggested for tumors composed predominately of clear cells, tumors with a significant papillary component, solid papillary renal cell carcinoma (RCC) versus metanephric adenoma versus Wilms tumor, tumors with oncocytic features, tumors with a predominant sarcomatoid pattern of growth, and distal nephron-like carcinomas. One of the challenges for the practicing general surgical pathologist is the availability of many of these markers. One other important recommendation from this review is the suggestion that PAX8 is the most useful immunohistochemical marker for establishing renal origin in metastatic lesions. Several immunohistochemical stains that are commonly used in present-day practice, including CD10, RCC, and Ksp-cadherin, may be supportive of metastatic renal cell carcinoma but are not as sensitive or specific as PAX8. Their use should therefore be limited.

For additional review regarding renal tumors with clear cell histology, I refer the readers to Reuter and Tickoo.[1]

M. L. Smith, MD

Reference

1. Reuter VE, Tickoo SK. Differential diagnosis of renal tumors with clear cell histology. *Pathology.* 2010;42:374-383.

6 Female Genital Tract

The role of immunohistochemistry in the evaluation of gynecologic pathology: a single institutional experience

Chamberlain BK, Fadare O, Desouki MM (Vanderbilt Univ Med Ctr, Nashville, TN; Univ of California San Diego)

Ann Diagn Pathol 19:88-90, 2015

Although morphology is the cornerstone of diagnostic pathology, it may be necessary to apply ancillary techniques, including immunohistochemistry (IHC) to resolve diagnostic problems. To provide some insights into IHC use in gynecologic (gyn) surgical pathology, we reviewed our institutional experience in using IHC during a 1-year period. A total number of 487 markers were ordered on 203 cases (2.4 markers/case). These 203 represented 4.8% of the 4216 gyn cases that were accessioned during the study period. Immunohistochemistry was used in 22 (9.3%) of 236 vulvar, 13 (9.2%) of 142 vaginal, 92 (5.9%) of 1557 cervical, 59 (3.5%) of 1698 uterine, 1 (0.3%) of 311 fallopian tube, and 16 (6.9%) of 232 ovarian specimens. The most common markers were p16 (n = 125), Ki-67 (n = 69), and p53 (n = 59). Immunohistochemistry proved to be a valuable tool in separating benign from dysplastic or malignant categories, or to increase diagnostic certainty in the latter category, in 131 (65%) of the 203 cases where IHC was requested, and 3.1% of all 4216 gyn cases examined. In the other 72 cases, IHC was utilized to histotype carcinomas, to define a site of origin for an established malignancy, or to assess the expression of predictive markers. Among 6 pathologists, years of practice and time spent on gyn service significantly affected IHC use, with less use with more than 10 years of practice and more than 10 weeks/year of service. This study documents IHC use at a tertiary care academic center and contributes data to define benchmarks for expected IHC use.

▶ Chamberlain et al show a pattern of immunohistochemistry (IHC) variability in the diagnosis of gynecologic pathology at a single institution. Imagine the variability among many institutions! These patterns reflect the lack of standardization among practicing physicians that is seen before concerted efforts to understand best practice. Ideally, there is a best IHC practice for all scenarios (eg, lack of diagnostic certainty, tumor classification, etc) that involves panel use and sequence and involves team efforts to define and work together. Our field is getting there, and these articles highlight our starting points.

S. Raab, MD

Endometrial stromal tumours revisited: an update based on the 2014 WHO classification

Ali RH, Rouzbahman M (Kuwait Univ, Safat)

J Clin Pathol 68:325-332, 2015

Endometrial stromal tumours (EST) are rare tumours of endometrial stromal origin that account for less than 2% of all uterine tumours. Recent cytogenetic and molecular advances in this area have improved our understanding of ESTs and helped refine their classification into more meaningful categories. Accordingly, the newly released 2014 WHO classification system recognises four categories: endometrial stromal nodule (ESN), low-grade endometrial stromal sarcoma (LGESS), highgrade endometrial stromal sarcoma (HGESS) and undifferentiated uterine sarcoma (UUS). At the molecular level, these tumours may demonstrate a relatively simple karyotype with a defining chromosomal rearrangement (as in the majority of ESNs, LGESSs and *YWHAE*-rearranged HGESS) or demonstrate complex cytogenetic aberrations lacking specific rearrangements (as in UUSs). Herein we provide an update on this topic aimed at the practicing pathologist.

▶ Ali and Rouzbahman provide an updated review of endometrial stromal tumors. This review provides important information on the gross appearance, histopathology, immunohistochemistry, and genetic findings of the 4 categories of stromal tumors. These tumors are rare, and the diagnosis generally does not need to depend on molecular analysis, although the 2014 World Health Organization classification system incorporates current molecular data. For additional reading, see reference list.[1,2]

S. Raab, MD

References

1. Stemme S, Ghaderi M, Carlson JW. Diagnosis of endometrial stromal tumors: a clinicopathologic study of 25 biopsy specimens with identification of problematic areas. *Am J Clin Pathol.* 2014;141:133-139.
2. Kurman RJ, Carcangiu ML, Herrington CS, Young RH. In: Lyon, France: IARC Press; 2014.

The Utility of Immunohistochemistry in the Differential Diagnosis of Gynecologic Disorders

Kaspar HG, Crum CP (Geisinger Health System, Wilkes-Barre, PA; Brigham and Women's Hosp, Boston, MA)

Arch Pathol Lab Med 139:39-54, 2015

Context.—Immunohistochemistry has assumed an increasing role in the identification and characterization of gynecologic disorders including lesions with deceptively bland morphology, uncommon and underdiagnosed neoplasms, and neoplasms with specific genetic alterations associated with overexpression or loss of expression of specific proteins. The diagnostic accuracy has been significantly improved owing to the discovery and increasing experience with the tumor-associated biomarkers, and the increasing demand for precise tumor classification to assess suitability for the expanding therapeutic modalities including clinical trials.

Objective.—To differentiate lesions of the gynecologic tract through the use of effective immunohistochemical panels.

Data Sources.—Literature review and authors' personal practice experience.

Conclusions.—The application of diagnostic and prognostic immunohistochemical panels has enabled pathologists to better guide therapeutic decisions and to better predict the clinical outcome. It is now well established that the use of ancillary testing, including immunohistochemistry, has a significant power in the identification, differentiation, and classification of reactive, premalignant, and malignant gynecologic disorders. This article discusses the utilities and pitfalls of the commonly used immunohistochemical markers in the context of overlapping morphologic features encountered in the uterus, ovaries, and fallopian tubes.

▶ Kaspar and Crum provide a superb summary of the use of immunohistochemical testing in the field of gynecologic surgical pathology. This summary is based on literature review (233 reports are referenced) and the authors' considerable experience. The authors describe specific scenarios in which the differential diagnosis consists of 2 or multiple entities. A challenge for the general pathologist is remembering (or even learning about) the studies reporting the sensitivity and specificity (especially in panel use) of newer antibodies. The authors also describe the clinical relevance in the separation of some entities. This article is worth keeping handy prior to immunohistochemical test ordering.

S. Raab, MD

Low Grade Serous Ovarian Carcinoma: From the molecular characterization to the best therapeutic strategy

Della Pepa C, Tonini G, Santini D, et al (Campus Bio-Medico Univ of Rome, Italy; et al)

Cancer Treat Rev 41:136-143, 2015

Low Grade Serous Ovarian Carcinoma, LGSOC, is certainly a rare disease, accounting for only a small proportion of all ovarian carcinomas, nevertheless in the last decade we have acquired many data about its molecular and clinical features and it has been largely accepted that it has distinct pathogenesis, genetic aberrations and clinical behavior compared to High Grade Serous Ovarian Carcinoma, HGSOC, which is the most common ovarian cancer histotype. A large number of series pointed out the high rate of KRAS and BRAF mutations in LGSOCs and Serous Borderline Tumors, SBLTs, in contrast with their rarity in HGSOC. Such finding, together with the recurrent observation of focus of LGSOC associated

TABLE 4.—LGSOC Compared to HGSOC. Differences Between the Two Subtypes Involve Molecular Profile as Well as Histology and Clinical Features

		HGSOC	LCSOC
Genes profiling	P53 mutation	Frequent (up to 73%)	Rare
	Genetic instability	High even at early stage	Absent
	KRAS mutation	Rare	Frequent (up to 63%)
	BRAF mutation	Rare	Frequent (up to 33%)
Histology	Nuclear atypia	Marked	Mild
	Mitotic index	High	Low
	Growth pattern	Large papillae	Mircopapillae
Clinical behavior	Age at diagnosis (median)	63 years	43 years
	ORR to platinum based CHT	High (up toi 80%)	Low (4%)
	Survival	24–63 months	81–126 months

Reprinted from Della Pepa C, Tonini G, Santini D, et al. Low grade serous ovarian carcinoma: from the molecular characterization to the best therapeutic strategy. *Cancer Treat Rev.* 2015;41:136-143, with permission from Elsevier.

with areas of SBLT in the same lesion, led to abandon the traditional histology classification, defining three types of serous carcinomas, in favor of a new dualistic grading system which recognizes only LG and HG carcinomas corresponding to distinct tumorigenesis pathways, the former based on KRAS/BRAF mutations and alteration of the MAP/ERK signaling, the latter characterized by early genetic instability and wild type status of KRAS and BRAF. LGSOC shows favorable overall survival, compared to general ovarian cancer population, but worrying resistance to conventional treatments. MEK inhibitors are emerging as active agents and may well represent an effective therapeutic strategy in the near future (Table 4).

▶ Della Pepa et al show how the intersection of the fields of diagnostic pathology, molecular pathology, clinical practice, and clinical outcomes research are transformational for patient care. Table 4 sums up the information supporting the separation of ovarian serous tumors into 2 types: high-grade serous ovarian carcinoma (HGSOC) and low-grade serous ovarian carcinoma (LGSOC). Traditional surgical pathology plays an important role and molecular pathology is playing an increasingly larger role. Specifically, through greater understanding of genetic abnormalities, the development of targeted treatments for both HGSOC and LGSOC are being studied and designed.

S. Raab, MD

Assessment of endometrial sampling as a predictor of final surgical pathology in endometrial cancer

Helpman L, Kupets R, Covens A, et al (Chaim Sheba Med Ctr, Ramat Gan, Israel; Sunnybrook Health Sciences Ctr, Toronto, Ontario, Canada)
Br J Cancer 110:609-615, 2014

Background.—The histology and grade of endometrial cancer are important predictors of disease outcome and of the likelihood of nodal involvement. In most centres, however, surgical staging decisions are based on a preoperative biopsy. The objective of this study was to assess the concordance between the preoperative histology and that of the hysterectomy specimen in endometrial cancer.

Methods.—Patients treated for endometrial cancer during a 10-year period at a tertiary cancer centre were identified from a prospectively collected pathological database. All pathology reports were reviewed to confirm centralised reporting of the original sampling or biopsy specimens; patients whose biopsies were not reviewed by a dedicated gynaecological pathologist at the treating centre were excluded. Surgical pathology data including histology, grade, depth of myometrial invasion, cervical stromal involvement and lymphovascular space invasion (LVSI) as well as preoperative histology and grade were collected. Preoperative and final tumour cell type and grade were compared and the distribution of other high-risk features was analysed.

Results.—A total of 1329 consecutive patients were identified; 653 patients had a centrally reviewed epithelial endometrial cancer on their original biopsy, and are included in this study. Of 255 patients whose biopsies were read as grade 1 (G1) adenocarcinoma, 45 (18%) were upgraded to grade 2 (G2) on final pathology, 6 (2%) were upgraded to grade 3 (G3) and 5 (2%) were read as a non-endometrioid high-grade histology. Overall, of 255 tumours classified as G1 endometrioid cancers on biopsy, 74 (29%) were either found to be low-grade (G1–2) tumours with deep myometrial invasion, or were reclassified as high-grade cancers (G3 or non-endometrioid histologies) on final surgical pathology. Despite these shifts, we calculate that omitting surgical staging in preoperatively diagnosed G1 endometrioid cancers without deep myometrial invasion would result in missing nodal involvement in only 1% of cases.

Conclusions.—Preoperative endometrial sampling is only a modest predictor of surgical pathology features in endometrial cancer and may underestimate the risk of disease spread and recurrence. In spite of frequent shifts in postoperative vs preoperative histological assessment, the

TABLE 1A.—Histological Features of Cases Grouped by Pre- and Post-Operative Histology (G1–3 Endometrioid, High Risk (HR), Non-Endometrioid Histological Subtypes)

Biopsy Histology Report	Hysterectomy Histology Report: G1 Endometrioid	G2 Endometrioid	G3 Endometrioid	HR Non-Endometrioid	Total
G1 endometrioid	199 (78%)	45 (18%)	6 (2%)	5 (2%)	255
G2 endometrioid	19 (15%)	74 (59%)	20 (16%)	12 (10%)	125
G3 endometrioid	1 (1%)	6 (7%)	57 (68%)	20 (24%)	84
HR non-endometrioid	1 (0.5%)	3 (1.6%)	9 (5%)	176 (93%)	189

Reprinted by permission from Macmillan Publishers Ltd. Helpman L, Kupets R, Covens A, et al. Assessment of endometrial sampling as a predictor of final surgical pathology in endometrial cancer. *Br J Cancer.* 2014;110:609-615, Copyright 2014.

TABLE 1B.—Detailed Histological Features of Cases Grouped by Pre- and Post-Operative Histology

	Hysterectomy Histology Report												
	G1 Endometrioid					G2 Endometrioid							
Biopsy Report	Total	DMI	CxSI	LVSI	LVSI/CxSI No DMI	Total	DMI	CxSI	LVSI	LVSI/CxSI No DMI	G3	HR	Total
G1 endometrioid	199 (78%)	44	17	31	15	45 (18%)	19	11	14	6	6 (2%)	5 (2%)	255
G2 endometrioid	19 (15%)	5	2	2	2	74 (59%)	21	19	23	18	20 (16%)	12 (10%)	125
G3 endometrioid	1 (1%)	0	0	0	0	6 (7%)	4	1	2	0	57 (68%)	20 (24%)	84
HR non-endometrioid	1 (0.5%)	0	1	0	1	3 (1.6%)	0	0	0	0	9 (5%)	176 (93%)	189

Abbreviations: CxSI = cervical stromal invasion; DMI = deep myometrial invasion; G1,2,3 = grade 1, 2 and 3 endometrioid adenocarcinoma of the endometrium; HR = non endometrioid high risk histologies, including serous endometrial cancer, clear cell adenocarcinoma and carcinosarcoma of the uterus; LVSI = lymphovascular space invasion.

predicted rate of missed nodal metastases with a selective staging policy remains low (Table 1A, Tables 1B).

▶ The findings by Helpman et al are similar to previously reported data that indicate an upgrading frequency of 16% to 40% from preoperatively diagnosed G1–2 endometrioid adenocarcinomas. Table 1 highlights both the upgrading and downgrading data from this study. The 2 major factors that contribute to changes in grade assessment are clinical sampling and interpretive variability (precision), and these factors are interrelated. Quality improvement initiatives would be different depending on the contribution that sampling and precision contribute to the overall difference in assessment. However, the authors indicate that omitting lymphadenectomy in low-risk endometrioid tumors, defined as tumors without deep myometrial invasion as assessed intraoperatively, would only fail to identify 1% of node-positive cases. See reference list for additional reading.[1,2]

S. Raab, MD

References

1. Leitao MM Jr, Kehoe S, Barakat RR, et al. Comparison of D&C and office endometrial biopsy accuracy in patients with FIGO grade 1 endometrial adenocarcinoma. *Gynecol Oncol.* 2009;113:105-108.
2. Nofech-Mozes S, Ismiil N, Dube V, et al. Interobserver agreement for endometrial cancer characteristics evaluated on biopsy material. *Obstet Gynecol Int.* 2012; 2012:414086.

7 Breast

Concomitant Detection of HER2 Protein and Gene Alterations by Immunohistochemistry (IHC) and Silver Enhanced In Situ Hybridization (SISH) Identifies HER2 Positive Breast Cancer with and without Gene Amplification

Varga Z, Tubbs RR, Moch H (Univ Hosp Zurich, Switzerland; Cleveland Clinic, OH)

PLoS One 9:e105961, 2014

Introduction.—HER2 status assessment became a mandatory test assay in breast cancer, giving prognostic and predictive information including eligibility for adjuvant anti-HER2 therapy. Precise and reliable assessment of HER2 status is therefore of utmost importance. In this study we analyzed breast cancer samples by a novel technology for concomitant detection of the HER2 protein and gene copy number.

Methods.—Tissue microarrays containing 589 invasive breast cancer samples were analyzed with a double immunohistochemistry (IHC) and silver labeled in situ hybridization (SISH) assay simultaneously detecting HER2 protein and gene copy number in the same tumor cells. This bright-field assay was analyzed using scores according to the modified ASCO guidelines and the results were correlated with patient prognosis.

Results.—Overall concordance rate between protein expression and the presence of gene amplification was 98%. Fifty-seven of 60 tumors (95%) with IHC score 3+, 6 of 10 tumors with IHC score 2+ (60%) and only 3 of 519 tumors (0.6%) with IHC score 0/1+ were amplified by SISH. Patients with gene amplification despite IHC score 0/1+ had a tendency for worse overall survival ($p = 0.088$, reaching nearly statistical significance) compared to IHC score 0/1+ without amplification. In contrast, there was no difference in overall survival in IHC score 3+/2+ tumors with and without gene amplification.

Conclusions.—The novel double IHC and SISH assay for HER2 is efficient in the identification of breast cancer with discordant HER2 protein and *HER2* gene status, especially for the prognostically relevant groups of *HER2* protein negative tumors with HER2 amplification and HER2 protein positive tumors without HER2 amplification. Breast cancer without HER2 amplification among IHC score 2+/3+ tumors (10% in our cohort) suggests that other mechanisms than gene amplification contribute to protein overexpression in these cells.

▶ In many settings in North America, HER2 status assessment in patients with breast cancer is performed through immunohistochemistry (IHC) testing and/or in situ hybridization testing, such as fluorescence in situ hybridization (FISH) testing. Varga et al simultaneously used double IHC and silver labeled in situ hybridization (SISH). Varga et al reported that HER2 gene amplification (independent from HER2 protein expression) in IHC scored 0/1+ cases correlated with a tendency to poorer overall survival. Varga et al indicated that the double IHC and SISH identified a prognostically relevant IHC 2+/3+ breast subgroup without HER2 amplification. These cases would not have been detected using FISH alone. For further reading, see reference list.[1,2]

S. Raab, MD

References

1. Gown AM, Goldstein LC, Barry TS, et al. High concordance between immunohistochemistry and fluorescence in situ hybridization testing for HER2 status in breast cancer requires a normalized IHC scoring system. *Mod Pathol.* 2008;21: 1271-1277.
2. Park K, Han S, Kim JY, Kim HJ, Kwon JE. Silver-enhanced in situ hybridization as an alternative to fluorescence in situ hybridization for assaying HER2 amplification in clinical breast cancer. *J Breast Cancer.* 2011;14:276-282.

Second opinion in breast pathology: policy, practice and perception

Geller BM, Nelson HD, Carney PA, et al (Univ of Vermont, Burlington; Oregon Health and Science Univ, Portland; et al)

J Clin Pathol 67:955-960, 2014

Aims.—To assess the laboratory policies, pathologists' clinical practice and perceptions about the value of second opinions for breast pathology cases among pathologists practising in the USA.

Methods.—Cross-sectional data were collected from 252 pathologists who interpret breast specimens in eight states using a web-based survey. Descriptive statistics were used to characterise findings.

Results.—Most participants had >10 years of experience interpreting breast specimens (64%), were not affiliated with academic centres (73%) and were not considered experts by their peers (79%). Laboratory policies mandating second opinions varied by diagnosis: invasive cancer 65%; ductal carcinoma in situ (DCIS) 56%; atypical ductal hyperplasia 36% and other benign cases 33%. 81% obtained second opinions in the absence of policies. Participants believed they improve diagnostic accuracy (96%) and protect from malpractice suits (83%), and were easy to obtain, did not take too much time and did not make them look less adequate. The most common (60%) approach to resolving differences between the first and second opinion is to ask for a third opinion, followed by reaching a consensus.

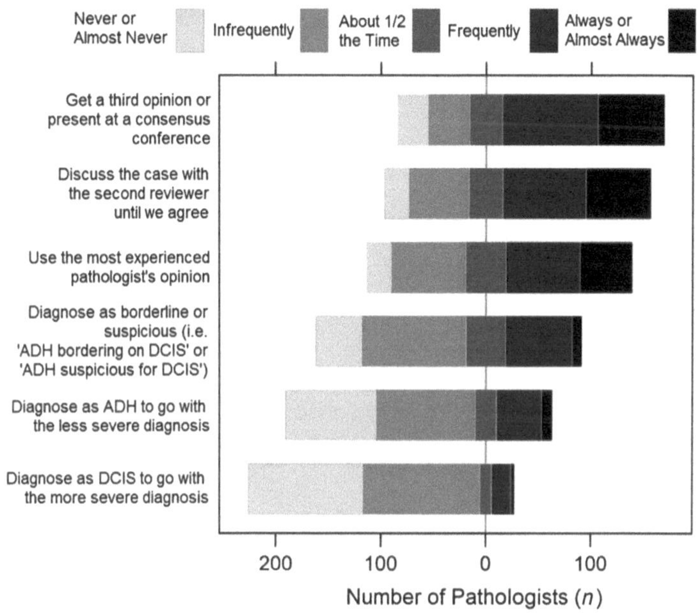

FIGURE 3.—Responses to questions about resolving differences between first and second opinions for a hypothetical case. (Reprinted from Geller BM, Nelson HD, Carney PA, et al. Second opinion in breast pathology: policy, practice and perception. *J Clin Pathol.* 2014;67:955-960, © 2014, American Society for Clinical Pathology.)

Conclusions.—Laboratory-based second opinion policies vary for breast pathology but are most common for invasive cancer and DCIS cases. Pathologists have favourable attitudes towards second opinions, adhere to policies and obtain them even when policies are absent. Those without a formal policy may benefit from supportive clinical practices and systems that help obtain second opinions (Fig 3).

▶ Geller et al report pathologist policies regarding the use of second opinions, how often they actually use second opinions, and their perception of ideal practice. Almost all pathologists believe that second opinions improve diagnostic accuracy, but policies vary among institutions for specific cases types that should be reviewed. Fig 3 is interesting in the variability of opinions based on resolving differences of opinion. For additional reading, please see reference list.[1,2]

S. Raab, MD

References

1. Oster N, Carney P, Allison K, et al. Development of a diagnostic test set to assess agreement in breast pathology: practical application of the guidelines for reporting reliability and agreement studies (GRRAS). *BMC Womens Health.* 2013;13:3.
2. Staradub V, Messenger K, Hao N, Wiley EL, Morrow M. Changes in breast cancer therapy because of pathology second opinions. *Ann Surg Oncol.* 2002;9:982-987.

Effects of tissue decalcification on the quantification of breast cancer biomarkers by digital image analysis

Gertych A, Mohan S, Maclary S, et al (Cedars-Sinai Med Ctr, Los Angeles, CA; et al)

Diagn Pathol 9:213, 2014

Background.—Recent technical advances in digital image capture and analysis greatly improve the measurement of protein expression in tissues. Breast cancer biomarkers provide a unique opportunity to utilize digital image analysis to evaluate sources of variability that are caused by the tissue preparation, in particular the decalcification treatment associated with the analysis of bone metastatic breast cancer, and to develop methods for comparison of digital data and categorical scores rendered by pathologists.

Methods.—Tissues were prospectively decalcified for up to 24 hours and stained by immunohistochemistry (IHC) for ER, PR, Ki-67 and p53. HER2 positive breast cancer sections were retrieved from the pathology archives, and annotated with the categorical HER2 expression scores from the pathology reports. Digital images were captured with Leica and Aperio slide scanners. The conversion of the digital to categorical scores was accomplished with a Gaussian mixture model and tested for accuracy by comparison to clinical scores.

Results.—We observe significant effects of the decalcification treatment on common breast cancer biomarkers that are used in the clinic. ER, PR and p53 staining intensities decreased 15–20%, whereas Ki-67 decreased >90% during the first 6 hrs of treatment and stabilized thereafter. In comparison with the Aperio images, pixel intensities generated by the Leica system are lower. A novel statistical model for conversion of digital to categorical scores provides a systematic approach for conversion of nuclear and membrane stains and demonstrated a high concordance with clinical scores.

Conclusion.—Digital image analysis greatly improves the quantification of protein expression in human tissues. Decalcification affects the accuracy of immunohistochemical staining results and cannot be reversed by image analysis. Measurement data obtained on a continuous scoring scale can be converted to categorical scores for comparison with categorical dataset that are generated by pathologists.

Virtual Slides.—The virtual slide(s) for this article can be found here: http://www.diagnosticpathology.diagnomx.eu/vs/13000_2014_213 (Fig 1).

▶ Gertych et al report that for breast cancer biomarkers, cancer cells show an intensity decrease or a decrease in cell positivity based on the length of time in decalcification (Fig 1). These data have relevance for bone tissues that show

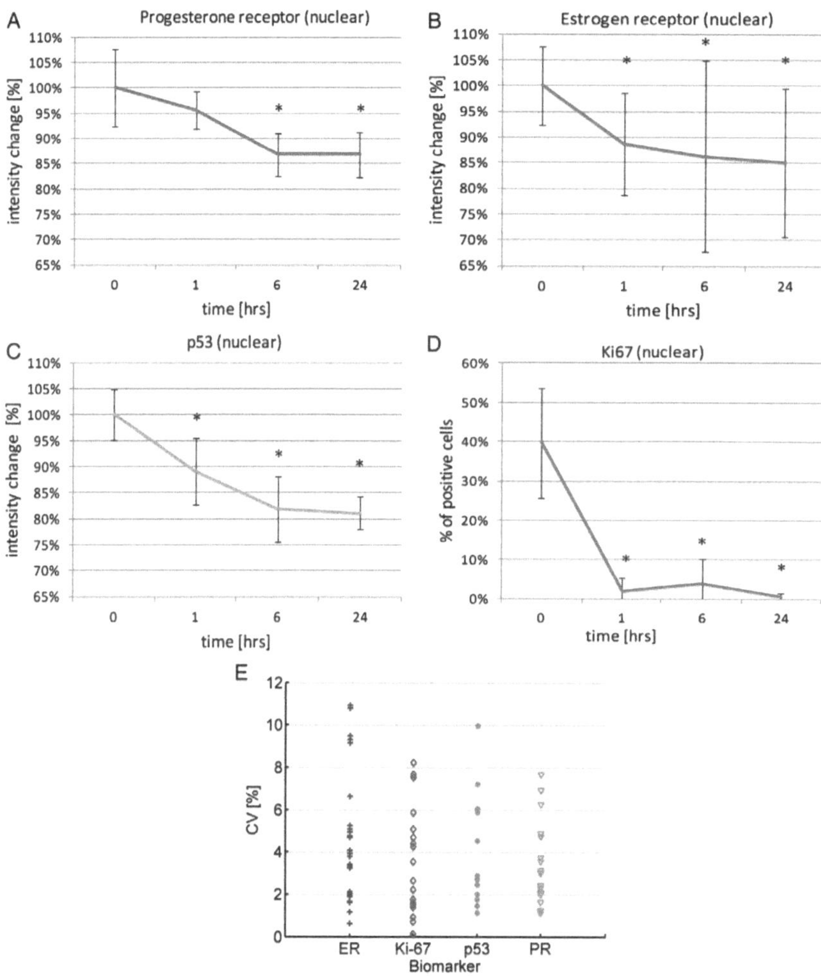

FIGURE 1.—Quantification of breast cancer biomarkers in tissues treated by decalcification: The study involved 9 cases and 5 fields per slide were measured at each time point. A - C) The average staining intensities at each time point across all slides are plotted on the Y-axis for the estrogen receptor (A), progesterone receptor (B) and p53 (C) and the % Ki-67 positive cells are platted in D. The X-axis indicates the time interval of the decalcification treatment. $*p < 0.005$ versus baseline. E) The %CV across 5 fields in each slide is shown for 29 slides stained for ER, 20 stained for PR, 12 stained for p53 and 18 stained for Ki-67. (Reprinted from Gertych A, Mohan S, Maclary S, et al. Effects of tissue decalcification on the quantification of breast cancer biomarkers by digital image analysis. *Diagn Pathol.* 2014;9:213, with permission from BioMed Central Ltd.)

metastatic disease. The authors describe a method for converting a continuous scoring scale to a categorical score, if necessary.

S. Raab, MD

Breast cancer detection in axillary sentinel lymph nodes: the impact of the method of pathologic examination

Calhoun BC, Chambers K, Flippo-Morton T, et al (Levine Cancer Inst, Charlotte, NC)

Hum Pathol 45:2497-2501, 2014

At Carolinas Medical Center, before 2008, axillary sentinel lymph nodes (SLNs) from breast cancer patients were evaluated with a single hematoxylin and eosin-stained slide. In 2008, the protocol changed to include a limited step sectioning at 500 μm. In this study, we compared the intraoperative and permanent section pathologic findings for SLN biopsies from 2006 to 2007 to those from 2009 to 2010. We hypothesized that evaluating 2 slides would increase the detection of micrometastases and isolated tumor cells (ITCs) on permanent sections and correspondingly decrease the sensitivity of intraoperative touch preparation cytology (IOTPC). From 2006 to 2007, 140 (23.5%) of 597 of SLN permanent sections contained tumor cells: 92 macrometastases (65.7%), 36 micrometastases (25.7%), and 12 ITCs 0.2 mm or less (8.6%). The sensitivity of IOTPC for 2006 to 2007 was 51.4% for any tumor cells and 71.7% for macrometastases. From 2009 to 2010, 160 (21.9%) of 730 SLN permanent sections were positive for any tumor cells: 76 macrometastases (47.5%), 55 micrometastases (34.4%), and 29 ITCs (18.1%). The sensitivity of IOTPC for 2009 to 2010 was 39.4% for any tumor cells and 76.3% for macrometastases. With limited step sectioning, we observed an approximately 10% increase in the detection of both micrometastases and ITCs in SLN. The increased detection of ITCs on permanent sections reached statistical significance (P =.018). However, under current clinical guidelines, patients with limited SLN involvement may not be required to undergo completion axillary lymph node dissection. The ability to detect SLN tumor deposits less than 2 mm must be balanced with the clinical utility of doing so.

▶ It is not surprising that a higher detection frequency is increased with increased sampling, through the cutting of an additional tissue section. From my calculation of the data, 8.0% and 11.5% of patients had a micrometastasis or isolated tumor cell (ITC) in 2006 to 2007 and 2008 to 2009, respectively. Both the frequency of positive micrometastasis and ITC increased. I agree that the utility of detecting ITC is controversial, as some argue that treatment should not be affected. Although the increase in the number of micrometastases was not statistically significant, additional studies might be warranted to determine if significance would be detected in a larger population, prior to discontinuing the practice of cutting 2 sections. For additional reading, see reference list.[1,2]

S. Raab, MD

References

1. Lyman GH, Giuliano AE, Somerfield MR, et al. American Society of Clinical Oncology guideline recommendations for sentinel lymph node biopsy in early-stage breast cancer. *J Clin Oncol*. 2005;23:7703-7720.

2. Viale G, Mastropasqua MG, Maiorano E, Mazzarol G. Pathologic examination of the axillary sentinel lymph nodes in patients with earlystage breast carcinoma: current and resolving controversies on the basis of the European institute of oncology experience. *Virchows Arch*. 2006;448:241-247.

A Targetable Androgen Receptor–Positive Breast Cancer Subtype Hidden Among the Triple-Negative Cancers

Safarpour D, Tavassoli FA (Yale Univ School of Medicine, New Haven, CT)
Arch Pathol Lab Med 139:612-617, 2015

Context.—Triple-negative breast cancer (TNBC) is a subgroup of breast cancers that by definition lack expression of estrogen receptor, progesterone receptor, and human epidermal growth factor receptor 2 (HER2). A diverse group of tumors, TNBC shares some morphologic and molecular features with basal-like breast cancer, a category of breast cancer defined by gene expression profiling. More likely to occur in young women and African Americans, TNBCs may exhibit aggressive behavior and are associated with poor prognosis despite their initial response to conventional chemotherapy. Because hormonal or HER2-targeted therapies are ineffective for these tumors, the main therapeutic option is systemic chemotherapy. Therefore, identification of new targets for therapy is urgently needed for this group.

Objective.—To review and present recent literature along with our own experience regarding the clinical and morphologic characteristics and the prevalence of androgen receptor (AR) expression in TNBC, and to discuss the potential use of AR as a therapeutic target for AR^+ TNBC.

Data Sources.—Data sources are published articles from peer-reviewed journals in PubMed (US National Library of Medicine).

Conclusions.—AR is the most commonly expressed hormone receptor among all breast carcinomas, with a prevalence of 25% to 75% among TNBCs. Therefore, we strongly support the routine assessment of AR in TNBC, and preferably in all breast carcinomas.

▶ Triple-negative breast cancers (TNBCs) are characterized by young age at diagnosis, early relapse and metastases, and poor prognosis compared with other types of breast carcinoma. Breast cancers developing in patients with BRCA1 mutations or dysfunction are often of the TNBC and basal-like breast cancer subtypes. Because TNBCs may express androgen receptor (AR), Safarpour and Tavassoli recommend routinely assessing for the presence for AR in TNBCs. Currently, targeted therapies are being explored that may address AR; therefore, this article calls our attention to potential changes in therapy (and laboratory testing) for this field. For further reading, see reference list.[1-3]

S. Raab, MD

References

1. Ogawa Y, Hai E, Matsumoto K, et al. Androgen receptor expression in breast cancer: relationship with clinicopathological factors and biomarkers. *Int J Clin Oncol.* 2008;13:431-435.

2. Alshenawy HA. Prevalence of androgen receptors in invasive breast carcinoma and its relation with estrogen receptor, progesterone receptor and Her2/neu expression. *J Egypt Natl Canc Inst.* 2012;24:77-83.
3. Yu Q, Niu Y, Liu N, et al. Expression of androgen receptor in breast cancer and its significance as a prognostic factor. *Ann Oncol.* 2011;22:1288-1294.

Estrogen Receptor Expression Is High but Is of Lower Intensity in Tubular Carcinoma Than in Well-Differentiated Invasive Ductal Carcinoma

Jorns JM, Thomas DG, Healy PN, et al (Univ of Michigan, Ann Arbor; et al)
Arch Pathol Lab Med 138:1507-1513, 2014

Context.—Tubular carcinoma (TC) is a rare, luminal A subtype of breast carcinoma with excellent prognosis, for which adjuvant chemotherapy is usually contraindicated.

Objective.—To examine the levels of estrogen receptor (ER) and progesterone receptor expression in cases of TC and well-differentiated invasive ductal carcinoma as compared to normal breast glands and to determine if any significant differences could be detected via molecular testing.

Design.—We examined ER and progesterone receptor via immunohistochemistry in tubular (N = 27), mixed ductal/tubular (N = 16), and well-differentiated ductal (N = 27) carcinomas with comparison to surrounding normal breast tissue. We additionally performed molecular subtyping of 10 TCs and 10 ductal carcinomas via the PAM50 assay.

Results.—Although ER expression was high for all groups, TC had statistically significantly lower ER staining percentage (ER%) (P = .003) and difference in ER expression between tumor and accompanying normal tissue (P = .02) than well-differentiated ductal carcinomas, with mixed ductal/tubular carcinomas falling between these 2 groups. Mean ER% was 79%, 87%, and 94%, and mean tumor-normal ER% differences were 13.6%, 25.9%, and 32.6% in tubular, mixed, and ductal carcinomas, respectively. Most tumors that had molecular subtyping were luminal A (9 of 10 tubular and 8 of 10 ductal), and no significant differences in specific gene expression between the 2 groups were identified.

Conclusions.—Tubular carcinoma exhibited decreased intensity in ER expression, closer to that of normal breast parenchyma, likely as a consequence of a high degree of differentiation. Lower ER% expression by TC may represent a potential pitfall when performing commercially available breast carcinoma prognostic assays that rely heavily on ER-related gene expression.

▶ Some cases of tubular carcinoma (TC) may be difficult to distinguish from mixed ductal/TCs by histological examination. Jorns et al remind us that other features, such as small size, lack of lymph node metastases, and the presence of flat epithelial atypia, are more likely seen in TC. Jorn et al also recommend that we carefully examine estrogen receptor (ER) reactivity patterns as an additional clue helpful in making the distinction. TCs more likely will exhibit an ER reactivity pattern of decreased intensity (compared with well-differentiated invasive ductal carcinoma of no special type) similar to normal breast parenchyma. This report promotes a subtle point in the art of breast cancer diagnosis. For further reading, see reference list.[1,2]

S. Raab, MD

References

1. Aulmann S, Elsawaf Z, Penzel R, Schirmacher P, Sinn HP. Invasive tubular carcinoma of the breast frequently is clonally related to flat epithelial atypia and low-grade ductal carcinoma in situ. *Am J Surg Pathol.* 2009;33:1646-1653.
2. Kunju LP, Ding Y, Kleer CG. Tubular carcinoma and grade 1 (welldifferentiated) invasive ductal carcinoma: comparison of flat epithelial atypia and other intra-epithelial lesions. *Pathol Int.* 2008;58:620-625.

8 Lung and Mediastinum

Pulmonary Adenocarcinoma With Signet Ring Cell Features: A Comprehensive Study From 3 Distinct Patient Cohorts

Boland JM, Wampfler JA, Jang JS, et al (Mayo Clinic, Rochester, MN)

Am J Surg Pathol 38:1681-1688, 2014

Comprehensive biological characteristics of pulmonary adenocarcinomas with signet ring cell features (SRC^+) are not well known. Herein, we systematically evaluated clinical and molecular features of SRC^+ cases with particular attention to smoking status. Surgically treated lung adenocarcinomas (n = 763) with follow-up ≥5 years in 3 cohorts were reviewed: all patients in 2006 to 2007 ("all-comers," n = 222; 168 ever-smokers), a never-smoker cohort (n = 266), and a cohort of ever-smokers (n = 275). SRC^+ tumors had ≥10% of SRCs agreed by 2 pathologists. SRC^+ cases were tested for rearrangement of *ALK* and *ROS1*, as well as 187 known mutations in 10 oncogenes including *EGFR, KRAS, BRAF, ERBB2, JAK2, AKT1, AKT2, KIT, MET,* and *PIK3CA*. Overall, 53 of 763 cases (7%) were SRC^+. In the 2006 to 2007 "all comer" cohort, 9% were SRC^+. In the never-smoker cohort, 9% were SRC^+. In the smoker cohort, 3% were SRC^+. Univariable analysis showed that SRC^+ never-smokers had shorter overall and disease-free survival ($P = 0.006$ and 0.0004, respectively), but the significance faded in the multivariable analysis. For the other 2 cohorts, crude 5-year survival was decreased by 6% to 27% in SRC^+ cases without reaching statistical significance. In SRC^+ tumors, *KRAS* mutation was most common (29%), followed by *ALK* (26%), *EGFR* (18%), *ROS1* (6%), *BRAF* (6%), and *PIK3CA* (3%). In summary, SRC^+ tumors in never-smokers had a worse survival by univariable analysis only. SRC^+ cases seemed enriched for ALK^+ and $ROS1^+$, and other mutations were generally in keeping with the patient's smoking status.

► The authors described their single-center experience with pulmonary adenocarcinoma showing signet ring cell features. Most pathologists associate signet ring cell carcinomas with a poor prognosis in aggressive clinical disease with most of their experience coming from signet ring cell carcinoma of the stomach. However, one of the surprising findings in this article is the lack of a worst prognosis for pulmonary adenocarcinoma showing signet ring cell features when analyzed with multivariate analysis including stage. It seems pulmonary adenocarcinoma with signet ring cell features presents at a higher stage and is thus associated with a more aggressive clinical course. One of the interesting aspects of signet ring cell carcinoma is how it might fit within the classification of lung adenocarcinoma in resectioned specimens, where signet ring cell carcinoma does not have a specific category. I suspect most pathologists would put signet ring cell carcinoma in the category of invasive mucinous adenocarcinoma. Further studies are required to analyze the correct area of classification for pulmonary signet ring cell adenocarcinoma.

This study also confirms what is already generally known—that mucinous adenocarcinomas of the lung show *KRAS* and *ALK* mutations more frequently than the other mutations. However, the low percentage (6%) of *ROS1* mutations is surprising. These findings raise the possibility of perhaps altered testing protocols for different pulmonary adenocarcinomas with regard to molecular studies for potential targeted therapies.

For additional reading on the classification of lung adenocarcinoma, I suggest Travis et al.[1]

M. L. Smith, MD

Reference

1. Travis WD, Brambilla E, Noguchi M, et al. International association for the study of lung cancer/American Thoracic Society/European Respiratory Society International Multidisciplinary Classification of Lung Adenocarcinoma. *J Thorac Oncol.* 2011;6:244-285.

Interobserver Variability for the WHO Classification of Pulmonary Carcinoids

Swarts DRA, van Suylen R-J, den Bakker MA, et al (Maastricht Univ Med Ctr, The Netherlands; Jeroen Bosch Hosp, 's-Hertogenbosch, The Netherlands; Maasstad Hosp, Rotterdam, The Netherlands; et al)
Am J Surg Pathol 38:1429-1436, 2014

Pulmonary carcinoids are neuroendocrine tumors histopathologically subclassified into typical (TC; no necrosis, <2 mitoses per 2 mm^2) and atypical (AC; necrosis or 2 to 10 mitoses per 2 mm^2). The reproducibility of lung carcinoid classification, however, has not been extensively studied and may be hampered by the presence of pyknotic apoptosis mimicking mitotic figures. Furthermore, prediction of prognosis based on histopathology varies, especially for ACs. We examined the presence of interobserver variation between 5 experienced pulmonary pathologists who reviewed 123 originally diagnosed pulmonary carcinoid cases. The tumors were subsequently redistributed over 3 groups: unanimously classified cases, consensus cases (4/5 pathologists rendered identical diagnosis), and disagreement cases (divergent diagnosis by ≥2 assessors). κ-values were calculated, and results were correlated with clinical follow-up and molecular data. When focusing on the 114/123 cases unanimously classified as pulmonary carcinoids, the interobserver agreement was only fair ($\kappa = 0.32$). Of these 114 cases, 55% were unanimously classified, 25% reached consensus classification, and for 19% there was no consensus. ACs were significantly more often in the latter category ($P = 0.00038$). The designation of TCs and ACs by ≥3 assessors was not associated with prognosis ($P = 0.11$). However, when disagreement cases were allocated on the basis of Ki-67 proliferative index (<5%; ≥5%) or nuclear orthopedia homeobox immunostaining (+; −), correlation with prognosis improved significantly ($P = 0.00040$ and 0.0024, respectively). In conclusion, there is a considerable interobserver variation in the histopathologic classification of lung carcinoids, in particular concerning ACs. Additional immunomarkers such as Ki-67 or orthopedia homeobox may improve classification and prediction of prognosis.

▶ In the most recent World Health Organization classification of tumors of the lung, pleura, thymus, and heart (edited by Travis et al 2014), it is recommended that low-grade neuroendocrine neoplasms of the lung be classified as either typical or atypical carcinoids. Terms used in the past such as well-differentiated neuroendocrine carcinoma or grade 1 neuroendocrine carcinoma are no longer recommended for clinical use. The distinction between typical and atypical carcinoid tumors is based primarily on the number of mitotic figures and the presence of necrosis. Because these tumors show otherwise similar architectural, gross, and imaging features, the distinction is primarily based on the histopathology. In contrast to neuroendocrine tumors of the gastrointestinal tract, it has yet to be recommended that an image analysis be performed for the accounting of Ki-67 positive cells. Instead, the classification is based primarily on mitotic figures. This article highlights some of the challenges with the interobserver variability in the classification of pulmonary carcinoid tumors. However, the present article does highlight the poor interobserver variability in the classification of pulmonary carcinoids and raises the possibility that perhaps using a Ki-67-based proliferative index may be a more reproducible mechanism for the classification of pulmonary carcinoids. I suspect the majority of neuroendocrine tumors throughout multiple organ systems will begin to move in this direction.

For additional reading regarding the use of Ki-67 in the evaluation of pulmonary carcinoids, I refer the reader to Warth et al.[1]

M. L. Smith, MD

Reference

1. Warth A, Fink L, Fisseler-Eckhoff A, et al. Interobserver agreement of proliferation index (Ki-67) outperforms mitotic count in pulmonary carcinoids. *Virchows Arch.* 2013;462:507-513.

Immunohistochemical study of 36 cases of pulmonary sarcomatoid carcinoma—sensitivity of TTF-1 is superior to napsin

Terra SBSP, Aubry MC, Yi ES, et al (Mayo Clinic, Rochester, MN)

Hum Pathol 45:294-302, 2014

Immunohistochemistry is often used to distinguish pulmonary sarcomatoid carcinoma from morphologic mimics. Napsin-A is a pulmonary adenocarcinoma marker, but literature on expression in sarcomatoid carcinoma is limited. Thirty-six cases of sarcomatoid carcinoma were stained for napsin, TTF-1, Oscar, CAM5.2, AE1/AE3, desmin, SMA, S-100, CK5/6, calretinin, D2-40, and WT1. Patients were 24 men and 12 women (mean, 70 years; range, 46-93). There were 27 pleomorphic carcinomas, 5 spindle cell carcinomas, 3 carcinosarcomas, and 1 giant cell carcinoma. Cases were positive for at least 1 keratin: AE1/3 was positive in all 36 cases; Oscar, in 34 cases (94%); and CAM5.2, in 32 cases (89%, weaker/more focal). Napsin was positive in 14 cases (39%): 8 diffuse, 3 focal, and 3 rare cells. TTF-1 was positive in 22 cases (61%): 15 diffuse, 3 focal, and 4 rare cells. No cases were napsin positive and negative for TTF-1. Variable staining for mesothelial markers was observed, including positivity for calretinin (12 cases, 33%), WT1 (6 cases, 17%), D2-40 (5 cases, 14%), and CK5/6 (9 cases, 25%). Mesenchymal markers were also sometimes positive (usually focal), including S-100 (4 cases, 11%), desmin (4 cases, 11%), and SMA (7 cases, 19%, 1 diffuse). In conclusion, TTF-1 is more sensitive than napsin for detection of sarcomatoid carcinoma, and no cases were positive for napsin but negative for TTF-1. CAM5.2 is less sensitive than AE1/AE3 and Oscar. Use of a thoughtful immunohistochemical panel is important in the evaluation of sarcomatoid carcinoma because mesothelial and mesenchymal markers can be expressed.

▶ Sarcomatoid malignancies of the peripheral lung/pleura/chest wall present great diagnostic challenge for the practicing surgical pathologist. Although sarcomatoid carcinomas of lung origin are most likely from a pure frequency perspective, it is the surgical pathologist's responsibility to exclude sarcomatoid mesothelioma, primary chest wall sarcomas, and metastatic sarcomas to the lung/pleura. Unfortunately, the available immunohistochemical studies, aside from keratin reactivity, lack in sensitivity and specificity, and even keratin reactivity may be seen in nearly 20% of primary chest wall sarcomas. Calretinin staining may be seen in both sarcomatoid carcinomas and sarcomatoid mesotheliomas as well as a minor component of primary chest wall sarcomas. Therefore, it would be helpful to have a more specific immunohistochemical stain for sarcomatoid carcinoma, seeing it as the most common sarcomatoid malignancy of the lungs, pleura, and chest wall. This article by Terra et al suggests that thyroid transcription factor (TTF) may be a useful initial marker when faced with the dilemma of a sarcomatoid malignancy of the peripheral lungs, chest wall, and pleura. TTF-1 is a fairly well-conserved transcriptional factor expressed in primary lung carcinomas and thyroid carcinomas. They found that 61% of sarcomatoid carcinomas of the lung expressed TTF-1. Thus, if a positive result is obtained, it is highly suggestive of a primary sarcomatoid carcinoma. Additional immunohistochemical studies of a large number of sarcomatoid mesotheliomas and primary chest wall sarcomas are required to evaluate the specificity of TTF-1 in this setting. In summary, a first panel of immunohistochemical stains to include AE1/AE3, desmin, S-100, and TTF-1 may be a reasonable initial approach when faced with this diagnostic dilemma.

For additional review of sarcomatoid neoplasms of the lung and pleura, I suggest the review by Travis.[1]

M. L. Smith, MD

Reference

1. Travis WD. Sarcomatoid neoplasms of the lung and pleura. *Arch Pathol Lab Med.* 2010;134:1645-1658.

Pulmonary Large Cell Carcinoma Lacking Squamous Differentiation Is Clinicopathologically Indistinguishable From Solid-Subtype Adenocarcinoma

Hwang DH, Szeto DP, Perry AS, et al (Brigham and Women's Hosp, Boston, MA; Banner MD Anderson Cancer Ctr, Gilbert, AZ; et al)

Arch Pathol Lab Med 138:626-635, 2014

Context.—Pulmonary large cell carcinoma (LCC) includes tumors not readily diagnosed as adenocarcinoma (ADC) or squamous cell carcinoma on morphologic grounds, without regard to immunophenotype, according to the World Health Organization (WHO). This ambiguous designation may cause confusion over selection of mutation testing and directed therapies. Several groups have proposed the use of immunohistochemistry (IHC) to recategorize LCC as ADC or squamous cell carcinoma; however, it remains unclear if strictly defined LCCs are a clinicopathologically distinct lung tumor subset.

Objective.—To compare the pathologic, molecular, and clinical features of 2 morphologically similar tumors: solid-subtype ADC and LCC.

Design.—Tumors were included on the basis of solid growth pattern; tumors with squamous or neuroendocrine differentiation were excluded. Solid ADC ($n = 42$) and LCC ($n = 57$) were diagnosed by using WHO criteria (5 intracellular mucin droplets in ≥ 2 high-power fields for solid ADC) and tested for *KRAS*, *EGFR*, and *ALK* alterations.

Results.—Both solid ADC and LCC groups were dominated by tumors with "undifferentiated"-type morphology and both had a high frequency of thyroid transcription factor 1 expression. *KRAS* was mutated in 38% of solid ADCs versus 43% of LCCs ($P = .62$). One *ALK*-rearranged and 1 *EGFR*-mutated tumor were detected in the solid ADC and LCC groups, respectively. There were no significant differences in clinical features or outcomes; the prevalence of smoking in both groups was greater than 95%.

Conclusions.—Other than a paucity of intracellular mucin, LCC lacking squamous or neuroendocrine differentiation is indistinguishable from solid-subtype ADC. We propose the reclassification of these tumors as mucin-poor solid adenocarcinomas (Tables 2 and 3).

▶ This article highlights and provides evidence for the most recent changes in the World Health Organization (WHO) classification for large cell carcinoma. In

TABLE 2.—Clinical Characteristics of Solid Adenocarcinoma (ADC) and Large Cell Carcinoma (LCC) Cohorts

	Solid ADC (n = 42)	LCC (n = 57)	*P* Value
Age, y, mean (range)	66.0 (36–86)	63.9 (38–86)	.35
Sex, No. (%)			
Male	18 (43)	28 (49)	.54
Female	24 (57)	29 (51)	
Smoking, No. (% of known)			
Ever (former/current)	34 (97)	53 (98)	>.99
Never	1 (3)	1 (2)	
Unknown	7	3	
Pack years, mean (range)	50.3 (5–168)	51.0 (15–100)	.92
Original diagnosis, No. (%)			
Large cell carcinoma	4 (10)	31 (54)	ND
Adenocarcinoma	36 (86)	16 (28)	
NSCLC	2 (5)	9 (16)	
Squamous cell carcinoma	0 (0)	1 (2)	
Stage at presentation, No. (%)			
Stage I	25 (60)	29 (51)	.54
Stage II	11 (26)	15 (26)	
Stage III/IV	6 (14)	13 (23)	
Treatment, No. (% of known)			
Resection alone	30 (71)	32 (62)	.15
Adjuvant chemotherapy	9 (21)	10 (19)	
Adjuvant radiation	0 (0)	6 (12)	
Adjuvant chemoradiation	3 (7)	4 (8)	
Unknown	0	5	

Abbreviations: ND, analysis not done; NSCLC, non–small cell lung cancer.

TABLE 3.—Morphologic and Immunohistochemical Characteristics of Solid Adenocarcinoma (ADC) and Large Cell Carcinoma (LCC)

	Solid ADC (n = 42)	LCC (n = 57)	*P* Value
Morphology, No. (%)			
Growth pattern			
Undifferentiated	41 (98)	52 (91)	.24
With palisading (% of UD)	9 (21)	1 (2)	.002
Basaloid	0 (0)	3 (5)	.26
Combined undifferentiated/basaloid	1 (2)	2 (4)	>.99
Clear cell features			
None	22 (52)	33 (58)	.27
Focal	15 (36)	22 (39)	
Extensive	5 (12)	2 (4)	
Immunohistochemistry, No. (%)			
TTF-1 +/ p63 –	25 (60)	37 (65)	.36
TTF-1 +/ p63 +	4 (10)	10 (18)	
TTF-1 –/ p63 –	11 (26)	9 (16)	
TTF-1 –/ p63 +/ p40 –	2 (5)	1 (2)	

Abbreviations: TTF-1, thyroid transcription factor 1; UD, undifferentiated.

the 2015 WHO classification of tumors of the lung, pleura, thymus, and heart (4th Edition), large cell carcinoma is defined as an undifferentiated non small cell carcinoma that lacks the cytologic, architectural, and immunohistochemical features of small cell carcinoma, adenocarcinoma, or squamous cell carcinoma. The diagnosis can only be made on resection specimens and requires immunohistochemistry for at least thyroid transcription factor 1 and P40. In the past, solid carcinomas lacking 5 or more mucin droplets were placed in the large cell carcinoma category regardless of immunohistochemistry. Using the prior classification system, as was done in this report, the authors found no significant difference with regard to smoking history, stage of presentation, treatment, and outcomes between these 2 subgroups of lung carcinoma (Table 2). In addition, no significant differences in molecular rearrangements were identified, with KRAS being the most common mutation identified in both subgroups. Table 3 highlights the morphologic and immunohistochemical features of the 2 groups of tumors involved in this study. As you can see, using the revised 2015 WHO classification, only 20 of these cases would currently be classified as large cell carcinoma while the remaining 79 would be reclassified as solid subtype adenocarcinoma based on the immunohistochemistry. Further studies are required to fully elucidate the clinical pathologic spectrum of large cell carcinoma as to whether this is truly a distinct entity when compared with solid subtype adenocarcinoma.

For additional review, I refer the reader to Travis et al.[1]

M. L. Smith, MD

Reference

1. Travis WD, Brambilla E, Noguchi M, et al. International association for the study of lung cancer/American thoracic society/European respiratory society international multidisciplinary classification of lung adenocarcinoma. *J Thorac Oncol.* 2011;6:244-285.

ALK **Rearrangement in a Large Series of Consecutive Non–Small Cell Lung Cancers: Comparison Between a New Immunohistochemical Approach and Fluorescence In Situ Hybridization for the Screening of Patients Eligible for Crizotinib Treatment**

Alì G, Proietti A, Pelliccioni S, et al (Azienda Ospedaliera Universitaria Pisana, Pisa, Italy; et al)

Arch Pathol Lab Med 138:1449-1458, 2014

Context.—Echinoderm microtubule associated protein-like 4–anaplastic lymphoma receptor tyrosine kinase (*EML4-ALK*) translocation has been described in a subset of patients with non–small cell lung cancer (NSCLC) and has been shown to have oncogenic activity. Fluorescence in situ hybridization (FISH) is used to detect ALK-positive NSCLC, but it is expensive, time-consuming, and difficult for routine application.

Objective.—To evaluate the potential role of immunohistochemistry (IHC) as a screening tool to identify candidate cases for FISH analysis and for ALK inhibitor therapy in NSCLC.

Design.—We performed FISH and IHC for *ALK* and mutational analysis for epidermal growth factor receptor (EGFR) and *KRAS* in 523 NSCLC specimens. We conducted IHC analysis with the monoclonal antibody D5F3 (Ventana Medical Systems, Tucson, Arizona) and a highly sensitive detection system. We also performed a MassARRAY-based analysis (Sequenom, San Diego, California) in a small subset of 11 samples to detect *EML4-ALK* rearrangement.

Results.—Of the 523 NSCLC specimens, 20 (3.8%) were positive for *ALK* rearrangement by FISH analysis. *EGFR* and *KRAS* mutations were identified in 70 (13.4%) and 124 (23.7%) of the 523 tumor samples, respectively. *ALK* rearrangement and *EGFR* and *KRAS* mutations were mutually exclusive. Of 523 tumor samples analyzed, 18 (3.4%) were ALK^{+} by IHC, 18 samples (3.4%) had concordant IHC and FISH results, and 2 ALK^{+} cases (0.3%) by FISH failed to show ALK protein expression. In the 2 discrepant cases, we did not detect any mass peaks for the *EML4-ALK* variants by MassARRAY.

Conclusions.—Our results show that IHC may be a useful technique for selecting NSCLC cases to undergo *ALK* FISH analysis.

▶ Advanced molecular studies for the tailoring of targeted therapies in lung cancer is one of the hottest topics in general surgical pathology at this time. Recent consensus recommendations have been made with regard to testing for potential targeted therapies.[1] For targeted molecular therapies to be efficacious in the treatment of lung cancer patients, 3 criteria must be met. The molecular target must be integral to tumor growth. The mutations must be testable either with traditional pathology testing procedures or with specialized molecular testing. There must be agents available that target the mutation and thus tumor growth. The previously mentioned recommendations suggest that there is no current evidence for immunohistochemistry for anaplastic lymphoma kinase (*ALK*) rearrangement at this time. However, this article makes a convincing case that screening patients for *ALK* rearrangements may be an effective strategy to incorporate into your oncology protocols. One of the important aspects to remember in molecular testing in lung cancer is that the mutations are generally mutually exclusive. This means that should the patient have a *KRAS*, for epidermal growth factor receptor (EGFR), or *ALK* mutation they will be negative for the other mutations. Therefore, ineffective immunohistochemical tests, as outlined in this article, may be useful in screening for patients with *ALK*-positive mutations. Another one of the challenges associated with molecular testing is the relatively low frequency of molecular abnormalities. *ALK* rearrangement testing was only identified in 3.8% of more than 500 specimens tested in the current material. EGFR is more common, found in 13.4% of cases, whereas *KRAS* was the most common mutation, found in 23.7% of cases. Unfortunately, there is no current effective therapy targeted at *KRAS* mutations; therefore, despite it being the most common mutation, no targeted therapies are available.

One thing to remember, however, when dealing with small biopsy specimens with a limited amount of tumor, is the material necessary for additional specialized molecular testing. Currently, EGFR testing is done via molecular polymerase chain reaction assays and generally requires approximately 300 tumor cells on the slide to have sufficient material. Of course, there are many other additional variables. Because traditionally recommended *ALK* testing is done via fluorescence in situ hybridization analysis, the number of cells required is only 50. These limitations should be kept in mind when evaluating poorly differentiated, non small cell lung cancer specimens with regard to additional immunohistochemical stands differentiating adenocarcinoma from squamous cell carcinoma. The recommendation is that any tumor that does not show squamous differentiation either by histology or by immunohistochemical studies should be tested for potential targeted therapies.

For additional reading on the consensus recommendations on molecular testing in lung cancer, I refer the reader to Lindeman et al.[1]

M. L. Smith, MD

Reference

1. Lindeman NI, Cagle PT, Beasley MB, et al. Molecular testing guideline for selection of lung cancer patients for EGFR and ALK tyrosine kinase inhibitors. Guidelines from the College of American pathologists, international association for the study of lung cancer, and association for molecular pathology. *Arch Pathol Lab Med.* 2013;137:828-860.

Surgical pathology of pleural coccidioidomycosis: a clinicopathological study of 36 cases

Shekhel TA, Ricciotti RW, Blair JE, et al (Univ of Arizona, Tucson; Mayo Clinic, Scottsdale, AZ; et al)

Hum Pathol 45:961-969, 2014

Most pulmonary coccidioidal infections are intraparenchymal; the pleurae are rarely involved. Pleuritis is a recognized complication of ruptured cavitary infections and occasionally occurs in other settings but has not been fully characterized. To define the clinical and histopathologic characteristics of pleural coccidioidomycosis as encountered by surgical pathologists, we reviewed the clinical history, imaging, and histology of 36 biopsy-, resection-, or autopsy-confirmed cases (with coccidioidal spherules present in pleural tissue; median age, 39 years; 22 men). These represented 7% of all pulmonary coccidioidal infections and showed 2 modes of presentation, including ruptured cavitary infection (26) and pleural-predominant disease with milder parenchymal involvement (10). Risk factors included immunodeficiency, smoking, and occupational exposure to soil. Common symptoms (median, 5 weeks) included cough (47%), chest pain (44%), and dyspnea (39%). Imaging often showed pleural adhesions (64%) and effusions (61%). Treatment included lobectomy or decortication, with antifungal medications. All cases showed granulomatous pleuritis. Both modes of presentation showed similar histologic features, including the

TABLE 3.—Histopathologic Features of the Pleura in Pleural Coccidioidomycosis

Feature	n (%, of 36 Cases)	Score (0-3+), Mean ± SD
Inflammatory infiltrates		
Neutrophils	19 (53)	0.8 ± 0.9
Abscess formation	7 (19)	0.2 ± 0.4
Lymphocytes	36 (100)	2.0 ± 0.6
Plasma cells	31 (86)	1.2 ± 0.8
Eosinophils	36 (100)	1.9 ± 0.9
Giant cells	30 (83)	0.8 ± 0.4
Granulomas	36 (100)	1.4 ± 0.8
PF, nonnecrotizing	8 (22)	
PF, necrotizing	14 (39)	
WF, nonnecrotizing	3 (8)	
WF, necrotizing	11 (31)	
Fibrin on pleural surface	31 (86)	1.6 ± 1.0
Pleural fibrosis	34 (94)	2.4 ± 0.9
Necrosis	25 (69)	1.1 ± 1.0
Mean spherule density		
<1 per 10 hpf	32 (89)	
1-10 per 10 hpf	2 (6)	
>10 per 10 hpf	2 (6)	

NOTE. Sums may not equal 100% due to rounding.
Abbreviations: PF, poorly formed; WF, well formed.
Reprinted from Human Pathology. Shekhel TA, Ricciotti RW, Blair JE, et al. Surgical pathology of pleural coccidioidomycosis: a clinicopathological study of 36 cases. *Hum Pathol.* 2014;45:961-969, with permission from Elsevier.

composition of inflammatory infiltrates, degree of fibrosis, and extent of necrosis. Spherules were usually few (mean density, <1/10 high-power field). Three deaths occurred (all with ruptured cavities); the remaining patients recovered. Differential diagnosis of pleural effusions should include coccidioidomycosis, particularly in endemic areas, even without significant intrapulmonary disease. Most cases of coccidioidomycotic pleuritis are encountered by pathologists after resection of ruptured cavities with decortication, but pleural-predominant infections may be biopsied for diagnostic purposes. Spherules are usually rare in pleural tissue, and liberal sampling, cultures, or serologic studies may be required to confirm the diagnosis (Table 3).

▶ Pleural biopsies are often challenging for the general surgical pathologist with respect to excluding the possibility of morbid mesothelioma. When densely fibrotic pleural biopsies are encountered, one should include the possibility of other etiologies for pleural fibrosis, including sarcoidosis and infectious etiologies, particularly in the setting of a chronic pleural effusion in the differential diagnosis. Most pathologists likely will think of sarcoidosis when they encounter granulomas within the pleura because of the typical lymphangitic distribution of pleural sarcoidosis. However, this report reviews in detail the clinical pathologic features of pleural coccidioidomycosis. This entity should be included in the differential diagnosis for any fibrotic or granulomatous pleural biopsies. Table 3 highlights the histopathological features of pleural coccidioidomycosis. It should be noted that 100% of their cases showed lymphocytes, eosinophils, and granulomas, with most granulomas showing central necrosis. However, up to 30% of the cases did not show necrotizing granulomas; therefore, the differential diagnosis with sarcoidosis would be distinctly more challenging. All cases showed spherules on Gomori methenamine silver (GMS) staining; however, most showed rare spherules, less than 1 per 10 high-power field. Therefore, it is reasonable to obtain multiple GMS stains, perhaps on multiple deeper levels, on pleural biopsies showing granulomatous inflammation, particularly if the patient has a history of travel or residence in affected areas, including Arizona and Southern California.

For a nice review of coccidioidomycosis, I refer the reader to Galgiani et al.[1]

M. L. Smith, MD

Reference

1. Galgiani JN, Ampel NM, Blair JE, et al. Coccidioidomycosis. *Clin Infect Dis.* 2005;41:1217-1223.

The Presence of Anti-HLA Donor-Specific Antibodies in Lung Allograft Recipients Does Not Correlate With C4d Immunofluorescence in Transbronchial Biopsy Specimens

Roberts JA, Barrios R, Cagle PT, et al (Houston Methodist Hosp, TX; et al)
Arch Pathol Lab Med 138:1053-1058, 2014

Context.—C4d immunofluorescence (IF) is a surrogate for development of donor-specific antibodies (DSAs) against human leukocyte antigen (HLA) class I and II antigens in kidney and heart biopsy specimens for monitoring of antibody-mediated (humoral) allograft rejection (AMR). Use of C4d IF in monitoring of lung allografts has shown conflicting results.

Objective.—To determine if C4d IF can be used as a reliable marker for AMR and if it correlates with the presence of DSAs and histologic findings on biopsy.

Design.—All transbronchial biopsies in lung allograft recipients, performed at our institution in a 3-year period, were reviewed. A cohort of 92 patients with 110 corresponding biopsies met the inclusion criteria of (1) having a resulted DSA within 2 weeks of biopsy and (2) having C4d immunofluorescence studies performed and confirmed.

Results.—Twenty-nine patients (31.5%) were positive for DSAs and 63 patients (68.5%) did not develop DSAs. Positive C4d capillary IF was seen in 18 of 110 total biopsy specimens (16.4%). Eight of these biopsy samples were from patients positive for DSAs and 10 were from patients negative for DSAs. The correlation coefficient between the presence of DSAs and C4d IF was 0.1628 ($P = .09$).

Conclusions.—A significant proportion of DSA-positive patients had negative C4d IF results and frequently have no histologic changes on biopsy specimens. DSA-negative patients can be positive for C4d and may show the same histologic changes as reported for DSA-positive patients. Diagnosis of AMR in lung may require a collaborative approach combining clinical data, DSA status, and histology.

▶ It is interesting that all solid organ transplants, including kidney, liver, pancreas, heart, and lung, are at risk for the development of antibody-mediated rejection. Antibody-mediated rejection is characterized by microvascular injury secondary to the activation of complement, usually due to the development of an antibody specifically directed at donor human leukocyte antigen class I or class II. Despite this overarching similarity among the organ systems, each organ system seems to go through a similar process of initially defining antibody-mediated rejection from a pathological perspective and then adding various qualifiers such as C4d immunofluorescence/immunohistochemical reactivity and the presence of donor-specific antibodies. It seems that the lung transplant group is reaching a point of requiring a collaborative approach to the diagnosis of antibody-mediated rejection to include donor-specific antibody status, evidence of complement activation on the biopsy, and evidence of pathological change on the biopsy. This is similar to the initial criteria defined for kidney allograft biopsies in the early 2000s. This article highlights some of the challenges associated with the various mechanisms to evaluate for donor-specific antibodies, the presence of complement activation in the microcirculation, and pathological changes on the biopsy. As has been seen in other organs, there is not 100% correlation between these 3 criteria; in fact, the correlation between donor-specific antibody and C4d reactivity by immunofluorescence in this cohort is particularly poor. These data suggest that the identification of true cases of antibody-mediated rejection in lung allografts may be more challenging when compared with other organ systems. Perhaps a scoring system that includes scores from all 3 domains (clinical, serologic, and pathologic) may be required for a more reproducible definition of antibody-mediated rejection within the lung.

For additional review of this topic, I refer the reader to Ionescu et al[1] and Yousem and Zeevi.[2]

M. L. Smith, MD

References

1. Ionescu DN, Girnita AL, Zeevi A, et al. C4d deposition in lung allografts is associated with circulating anti-HLA alloantibody. *Transpl Immunol.* 2005;15:63-68.
2. Yousem SA, Zeevi A. The histopathology of lung allograft dysfunction associated with the development of donor-specific HLA alloantibodies. *Am J Surg Pathol.* 2012;36:987-992.

Lung Tumors Masquerading as Desquamative Interstitial Pneumonia (DIP): Report of 7 Cases and Review of the Literature

Raparia K, Ketterer J, Dalurzo ML, et al (Northwestern Univ, Chicago, IL; Mayo Clinic, Scottsdale, AZ; Italian Hosp of Buenos Aires, Argentina)
Am J Surg Pathol 38:921-924, 2014

Malignant tumors in the lung (both primary and metastatic) rarely may be associated with markedly discohesive tumor cells, resulting in airspace filling reminiscent of "desquamative interstitial pneumonia" (DIP) on histopathology evaluation. A peculiar aspect of this growth pattern is the relatively bland appearance of the tumor cells, in many cases simulating benign alveolar macrophages at scanning magnification. We searched the Charles Carrington Memorial consultation files in the Department of Laboratory Medicine and Pathology at Mayo Clinic Arizona for instances of malignant tumors in lung simulating DIP, from 1992 to 2011. We identified 7 cases involving transbronchial biopsies, needle core samples, or resected lung specimens. Clinical, histopathologic, and immunohistochemical analyses of these 7 patients were performed, including detailed morphometric analysis of the individual tumor cells using calibrated measurement tools on digital images. We compared the results with those of a control group of 4 patients with benign DIP-macrophage reactions in smoking-related lung disease. The study group comprised 5 male and 2 female patients, 48 to 86 years in age (median: 67 y). The radiologic findings included lobar consolidation, localized ground-glass opacities, and 1 or more nodules. None of the patients had typical bilateral infiltrates of DIP. Microscopically, the lung parenchyma was dominated by the presence of prominent tumor cells filling alveolar spaces. Four patients had primary lung carcinoma (adenocarcinoma), whereas 3 had metastases from other

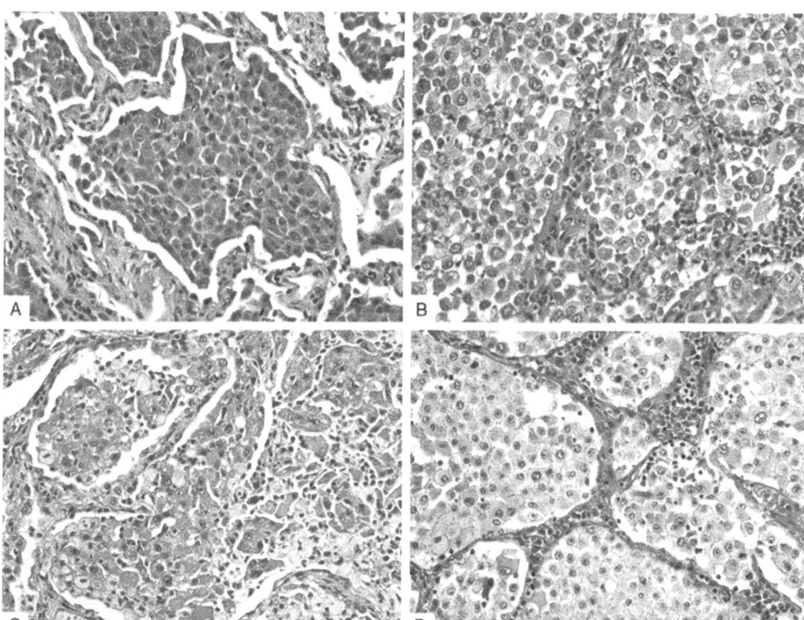

FIGURE 1.—DIP-pattern. A, Pigmented "smokers-type" alveolar macrophages filling alveolar spaces. B, Pulmonary adenocarcinoma. C, Metastatic renal cell carcinoma. D, Metastatic melanoma. Hematoxylin and eosin stains. (Reprinted from Raparia K, Ketterer J, Dalurzo ML, et al. Lung tumors masquerading as desquamative interstitial pneumonia (DIP): report of 7 cases and review of the literature. *Am J Surg Pathol.* 2014;38:921-924.)

sites, including a melanoma. Immunohistochemical staining studies were performed on 6 of 7 cases to establish the diagnosis. Nuclear diameter, cytoplasmic diameter, and nuclear/cytoplasmic (N/C) ratios in patient and control groups were compared using the Wilcoxon rank sum test. No significant difference in the diameters of nucleus and cytoplasm between cases and control groups ($P = 0.3447$ and 0.7055, respectively) was seen, and only a marginally significant difference in N/C ratios ($P = 0.0890$) was seen. A more complex analysis, generalized estimating equation analysis, showed a significant difference in N/C ratio between the 2 groups ($P = 0.0278$). A "DIP-growth pattern" of malignant tumors in the lung is presented. Although the N/C ratio differences approached statistical significance when compared with controls, the key to diagnosis is the recognition of the malignant cytology of the tumor nuclei. Immunohistochemical studies (keratin or other markers) are helpful in establishing an accurate diagnosis in this setting (Fig 1).

▶ The authors present a rare but challenging pitfall in the interpretation of lung biopsy specimens in the form of neoplasms masquerading as desquamative interstitial pneumonia. Fig 1 highlights the morphologic similarities between typical smokers-type macrophages in the setting of desquamative interstitial pneumonia (panel A) and a "pseudo Desquamative Interstitial Pneumonia (DIP) pattern" in different neoplastic settings (panels B, C, and D). A unique feature of this report was the investigation as to the nuclear cytoplasmic ratio and whether that could be a helpful differentiating feature to distinguish true DIP from neoplasms masquerading as DIP. I am surprised by the results that there was no statistical significance. However, this is probably related to the low power of the study (only 7 patients). One question raised by this study is whether the cases of pulmonary adenocarcinoma had other histologic areas within the samples that showed more typical patterns such as acinar, lepidic, or micropapillary. In my experience, it is not uncommon to have micropapillary cells that are fairly discohesive and may fill the alveolar spaces. Another important clue to a neoplasm, compared with DIP, is the lack of the brown tinge to the cells within the alveolar spaces, a characteristic feature in smoking-related interstitial lung disease, including respiratory bronchiolitis and desquamative interstitial pneumonia. On resection specimens for neoplasm, this differential diagnosis is likely fairly straightforward. However, this pattern of neoplastic infiltration could be particularly treacherous on the transbronchial biopsy specimen.

For additional reading on alveolar filling patterns of lung carcinoma, I refer the reader to Yousem.[1]

M. L. Smith, MD

Reference

1. Yousem SA. Peripheral squamous cell carcinoma of the lung: patterns of growth with particular focus on air space filling. *Human Pathology*. 2009;40:861-867.

Approach to Lung Biopsies From Patients With Pneumothorax

Schneider F, Murali R, Veraldi KL, et al (Univ of Pittsburgh Medical Ctr, PA; Human Oncology and Pathogenesis Program Memorial Sloan-Kettering Cancer Ctr, NY; et al)

Arch Pathol Lab Med 138:257-265, 2014

Context.—Patients with pneumothorax occasionally require limited lung resections to control persistent air leaks. In some patients, especially smokers, histopathologic findings suggest that a ruptured bulla or bleb caused the pneumothorax. Other patients only exhibit histopathologic changes related to the physical trauma of acute, and likely occult recurrent, peripheral lung injury in the setting of "spontaneous," or idiopathic, lung rupture. Sometimes, pneumothorax occurs secondary to an underlying localized or diffuse parenchymal lung disease. A comprehensive description of the morphologic findings that may be seen in these specimens will help the surgical pathologist distinguish patients with more common and indolent occurrences of pneumothorax from those requiring additional workup or treatment.

Objective.—To develop a diagnostic approach for surgical pathologists encountering lung specimens obtained in the context of pneumothorax repair.

Data Sources.—Literature review and consultation experience of the authors.

Conclusions.—Two general categories of histopathologic changes can be identified: (1) nonspecific changes, reflecting the lung's acute and chronic response to localized injury, and (2) changes suggesting an underlying lung disease that may have played an etiologic role in the development of pneumothorax. The latter changes are important to recognize because they may require additional workup or treatment of clinically occult lung disease. Difficulty arises when nonspecific histopathologic changes overlap with those of an underlying lung disease. Awareness of these diagnostic challenges and pitfalls, together with clinicoradiographic correlation, is essential in these situations and will help guide the surgical pathologist toward an accurate diagnosis and the appropriate management of clinically occult disease (Fig 2 and Table 2).

▶ The authors provide a comprehensive analysis of the various pathologies seen in the setting of patients with pneumothorax. This is an excellent review that should be readily available for the general surgical pathologist reviewing lung biopsy specimens. Table 2 highlights the variety of changes seen in the setting of pneumothorax, which include changes within the pleura and lung parenchyma. In addition, the authors provide an algorithmic approach to the surgical pathology specimen in patients with a history of pneumothorax (Fig 2). One of the major challenges is that patients with pneumothorax can develop subpleural fibrosis as well as associated fibroblast foci. In limited biopsy specimens, this finding may be interpreted as a fibrosing lung disease with fibroblast foci, including usual interstitial pneumonia pattern. It would be a major pitfall if the patient

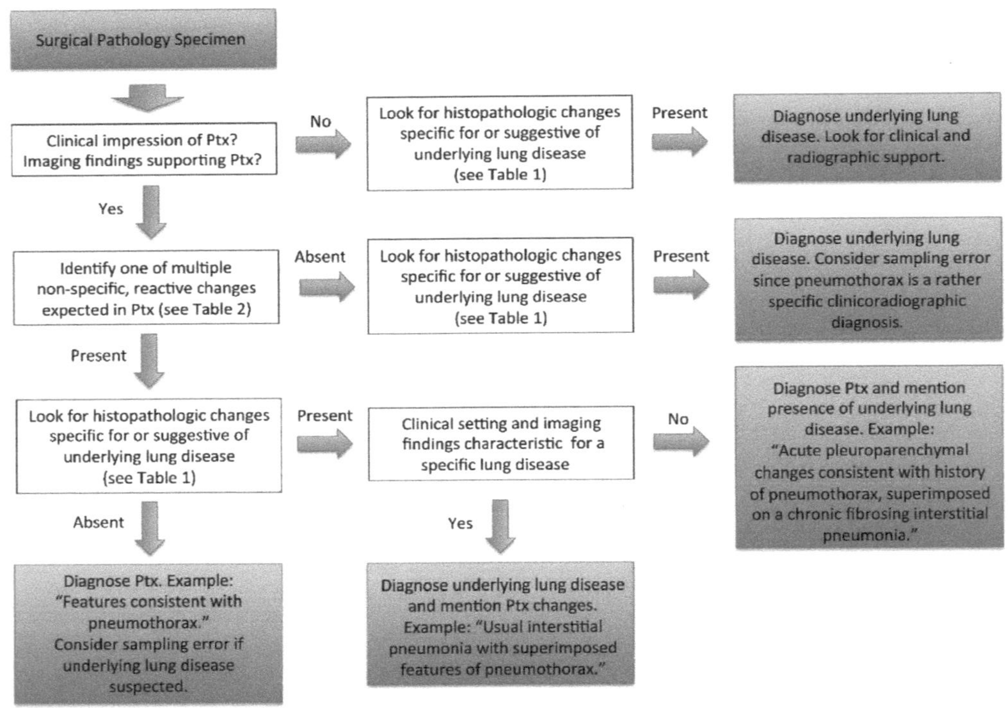

FIGURE 2.—Pathologists interpreting pneumothorax specimens should identify the (nonspecific) features expected in such samples, followed by a search (both in the submitted tissue and by correlation with clinical and radiologic findings) for underlying lung disease or evidence of other potential etiologies of the pneumothorax. Sampling error needs to be considered if clinical or radiographic features do not support the histopathologic changes seen. Abbreviation: Ptx, pneumothorax. (Reproduced with permission of College of American Pathologists from Schneider F, Murali R, Veraldi KL, et al. Approach to lung biopsies from patients with pneumothorax. *Arch Pathol Lab Med.* 2014;138:257-265; permission conveyed through Copyright Clearance Center, Inc.)

TABLE 2.—Nonspecific Histopathologic Features Seen in Surgical Specimens From Patients With Pneumothorax[a]

Changes in pleura
Eosinophilic pleuritis[9,11]
Fibrinous exudate (can be therapy related[90])
Columnar, squamous, or mucous cell metaplasia of pleura[91–93]
Mesothelial hyperplasia[13]
Changes in lung
Subpleural fibrosis
Vasculopathy[8]
Eosinophilic infiltration of vessels[10]
Arteriovenous malformation–like vascular lesion[94]
Fibroblastic foci[25]
Atelectasis
Fluid accumulation
Bronchiolar, alveolar, and mesothelial cell proliferation[13]
Exuberant type II pneumocyte hyperplasia[95]
Changes in pleura and lung
Eosinophilic pneumonia–like changes with eosinophilic pleuritis
Chronic inflammation[13]
Hemosiderin deposition

Editor's Note: Please refer to original journal article for full references.
[a]Specific histopathologic features often associated with disease etiology are described in Table 1.
Reproduced with permission of College of American Pathologists from Schneider F, Murali R, Veraldi KL, et al. Approach to lung biopsies from patients with pneumothorax. *Arch Pathol Lab Med.* 2014;138:257-265; permission conveyed through Copyright Clearance Center, Inc.

simply has a recurrent pneumothorax. Close correlation with the radiographic imaging study is essential to help avoid this common challenge. In some cases, it may be impossible to separate the changes associated with the pneumothorax from a potential underlying interstitial lung disease. In these settings, the multidisciplinary discussion is essential for correct patient classification. For additional review of this article, I refer the reader to Fraire.[1]

M. L. Smith, MD

Reference

1. Fraire A. Histopathology of pneumothorax: potential diagnostic pitfalls. *Arch Pathol Lab Med.* 2007;131:848-849.

Clinicopathologic features associated with relapse in cryptogenic organizing pneumonia

Nishino M, Mathai SK, Schoenfeld D, et al (Massachusetts General Hosp, Boston)
Hum Pathol 45:342-351, 2014

Organizing pneumonia (OP) is a histopathologic pattern of response to lung injury. Fibrin is a marker of acute microvascular injury, and variable amounts of intraalveolar fibrin are seen in OP; however, its relevance to clinical outcomes is unclear. We examined lung wedge biopsies of 26 patients with cryptogenic organizing pneumonia (COP), assessed the amount of fibrin associated with airspace organization, and correlated fibrin levels with other histologic, clinical, and radiographic findings. Seven patients with COP had disease relapse. Patients with multifocal fibrin deposits or acute fibrinous and organizing pneumonia (collectively, "high fibrin") showed a higher rate of OP relapse compared to those with no or focal fibrin (60% versus 6%, $P < .05$). Patients with radiographic evidence of disease involving all three lung zones (upper, middle, and lower) also showed higher rates of relapse compared to those in whom disease was limited to one or two zones (41% versus 0%, $P = .055$). In patients with both pathologic evidence of high fibrin and radiographic evidence of three-zone disease, OP relapse could be predicted with a sensitivity of 86% and specificity of 84% (positive predictive value of 67% and negative predictive value of 94%). The presence of high levels of intraalveolar fibrin in lung biopsies and radiographic evidence of disease involving all three lung zones is associated with increased risk of relapse in patients with COP, and these features may help identify patients who may benefit from more intensive steroid therapy.

▶ The authors review their experience with the so-called cryptogenic organizing pneumonia and investigate the biopsies for histopathologic features that might predict relapse. Of particular importance to the clinical significance of this article is the way in which the cohort with so-called cryptogenic organizing pneumonia was developed. The authors initially searched their database for surgical pathology reports with the terminology "organizing pneumonia." Then cases with other pathological features such as hyaline membranes were excluded. In addition, patients with other clinical or serologic evidence of an alternative diagnosis were excluded, including viral studies and serologic studies for collagen vascular disease. The remaining 26 patients with organizing pneumonia on biopsy were designated as cryptogenic organizing pneumonia. This is important because it is highly likely that not all cases of organizing pneumonia without a definitive etiology from a clinical or pathological perspective actually represent the idiopathic syndrome cryptogenic organizing pneumonia. Cryptogenic organizing pneumonia is typically associated with a good prognosis and prompt steroid response. In our consultative practice when we see an organizing pneumonia that is generally air-space centered but contains abundant fibrin, we do not favor a diagnosis of cryptogenic organized pneumonia. The data from this article would support that distinction in that patients with abundant fibrin tended to be more likely to relapse and behave clinically as a disease process other than cryptogenic organizing pneumonia. One etiologic possibility for the cases of organizing pneumonia with abundant fibrin is aspiration. The authors considered this possibility but did not exclude patients unless a definitive foreign material was identified in the biopsy. It should be noted that repeated aspiration of saliva can result in an organizing pneumonia with fibrin and may not show definitive foreign material. Therefore, some of these cases with organizing pneumonia and abundant fibrin may represent recurrent, perhaps subclinical aspiration-related organizing pneumonia.

For additional review on this topic, I refer the reader to the article by Drakopanagiotakis et al.[1]

M. L. Smith, MD

Reference

1. Drakopanagiotakis F, Paschalaki K, Abu-Hijleh M, et al. Cryptogenic and secondary organizing pneumonia: clinical presentation, radiographic findings, treatment of response and prognosis. *Chest.* 2011;139:893-900.

Prognostic Significance of Adenocarcinoma In Situ, Minimally Invasive Adenocarcinoma, and Nonmucinous Lepidic Predominant Invasive Adenocarcinoma of the Lung in Patients With Stage I Disease

Kadota K, Villena-Vargas J, Yoshizawa A, et al (Memorial Sloan-Kettering Cancer Ctr, NY; Shinshu Univ Hosp, Matsumoto, Japan; et al)

Am J Surg Pathol 38:448-460, 2014

According to the IASLC/ATS/ERS classification, the lepidic predominant pattern consists of 3 subtypes: adenocarcinoma in situ (AIS), minimally invasive adenocarcinoma (MIA), and nonmucinous lepidic predominant invasive adenocarcinoma. We reviewed tumor slides from 1038 patients with stage I lung adenocarcinoma, recording the percentage of each histologic pattern and measuring the invasive tumor size. Tumors were classified according to the IASLC/ATS/ERS classification: 2 were AIS, 34 MIA, and 103 lepidic predominant invasive. Cumulative incidence of recurrence (CIR) was used to estimate the probability of recurrence. Patients with AIS and MIA experienced no recurrences. Patients with lepidic predominant invasive tumors had a lower risk for recurrence (5-y CIR, 8%) than nonlepidic predominant tumors (n = 899; 19%; $P = 0.003$). Patients with >50% lepidic pattern tumors experienced no recurrences (n = 84), those with >10% to 50% lepidic pattern tumors had an intermediate risk for recurrence (n = 344; 5-y CIR, 12%), and those with ≤10% lepidic pattern tumors had the highest risk (n = 610; 22%; $P < 0.001$). CIR was lower for patients with ≤2 cm tumors than for those with >2 to 3 cm tumors (for both total and invasive tumor size), with the difference more pronounced for invasive tumor size (5-y CIR, 13% vs. 21% [total size; $P = 0.022$] and 12% vs. 27% [invasive size; $P < 0.001$]). Most patients with lepidic predominant adenocarcinoma who experienced a recurrence had potential risk factors, including sublobar resection with close margins (≤0.5 cm; n = 2), 20% to 30% micropapillary component (n = 2), and lymphatic or vascular invasion (n = 2). It therefore may be possible to identify lepidic predominant adenocarcinomas that carry a low or high risk for recurrence.

► The latest multidisciplinary classification of lung adenocarcinoma,[1] published in 2011, proposed several new terms for the classification of pulmonary adenocarcinoma, including "adenocarcinoma in situ," "minimally invasive adenocarcinoma," and "nonmucinous lepidic-predominant invasive adenocarcinoma." This classification system recommended the cessation of the use of the term "bronchioalveolar carcinoma" and has generated much confusion on the part of the general surgical pathologist. In particular, the diagnosis of adenocarcinoma in situ and minimally invasive adenocarcinoma seems daunting in the context of both needle core biopsy specimens and resection specimens because it is difficult to precisely delineate the areas of invasion within these tumors. Although this article seeks to show the prognostic differences in these different classification systems, in my opinion, one of the most interesting findings is the relative frequency of these new diagnostic entities. More than 1000 lung adenocarcinomas were evaluated, and only 2 were classified as adenocarcinoma in situ, whereas 34 were classified as minimally invasive adenocarcinoma. At the rate of $<0.2\%$, a diagnosis of adenocarcinoma in situ is exceedingly uncommon and likely should rarely be used by the general surgical pathologist. The distinction between minimally invasive adenocarcinoma and nonmucinous lepidic predominant invasive adenocarcinoma has been arbitrarily set at >5 mm of stromal invasion. Because this is not reproducible, it is also challenging to make a definitely diagnosis of minimally invasive adenocarcinoma. Therefore, in our practice, we routinely use the term "invasive adenocarcinoma, acinar and lepidic predominant." Of the 103 patients with lepidic-predominant invasive adenocarcinoma, only 4 recurrences were noted over the nearly 10 years of follow-up. That is in contrast to no recurrences noted in the adenocarcinoma/minimally invasive adenocarcinoma cohort, which was only 36 total patients.

For additional review of the most recent classification of pulmonary adenocarcinoma, I refer the reader to the following consensus document by Travis et al.[1]

M. L. Smith, MD

Reference

1. Travis WD, Brambilla E, Noguchi M, et al. International association for the study of lung cancer/American thoracic society/European respiratory society international multidisciplinary classification of lung adenocarcinoma. *J Thorac Oncol.* 2011;6:244-285.

Banff 2013 Meeting Report: Inclusion of C4d-Negative Antibody-Mediated Rejection and Antibody-Associated Arterial Lesions

Haas M, as the Banff meeting report writing committee (Cedars-Sinai Med Ctr, Los Angeles, CA; et al)

Am J Transplant 14:272-283, 2014

The 12th Banff Conference on Allograft Pathology was held in Comandatuba, Brazil, from August 19–23, 2013, and was preceded by a 2-day Latin American Symposium on Transplant Immunobiology and Immunopathology. The meeting was highlighted by the presentation of the findings of several working groups formed at the 2009 and 2011 Banff meetings to: (1) establish consensus criteria for diagnosing antibody-mediated rejection (ABMR) in the presence and absence of detectable C4d deposition; (2)

TABLE 1.—Summary of Findings of Banff Working Groups

Working Group	Isolated v	Glom. Lesions	Fibrosis	Implantation Biopsy	Polyoma	C4d– ABMR	BIFQUIT
Leader	Banu Sis	Banu Sis	A. Brad Farris	Helen Liapis	Volker Nickeleit	Mark Haas	Michael Mengel
Issues to address	Do these truly represent acute rejection?	Improve inter-observer agreement in scoring of g, cg	Optimize inter-observer agreement in assessment of IF/TA	Inter-observer variability and clinical correlations in wedge vs. core biopsies; frozen vs. paraffin sections	Develop a clinically relevant morphologic classification for polyoma virus nephropathy (PVN)	Consensus criteria for introduction into Banff ABMR classification	Quality assurance trials for C4d and polyoma stains
Group findings	Isolated v shows comparable response to treatment and graft survival as v lesions with i and t. Thus, most isolated v lesions should be reported as type 2 (or 3) acute TCMR. Although C4d + cases were excluded, 11% and 13%, respectively, of isolated v biopsies were associated with anti-Class I and anti-Class II DSA. Therefore, some isolated v lesions appear to represent acute ABMR or mixed ABMR+TCMR	Revised definition for g (requires endothelial swelling and capillary occlusion). Revised threshold for cg to optimize inter-observer agreement and correlation with C4d, DSA and molecular markers of ABMR, although kappa values for g and cg scoring were fair and moderate, respectively	% Abnormal cortex better than % cortex occupied by fibrous tissue with respect to inter-observer agreement, although kappa value only fair	Frozen section wedge biopsy shows adequate inter-observer agreement, better for glomerular than vascular and tubule-interstitial parameters. Digital images adequate for interpretation	3 Stage scoring for PVN (1, 2, 3) based on % infected (SV40+) tubules and ci score. PVN3 lesions correlated with higher serum creatinine at the time of biopsy and 12 months postbiopsy and were strongly correlated with graft loss	Determined consensus criteria for C4d– ABMR to be incorporated into Banff classification (see Table 2)	Results from the first BIFQUIT C4d trial (Banff Initiative for Quality Assurance in Transplantation) have been published (1) and revealed significant inter-institutional variability for C4d immunohistochemistry

(*Continued*)

TABLE 1. *(continued)*

Working Group	Isolated v	Glom. Lesions	Fibrosis	Implantation Biopsy	Polyoma	C4d– ABMR	BIFQUIT
Future plans	Publish findings—examine isolated v lesions in a cohort including C4d + biopsies	Publish findings—validate new criteria as predictors of graft outcomes	Publish findings—explore possible methods to improve inter-observer agreement	Studies in a larger cohort to examine correlation between biopsy findings and DGF, SCr levels at 6 and 12 months	Publish findings—validation studies in other patient/biopsy cohorts	Correlate new diagnostic categories with clinical outcomes in patients with recurrent versus *de novo* DSA	Follow-up trials with the aim to establish ongoing QA activities for ancillary diagnostic testing in transplantation pathology

ABMR, antibody-mediated rejection; cg, Banff chronic glomerulopathy score; DGF, delayed graft function; DSA, donor-specific antibody; g, Banff glomerulitis score; i, Banff interstitial inflammation score; IF/TA, interstitial fibrosis and tubular atrophy; SCr, serum creatinine; t, Banff tubulitis score; TCMR, T cell–mediated rejection; v, Banff arteritis score.

Reprinted from Haas M, as the Banff meeting report writing committee. Banff 2013 meeting report: inclusion of c4d-negative antibody-mediated rejection and antibody-associated arterial lesions. *Am J Transplant*. 2014;14:272–283, with permission from American Journal of Transplantation and John Wiley and Sons, www.interscience.wiley.com.

TABLE 2.—Revised (Banff 2013) Classification of Antibody-Mediated Rejection (ABMR) in Renal Allografts

Acute/active ABMR; all three features must be present for diagnosis[1,2]

1. Histologic evidence of acute tissue injury, including one or more of the following:
   - Microvascular inflammation (g >0[3] and/or ptc >0)
   - Intimal or transmural arteritis (v >0)[4]
   - Acute thrombotic microangiopathy, in the absence of any other cause
   - Acute tubular injury, in the absence of any other apparent cause
2. Evidence of current/recent antibody interaction with vascular endothelium, including at least one of the following:
   - Linear C4d staining in peritubular capillaries (C4d2 or C4d3 by IF on frozen sections, or C4d >0 by IHC on paraffin sections)
   - At least moderate microvascular inflammation ([g + ptc] ≥2)[5]
   - Increased expression of gene transcripts in the biopsy tissue indicative of endothelial injury, if thoroughly validated[6]
3. Serologic evidence of donor-specific antibodies (DSAs) (HLA or other antigens)

Chronic, active ABMR; all three features must be present for diagnosis[1,7]

1. Morphologic evidence of chronic tissue injury, including one or more of the following:
   - Transplant glomerulopathy (TG) (cg >0)[8], if no evidence of chronic thrombotic microangiopathy
   - Severe peritubular capillary basement membrane multilayering (requires EM)[9]
   - Arterial intimal fibrosis of new onset, excluding other causes[10]
2. Evidence of current/recent antibody interaction with vascular endothelium, including at least one of the following:
   - Linear C4d staining in peritubular capillaries (C4d2 or C4d3 by IF on frozen sections, or C4d >0 by IHC on paraffin sections)
   - At least moderate microvascular inflammation ([g + ptc] ≥2)[5]
   - Increased expression of gene transcripts in the biopsy tissue indicative of endothelial injury, if thoroughly validated[6]
3. Serologic evidence of DSAs (HLA or other antigens)

C4d staining without evidence of rejection; all three features must be present for diagnosis[11]

1. Linear C4d staining in peritubular capillaries (C4d2 or C4d3 by IF on frozen sections, or C4d >0 by IHC on paraffin sections)
2. g = 0, ptc = 0, cg = 0 (by light microscopy and by EM if available), v = 0; no TMA, no peritubular capillary basement membrane multilayering, no acute tubular injury (in the absence of another apparent cause for this)
3. No acute cell-mediated rejection (Banff 97 type 1A or greater) or borderline changes

cg, Banff chronic glomerulopathy score; EM, electron microscopy; ENDAT, endothelial activation and injury transcript; g, Banff glomerulitis score; GBM, glomerular basement membrane; IF, immunofluorescence; IHC, immunohistochemistry; ptc, peritubular capillary; TCMR, T cell–mediated rejection; v, Banff arteritis score.

[1]For all ABMR diagnoses, it should be specified in the report whether the lesion is C4d-positive (C4d2 or C4d3 by IF on frozen sections; C4d >0 by IHC on paraffin sections) or without evident C4d deposition (C4d0 or C4d1 by IF on frozen sections; C4d0 by IHC on paraffin sections).

[2]These lesions may be clinically acute, smoldering or subclinical. Biopsies showing two of the three features, except those with DSA and C4d without histologic abnormalities potentially related to ABMR or TCMR (C4d staining without evidence of rejection; see footnote 11, below) may be designated as "suspicious" for acute/active ABMR.

[3]Recurrent/*de novo* glomerulonephritis should be excluded.

[4]It should be noted that these arterial lesions may be indicative of ABMR, TCMR or mixed ABMR/TCMR. "v" lesions are only scored in arteries having a continuous media with two or more smooth muscle layers.

[5]In the presence of acute TCMR, borderline infiltrates or evidence of infection, ptc ≥2 alone is not sufficient to define moderate microvascular inflammation and g must be ≥1.

[6]At present the only validated molecular marker meeting this criterion is ENDAT expression (4), and this has only been validated in a single center (University of Alberta). The use of ENDAT expression at other centers or other test(s) of gene expression within the biopsy as evidence of ABMR must first undergo independent validation as was done for ENDAT expression by Sis et al (4).

[7]Lesions of chronic, active ABMR can range from primarily active lesions with early TG evident only by EM(cg1a) to those with advanced TG and other chronic changes in addition to active microvascular inflammation. In the absence of evidence of current/recent antibody interaction with the endothelium (those features in the Second Section), the term active should be omitted; in such cases DSA may be present at the time of biopsy or at any previous time posttransplantation.

[8]Includes GBM duplication by EM only (cg1a) or GBM double contours by light microscopy.

[9]≥7 layers in one cortical peritubular capillary and ≥5 in two additional capillaries (17), avoiding portions cut tangentially.

[10]While leukocytes within the fibrotic intima favor chronic rejection, these are seen with chronic TCMR as well as chronic ABMR, and are therefore helpful only if there is no history of TCMR. An elastic stain may be helpful as absence of elastic lamellae is more typical of chronic rejection and multiple elastic lamellae are most typical of arteriosclerosis, although these findings are not definitive.

[11]The clinical significance of these findings may be quite different in grafts exposed to anti-blood-group antibodies (ABO-incompatible allografts), where they do not appear to be injurious to the graft (18,19) and may represent accommodation. However, with anti-HLA antibodies such lesions may progress to chronic ABMR (20) and more outcome data are needed.

develop consensus definitions and thresholds for glomerulitis (g score) and chronic glomerulopathy (cg score), associated with improved inter-observer agreement and correlation with clinical, molecular and serological data; (3) determine whether isolated lesions of intimal arteritis ("isolated v") represent acute rejection similar to intimal arteritis in the presence of tubulointerstitial inflammation; (4) compare different methodologies for evaluating interstitial fibrosis and for performing/evaluating implantation biopsies of renal allografts with regard to reproducibility and prediction of subsequent graft function; and (5) define clinically and prognostically significant morphologic criteria for subclassifying polyoma virus nephropathy. The key outcome of the 2013 conference is defining criteria for diagnosis of C4d-negative ABMR and respective modification of the Banff classification. In addition, three new Banff Working Groups were initiated (Tables 1 and 2).

▶ This report nicely summarizes the 2013 Banff meeting on allograft pathology. Several important updates were given at this meeting, including changes to classification systems used by general surgical pathologists. Table 1 shows a summary of the findings from different Banff working groups. Highlights from this table include the finding that isolated v lesions (endothelialitis and the absence of interstitial information and tubulitis) show similar prognosis and outcomes as v lesions and association with interstitial information and tubulitis and should, therefore, be reported and treated as acute cellular rejection. In addition, the glomerulitis score was revised to require endothelial swelling and capillary occlusion. The chronic glomerular change (CG score) was also updated. Finally, results from the BIFQUIT trial were published and showed fairly dramatic interinstitutional variability for C4d immunohistochemistry. Therefore, a recommendation for a possible ongoing quality assessment program was provided.[1] However, the largest changes arising from the 2013 Banff conference had to do with dramatic alterations to the classification of antibody-mediated rejection to include the possibility of C4d-negative antibody-mediated rejection as well as large vascular lesions within the criteria for antibody-mediated rejection. Table 2 highlights the main changes. For additional review of this topic, I refer the reader to Mengel et al[1] and Haas.[2]

M. L. Smith, MD

References

1. Mengel M, Chan S, Climenhaga J, et al. Banff initiative for quality assurance and transplantation (BIFQUIT): reproducibility of C4d immunohistochemistry in kidney allografts. *Am J Transplant.* 2013;13:1235-1245.
2. Haas M. Pathology of C4d-negative antibody-mediated rejection in renal allografts. *Curr Opin Organ Transplant.* 2013;18:319-326.

p16 FISH Deletion in Surface Epithelial Mesothelial Proliferations Is Predictive of Underlying Invasive Mesothelioma

Hwang H, Tse C, Rodriguez S, et al (PhenoPath Laboratories, Seattle, WA; et al)
Am J Surg Pathol 38:681-688, 2014

An atypical mesothelial proliferation along the pleural or peritoneal surface without evidence of invasive tumor poses a diagnostic challenge. Homozygous deletion of p16 (CDKN2A) by fluorescence in situ hybridization (FISH) has been shown to be a good marker of malignancy in mesothelial proliferations, but correlations of p16 status between atypical surface proliferations and underlying mesothelioma have not been described. We used p16 FISH to investigate 11 pleural and 7 peritoneal mesotheliomas that had both an invasive component and a separate surface mesothelial proliferation. In 5/11 pleural samples and 1/7 peritoneal samples, the invasive mesotheliomas showed homozygous deletion of p16 (all cases in excess of 90% of cells deleted); the surface proliferation in all 6 cases with deletion in the invasive tumor was also p16 deleted. Conversely, the 12 tumors that did not show p16 deletion in the invasive compartment also did not have deletion in the surface component. We conclude that (1) surface mesothelial proliferations near invasive mesotheliomas show the same pattern of p16 by FISH as the underlying tumor and may represent in situ disease or growth of the underlying mesothelioma along the serosal surface; (2) p16 deletion in mesothelial surface proliferations is strongly associated with p16 deletion in underlying mesotheliomas, and biopsies consisting of

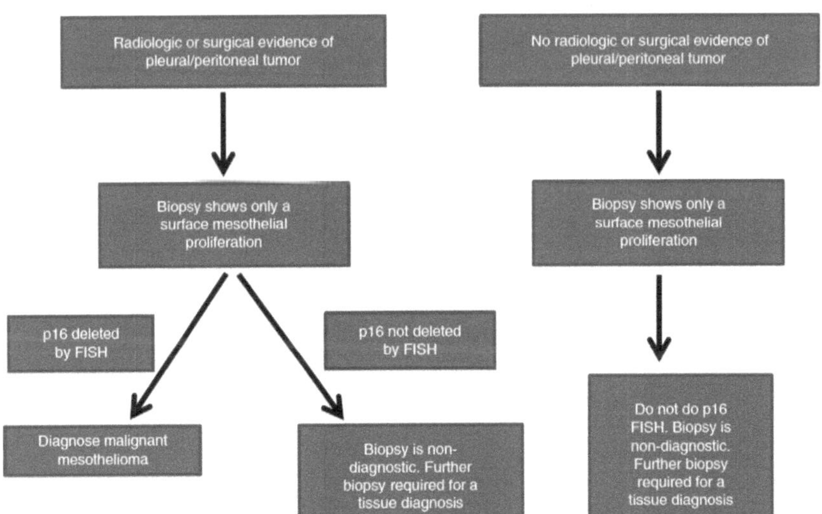

FIGURE 4.—Diagnostic algorithm for using p16 FISH on biopsies with only a surface mesothelial proliferation. (Reprinted from Hwang H, Tse C, Rodriguez S, et al. p16 FISH deletion in surface epithelial mesothelial proliferations is predictive of underlying invasive mesothelioma. *Am J Surg Pathol.* 2014;38:681-688, with permission from Lippincott Williams & Wilkins.)

pure surface mesothelial proliferations that are p16 deleted allow a diagnosis of mesothelioma without an additional biopsy if there is clinical (thoracosopic/laparoscopic) or radiologic evidence of diffuse pleural or peritoneal tumor; (3) however, the absence of p16 deletion in surface proliferations does not rule out underlying invasive mesothelioma (Fig 4).

▶ The distinction between benign mesothelial proliferations and malignant mesothelioma is one of the most challenging diagnostic dilemmas faced by general surgical pathologists. Although many cases are relatively straightforward in that there is clear evidence of cytologic malignancy or clear architectural evidence of malignancy in the form of invasion into underlying soft tissue, approximately one-third of cases remain challenging because of the absence of definitive features of malignant mesothelioma. In these cases, it is not uncommon to use additional special studies to help arrive at a definitive diagnosis. Most of these studies are related to the distinction between malignant mesothelial cells vs malignant epithelial cells in the differential diagnosis of malignant mesothelioma vs poorly differentiated pulmonary adenocarcinoma. There are very few clinically available diagnostic tools to help with the identification of malignancy. The authors present the possibility of using p16 homozygous deletion by fluorescence in situ hybridization (FISH) studies as a way to evaluate for malignant mesothelioma. Fig 4 proposes a diagnostic algorithm for the use of p16 FISH on biopsies showing only a mesothelial surface proliferation. One of the important features to understand in this setting is the radiologic and surgical evidence of a pleural or peritoneal tumor. In the absence of a bulky mass lesion, any mesothelial proliferation, if not cytologically malignant or showing invasion of soft tissue, cannot be diagnosed as malignant mesothelioma. However, the authors propose that in the setting of a bulky pleural lesion and a biopsy result showing a mesothelial proliferation, the presence of p16 deletion by FISH studies is supportive of a diagnosis of mesothelioma. Notably absent from this article is the absence of homozygous p16 deletion and mesothelial proliferations that are not associated with an underlying malignant mesothelioma. In my opinion, this information is essential before the clinical use of p16. It should also be noted that the sensitivity of homozygosity of p16 deletion in cases showing an underlying malignant mesothelioma is relatively low (only 6 of 18 biopsies, 33%). Additional considerations when faced with an atypical mesothelial surface proliferation are the medical-legal aspects. I suspect a diagnosis based purely on homozygosity for p16 deletion by FISH studies would be strongly questioned in the medical-legal realm.

A recent consensus statement from the International Mesothelioma Interest Group nicely reviews the criteria for a diagnosis of malignant mesothelioma and I refer the reader to Husain et al.[1]

M. L. Smith, MD

Reference

1. Husain AN, Colby T, Ordonez N, et al. Guidelines for a pathologic diagnosis of malignant mesothelioma: 2012 update of the consensus statement from the International Mesothelioma Interest Group. *Arch Pathol Lab Med.* 2013;137:647-667.

9 Cardiovascular

Sudden Cardiac Death: A Modern Pathology Approach to Hypertrophic Cardiomyopathy

Kocovski L, Fernandes J (McMaster Univ, Hamilton, Ontario, Canada; Hamilton General Hosp, Ontario, Canada)
Arch Pathol Lab Med 139:413-416, 2015

Hypertrophic cardiomyopathy is one of the most common causes of sudden cardiac death among young adults and adolescents. Unfortunately, the first manifestation of the condition may be sudden death during exertion, such as sporting activities. Other clinical symptoms include exertional dyspnea, angina, and syncope. Postmortem examination often reveals asymmetrical septal thickening and mural plaque formation in the left ventricular outflow tract. Histologic analysis shows cardiac myocyte hypertrophy, myofiber disarray, and interstitial and replacement fibrosis. Molecular analysis for known genetic abnormalities is essential to genetic counseling of living relatives of decedents to assess and reduce the risk of sudden cardiac death from hypertrophic cardiomyopathy.

► Kocovski and Fernandes provide a nice overview of hypertrophic cardiomyopathy as a cause of sudden cardiac death in young adults and adolescents. For a patient who has died from a sudden cardiac death, current recommendations include collection of tissue samples for molecular testing/DNA analysis. The pathologist would obtain whole blood in EDTA tubes; blood spot card, such as fast technology for analysis of nucleic acids card; or frozen sample of heart, liver, or spleen. Paraffin-embedded tissues also may be used but have lower yield and lower accuracy. Genetic testing may assist in the genetic counseling of living relatives. For additional reading, see reference list.[1,2]

S. Raab, MD

References

1. Ackerman MJ, Priori SG, Willems S, et al; Heart Rhythm Society, European Heart Rhythm Association. HRS/EHRA expert consensus statement on the state of genetic testing for the channelopathies and cardiomyopathies [published correction appears in Europace. 2012;14(2):277]. *Europace*. 2011;13:1077-1109.
2. Frustaci A, Russo MA, Chimenti C. Diagnostic contribution of left ventricular endomyocardial biopsy in patients with clinical phenotype of hypertrophic cardiomyopathy. *Hum Pathol*. 2013;44:133-141.

Pathologic diagnosis of antibody-mediated rejection in endomyocardial biopsy after heart transplantation based on renewed International Society for Heart and Lung Transplantation criteria

Szymańska S, Grajkowska W, Pronicki M (The Children Memorial Health Inst, Warsaw, Poland)

Pol J Pathol 65:176-181, 2014

Heart transplantation is a well-established life-saving treatment for patients presenting with end-stage cardiac failure. Despite improved efficacy of the procedure, allograft rejection continues to be a major cause of mortality and morbidity in cardiac allograft patients. Although acute cellular rejection (ACR) is quite unusual nowadays, acute antibody-mediated rejection (AMR) remains a significant problem. The role of pathologists in detection of AMR is very important, especially in sub-clinical cases. In 1990, histologic hallmarks of AMR were first stated by International Society for Heart and Lung Transplantation (ISHLT) and detailed histopathologic features and immunopathologic criteria were established in 2005. Recently (2013) ISHLT revised nomenclature and classification of AMR. Aim of this paper was to present practical changes coming from new criteria as well as to highlight difficulties concerning AMR assessment in endomyocardial biopsies (EMB).

▶ Szymańska et al provide a Polish perspective on the pathologic diagnosis of antibody-mediated rejection (AMR) in endomyocardial biopsies. Table 1 from the original article highlights the 2013 International Society for Heart and Lung Transplantation (ISHLT) Working Formulation for standardization of nomenclature in the pathologic diagnosis of AMR in heart transplantation.[1] The new ISHLT criteria for the pathologic assessment of AMR stated that clinical dysfunction or positive donor-specific antibodies are no longer obligatory for a firm humoral rejection diagnosis.[2]

S. Raab, MD

References

1. Berry GJ, Burke MM, Andersen C, et al. The 2013 International Society for Heart and Lung Transplantation Working Formulation for standarization of nomenclature in the pathologic diagnosis of antibody-mediated rejection in heart transplantation. *J Heart Lung Transplant.* 2013;32:1147-1161.
2. Fedrigo M, Gambino A, Benazzi E, et al. Role of morphologic parameters on endomyocardial biopsy to detect sub-clinical antibody-mediated rejection in heart transplantation. *J Heart Lung Transplant.* 2011;12:1381-1388.

10 Gastrointestinal System

Diagnosis of inflammatory bowel disease: Potential role of molecular biometrics

M'Koma AE (Meharry Med College School of Medicine, Nashville, TN)

World J Gastrointest Surg 6:208-219, 2014

Accurate diagnosis of predominantly colonic inflammatory bowel disease (IBD) is not possible in 30% of patients. For decades, scientists have worked to find a solution to improve diagnostic accuracy for IBD, encompassing Crohn's colitis and ulcerative colitis. Evaluating protein patterns in surgical pathology colectomy specimens of colonic mucosal and submucosal compartments, individually, has potential for diagnostic medicine by identifying integrally independent, phenotype-specific cellular and molecular characteristics. Mass spectrometry (MS) and imaging (I) MS are analytical technologies that directly measure molecular species in clinical specimens, contributing to the in-depth understanding of biological molecules. The biometric-system complexity and functional diversity is well suited to proteomic and diagnostic studies. The direct analysis of cells and tissues by Matrix-Assisted-Laser Desorption/Ionization (MALDI) MS/IMS has relevant medical diagnostic potential. MALDI-MS/IMS detection generates molecular signatures obtained from specific cell types within tissue sections. Herein discussed is a perspective on the use of MALDI-MS/IMS and bioinformatics technologies for detection of molecular-biometric patterns and identification of differentiating proteins. I also discuss a perspective on the global challenge of transferring technologies to clinical laboratories dealing with IBD issues. The significance of serologic-immunometric advances is also discussed.

► The differentiation between ulcerative colitis and Crohn's disease depends on a proper assessment of clinical, radiologic, endoscopic, and surgical pathology findings. M'Koma indicates that approximately 15% of inflammatory bowel disease (IBD) is indistinguishable, even after assessment of all the clinical and pathologic factors. M'Koma reports that in another 15% of colonic IBD cases that undergo pouch surgery based on an ulcerative colitis pathologic diagnosis, the original ulcerative colitis diagnosis will be changed to Crohn's colitis based on the postoperative follow-up. One-half of these patients will require pouch excision or diversion. M'Koma provides an overview of molecular biometrics as a tool to better classify patients with inflammatory bowel disease, which will lead to the clinical laboratory playing an important role in diagnosis. For the practicing pathologist, the use of published criteria for the separation of ulcerative colitis and Crohn's colitis becomes critical as a first step in diagnosis, as we need to recognize the indeterminate and the diagnostically challenging cases. See reference list for further reading.[1-3]

S. Raab, MD

References

1. Griffiths AM. Challenging question: can we diagnose Crohn's disease without histology? *Dig Dis.* 2013;31:202-206.
2. Stange EF, Travis SP, Vermeire S, et al. European evidence-based consensus on the diagnosis and management of ulcerative colitis: definitions and diagnosis. *J Crohns Colitis.* 2008;2:1-23.
3. Van Assche G, Dignass A, Reinisch W, et al. The second European evidence-based consensus on the diagnosis and management of Crohn's disease: special situations. *J Crohns Colitis.* 2010;4:63-101.

Challenges Posed to Pathologists in the Detection of *KRAS* Mutations in Colorectal Cancers

Dudley J, Tseng L-H, Rooper L, et al (Johns Hopkins Univ School of Medicine, Baltimore, MD)
Arch Pathol Lab Med 139:211-218, 2015

Context.—Detection of *KRAS* mutation is mandatory to predict response to anti-epidermal growth factor receptor monoclonal antibodies in patients with metastatic colorectal cancers.

Objective.—To demonstrate challenges posed to pathologists in the clinical detection of *KRAS* mutations in colorectal cancers.

Design.—In this retrospective analysis for quality assessment of the pyrosequencing assay, we survey the characteristics of 463 formalin-fixed, paraffin-embedded neoplastic tissues submitted for *KRAS* mutation detection during a 26-month period.

Results.—The *KRAS* mutation was detected in 39.2% of tumors. This included 2 tumors with complex pyrograms (GGT > GAG at codon 12 and GGC > GTT at codon 13, as resolved by a Pyromaker software program) and 3 tumors with an indeterminate percentage of mutant alleles (defined as 4% to 5% and confirmed by a next-generation sequencing platform). Among the 25 specimens (5.5%) with fewer than 20% tumor cells, 22 were resected after chemotherapy/radiation. Significant depletion of tumor cells was observed in rectal cancers resected after neoadjuvant therapy (31.0%) versus those without previous treatment (0%) ($P = .01$). We also explore other specimens with low tumor cellularity and potential causes of discrepancy between the estimated tumor cell percentage and detected mutant allele frequency, such as intratumor heterogeneity of *KRAS* mutation.

Conclusions.—Neoadjuvant therapy may deplete tumor cells and confound the molecular diagnosis of *KRAS* mutations. Accurate detection of specimens with poor tumor cellularity requires the appropriate selection of neoplastic tissues, evaluation of tumor cellularity, use of assays with high sensitivity, and prospective quality assessment.

▶ Dudley et al describe several factors that affect the quality of samples obtained for testing for *KRAS* mutation in colorectal cancers. In general, pretreatment biopsy tissues are the best choice for *KRAS* mutation assessment. The pathologist plays a critical role in the assessment of tissues and, in general, should determine the areas of manual macrodissection to enrich tumor cellularity, especially in samples that are obtained after neoadjuvant chemotherapy and radiation therapy.

S. Raab, MD

Association between *Helicobacter pylori* and Barrett's Esophagus: A Case–Control Study

Fischbach LA, Graham DY, Kramer JR, et al (Univ of North Texas Health Science Ctr, Fort Worth; Michael E. DeBakey VA Med Ctr, Houston, TX; et al)
Am J Gastroenterol 109:357-368, 2014

Objectives.—The estimated association between *Helicobacter pylori* and Barrett's esophagus (BE) has been heterogenous across previous studies. In this study, we aimed to examine the association between *H. pylori* and BE and to identify factors that may explain or modify this association.

Methods.—We conducted a case–control study in which we used screening colonoscopy controls recruited from primary care clinics as our primary control group in order to minimize selection bias. All participants underwent an esophagogastroduodenoscopy with gastric mapping biopsies. We used logistic regression to obtain odds ratios (ORs) and 95% confidence intervals (CIs) to estimate the association between *H. pylori* and BE while controlling for confounders.

Results.—We identified 218 cases and 439 controls. The overall OR for the association between *H. pylori* and BE after controlling for age and white race was 0.55 (95% CI: 0.35–0.84). We observed an even stronger inverse association (OR: 0.28; 95% CI: 0.15, 0.50) among participants with corpus atrophy or antisecretory drug use ≥1 time per week (factors thought to lower gastric acidity), and no inverse association in patients without these factors (OR: 1.32; 95% CI: 0.66, 2.63).

Conclusions.—The association between *H. pylori* and a decreased risk for BE appears to occur in patients with factors that would likely lower gastric acidity (corpus atrophy or taking antisecretory drugs at least once a week).

▶ Barrett's esophagus (BE) is a precancerous lesion for esophageal adenocarcinoma, although the pathway leading to BE has not been known. Fischbach et al found that the absence of *Helicobacter pylori infection* was associated with BE, and this was especially associated with patients with corpus atrophy or using antisecretory medications. This finding has important ramifications for pathology practices in their evaluation of gastric biopsy specimens for *H. pylori* infection and the presence of corpus atrophy. For further reading, see reference list.[1-3]

S. Raab, MD

References

1. Brown LM, Devesa SS, Chow WH. Incidence of adenocarcinoma of the esophagus among white Americans by sex, stage, and age. *J Natl Cancer Inst*. 2008;100: 1184-1187.
2. Moghissi K, Sharpe DA, Pender D. Adenocarcinoma and Barrett's oesophagus. A clinicopathological study. *Eur J Cardiothorac Surg*. 1993;7:126-131.
3. Raghunath A, Hungin PS, Wooff D, Childs S. Prevalence of *Helicobacter pylori* in patients with gastro-oesphageal reflux disease: systematic review. *BMJ*. 2003;326: 736-739.

Guidelines for Diagnosis and Treatment of Carcinoma of the Esophagus April 2012 edited by the Japan Esophageal Society

Kuwano H, Nishimura Y, Oyama T, et al (Gunma Univ Graduate School of Medicine, Maebashi, Japan; Kinki Univ Faculty of Medicine, Osaka-Sayama, Japan; Saku Central Hosp, Nagano, Japan; et al)

Esophagus 12:1-30, 2015

Background.—Guidelines were established by the Japan Esophageal Society for the diagnosis and treatment of esophageal carcinoma. These present standard practices in diagnosing and treating these cases to improve the safety and results of treatment, reduce costs and resource use, and relieve patient anxiety.

Epidemiology and Diagnosis.—Japan has seen an increased incidence of esophageal carcinoma among men but a leveling off in women. However, mortality has plateaued in men but is falling in women. The disorder is more common in patients in their 60s and 70s, more commonly affects the middle thoracic esophagus, and is most often squamous cell carcinoma. Synchronous or metachronoous multiple carcinoma is often seen.

Various diagnostic imaging procedures are used to determine depth of tumor invasion, whether the lymph nodes are involved, and distant metastasis. Therapeutic strategies are based on the malignancy's grade and the patient's general condition. Options include endoscopic treatment, such as endoscopic resection (ER), photodynamic therapy, and argon plasma coagulation. Other contributing factors are the location and extent of the lesion, depth of invasion, and the institution providing the treatment.

Treatment.—For cervical esophageal carcinoma, resection, larynx-conserving surgery, laryngopharyngoesophagectomy (combined laryngectomy), lymph node dissection, and reconstructive surgery must be considered. For thoracic esophageal carcinoma, resection, endoscopic esophagectomy and reconstruction, and lymph node dissection are options.

In addition, treatment is differentiated by whether the region of the thoracic region involved–upper, middle, or lower. Three routes (the antethoracic, retrosternal, and posterior mediastinal) are available for reconstructive efforts, and grafts may come from the stomach, colic and ileocolic, or jejunal areas. For abdominal esophageal carcinoma, the most common surgical treatment is resection plus lymph node dissection, with reconstruction through intrathoracic or esophagogastric anastomosis.

If the patient's condition or the specific cancer complicates standard surgical approaches, transhiatal esophagectomy or bypass surgery are options. Salvage surgery to address residual or recurrent tumor after definitive chemoradiotherapy poses a greater risk for patients than general surgery. Often the resection is noncurative and carries a poor prognosis, but when the resection is curative, the prognosis improves. Salvage surgery is the only curative treatment for recurrent or residual tumor.

Unresectable advanced carcinomas receive radiotherapy, chemotherapy, or chemoradiotherapy to improve the resection rate and long-term follow-up results by reducing primary lesion size and controlling lymph node metastasis and micrometastasis. However, drug resistance may occur, local control may be delayed so that metastatic spread is unchecked, and radiotherapy may increase the difficulty of surgical approaches and postoperative risk level. The value of adjuvant therapy after surgery for esophageal carcinoma is not yet determined.

Other Concerns.—Barrett's esophagus and Barrett's carcinoma can also occur. Treatment is designed to complement the approach to squamous cell carcinoma at the same level, with endoscopic resection for lesions confined to the lamina propria mucosae.

Esophageal carcinoma is often accompanied by carcinoma of other structures or organs, especially the head and neck, stomach, and lungs. Double carcinoma refers to the presence of two primary carcinomas in different organs. Head and neck carcinomas may occur most frequently with esophageal carcinoma, with gastric carcinoma also often seen. Smoking is a common risk factor for both esophageal carcinoma and gastric carcinoma.

Follow-up observation after treatment of esophageal carcinoma is designed for the early detection and treatment of recurrence or multiple esophageal carcinomas and double carcinomas involving other organs. General management of the patient is enhanced by monitoring and maintaining the patient's quality of life, which is often severely compromised by esophageal cancer. Should recurrent cancer be detected, it may be curable depending on the type of recurrence; aggressive treatment may be desirable to suppress tumor aggravation and improve quality of life. Palliative medical treatment begins when the patient is first diagnosed and is provided during daily clinical practice through a team approach. The goal is to address difficulty swallowing caused by esophageal stenosis, malnutrition, other symptoms related to the primary tumor or to distant metastasis, and hypercalcemia.

In Europe and North America, most esophageal lesions involve the lower esophagus and are adenocarcinomas, dictating a different method of

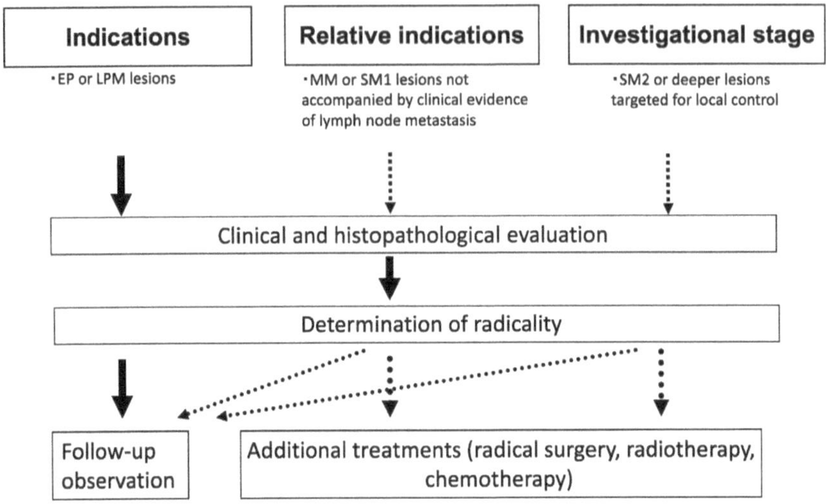

FIGURE 3.—Indications for endoscopic resection. (Reprinted from Kuwano H, Nishimura Y, Oyama T, et al. Guidelines for diagnosis and treatment of carcinoma of the esophagus April 2012 edited by the Japan esophageal society. *Esophagus*. 2015;12:1-30, with permission from The Japan Esophageal Society and Springer Japan.)

treatment and having differing results. Treatment is more often transhiatal esophagectomy, with lymph node dissection limited to the middle and lower mediastinum. Neoadjuvant chemotherapy is restricted to carcinomas of the lower esophagus and esophagogastric junction, with chemoradiotherapy employed for other esophageal carcinomas (Fig 3).

▶ Kuwano et al provide an update on the diagnosis and treatment of esophageal carcinoma from a Japanese perspective. The link between the pathology and the clinical perspectives is interesting, as it highlights the differences in treatment based on the pathology diagnosis and the interplay between multiple medical fields (eg, pathology, surgery, medicine, oncology, and radiology). Fig 1 in the original article shows the algorithm for treatment, which illustrates the treatments for different disease stages. The article contains several pointers for pathologists, such as Fig 3, which depicts gross examination and sectioning protocols, based on adequate and small resection margins.

S. Raab, MD

Utility of ancillary stains for *Helicobacter pylori* in near-normal gastric biopsies

Panarelli NC, Ross DS, Bernheim OE, et al (Weill Cornell Med College, NY)
Hum Pathol 46:397-403, 2015

Documentation of *Helicobacter pylori* infection and eradication is important, prompting some clinicians and pathologists to request ancillary stains on all gastric samples that do not demonstrate *H. pylori* on initial histologic review. Studies evaluating the utility of ancillary stains in patients with minimal inflammation are lacking. We used Giemsa, Warthin-Starry, acridine orange, and immunohistochemical stains to search for organisms in 56 patients with biochemical evidence of *H. pylori* infection (positive Campylobacter-like organism test) and gastric mucosal samples interpreted to be *H. pylori* negative by hematoxylin and eosin (H&E). We correlated the findings with severity of inflammation and patients' histories of medication use. Nineteen (34%) patients had histologically normal mucosae, 22 (39%) had chronic inflammation with or without focal activity, and 15 (27%) had chemical gastropathy. Fifty (89%) cases were negative for *H. pylori* with additional stains, and 6 contained bacteria that were detected with all 4 ancillary stains and on retrospective review of H&E stained sections that also showed chronic inflammation. Eleven (20%) patients were taking proton pump inhibitors, and 4 (7%) had previously received *H. pylori* eradication therapy. We conclude that H&E stains demonstrate *H. pylori* in most infected patients, so preemptive stain requests are largely unnecessary. Failure to identify bacteria by H&E evaluation generally reflects their absence in biopsy material, even among *Campylobacter*-like organism test—positive patients. However, organisms may be overlooked in patients with mild inflammation and in those receiving proton pump inhibitor or antibiotic therapy, so one should consider ordering ancillary stains to enhance detection of bacteria in these settings.

▶ More than 95% of gastric biopsy samples that contain *Helicobacter pylori* also show chronic or chronic active gastritis. Should we order ancillary stains in cases in which we do not see inflammation? The findings of Panarelli et al indicate that we may overlook organisms on a hematoxylin and eosin stain if chronic inflammation is slight or patients have a normal biopsy result and are receiving proton pump inhibitor or antibiotic therapy. Consequently, this may indicate that we may want to first reevaluate for the presence of chronic inflammation and then look at the clinical history. Note that this article focused only on patients with biochemical evidence of *H pylori* infection and not all patterns. For further reading, see reference list.[1,2]

S. Raab, MD

References

1. Smith SB, Snow AN, Perry RL, Qasem SA. *Helicobacter pylori*: to stain or not to stain? *Am J Clin Pathol.* 2012;137:733-738.
2. Batts KP, Ketover S, Kakar S, et al. Appropriate use of special stains for identifying *Helicobacter pylori*: recommendations from the Rodger C haggitt gastrointestinal pathology society. *Am J Surg Pathol.* 2013;37:e12-22.

Traditional serrated adenomas (TSAs) admixed with other serrated (so-called precursor) polyps and conventional adenomas: a frequent occurrence

Chetty R, Hafezi-Bakhtiari S, Serra S, et al (Univ Health Network and Univ of Toronto, Ontario, Canada; et al)

J Clin Pathol 68:270-273, 2015

Background.—Traditional serrated adenoma (TSA) is a very characteristic type of serrated polyp that has a predilection for the left colon. Recent molecular advances have shown two molecular phenotypes of TSA: one associated with BRAF mutations and the other with KRAS mutations. The former is associated with hyperplastic polyps (HPs) and sessile serrated adenomas (SSAs), while the latter is associated with more conventional adenomatous dysplasia.

Aims.—The association of TSAs with so-called precursor lesions (HPs and SSAs) is not well recognised and the purpose of this study was to explore the coexistent presence of HPs, SSAs and adenomatous polyps within a large cohort of TSAs.

Methods.—In total 149 TSAs were examined for the presence of HP, SSA and adenomatous polyps.

Results.—Seen in 83 men and 65 women ranging in age from 32 to 89 years and 127 were left sided with 22 in the right colon. Seventy-eight of the 149 TSAs showed evidence of another polyp (52.34%): 32 were low-grade tubular/tubulovillous adenomas (TAs/TVAs; 41%), 28 were HPs (36%) and 18 were SSAs (23%). Eleven of the 22 right-sided TSAs were associated with a precursor lesion (1 HP and 7 SSA). In addition, five TSAs showed more than one polyp type: TSA with TA/TVA and HP (3); TSA with TA/TVA and SSA (2). The TAs/TVAs were adjacent to the TSA but occurred as a separate discrete polyp, while HPs and SSAs were intermingled with the TSA and present at the base and surface of the lesion.

Conclusions.—More than 50% of TSAs are associated with a precursor lesion or adjacent TA/TVA. Their recognition is important as this may have surveillance and management ramifications.

▶ Chetty et al reported that at least 50% of traditional serrated adenomas (TSAs) are associated with areas of hyperplastic polyp, sessile serrated adenoma, or tubular or tubulovillous adenoma. Documentation of the occurrence of precursor lesions and adenomatous polyps are important for the practicing pathologist, as these findings may impact future management protocols. The clinicians indicate that if adenomatous polyps or conventional adenomatous areas are noted within a TSA, a KRAS mutation is likely to be operative. For further reading, see reference list.[1,2]

S. Raab, MD

References

1. Kim M-J, Lee E-J, Suh J-P, et al. Traditional serrated adenoma of the colorectum: clinicopathologic implications and endoscopic findings of the precursor lesions. *Am J Clin Pathol.* 2013;140:898-911.
2. Kim K-M, Lee EJ, Kim Y-H, Chang DK, Odze RD. KRAS mutations in traditional serrated adenomas from Korea herald an aggressive phenotype. *Am J Surg Pathol.* 2010;34:667-675.

HER2/neu Testing in Gastric Cancer by Immunohistochemistry: Assessment of Interlaboratory Variation

Sheffield BS, Garratt J, Kalloger SE, et al (Univ of British Columbia, Vancouver, Canada; et al)

Arch Pathol Lab Med 138:1495-1502, 2014

Context.—Immunohistochemical (IHC) testing for HER2/neu is becoming the standard of care for guiding adjuvant treatment of gastric carcinoma with trastuzumab.

Objective.—To assess interlaboratory variation in IHC staining and interpretation across multiple laboratories.

Design.—A tissue microarray consisting of 45 cores from 28 gastric cancers was distributed to 37 laboratories for HER2/neu assessment. The IHC results were compared against expert scores at an academic institution and correlated with in situ hybridization results from the originating specimen. Interlaboratory agreement was calculated using Cohen κ statistic.

Results.—The survey demonstrated several variations in IHC methods, including the primary antibodies in use. There was excellent agreement among laboratories in HER2/neu^{+} (IHC 3^{+}) cases ($\kappa = 0.80 \pm 0.01$) and very good agreement among laboratories in HER2/neu^{+} (IHC 0 or 1^{+}) cases ($\kappa = 0.58 \pm 0.01$). Less agreement was observed among laboratories when scoring equivocal (IHC 2^{+}) cases ($\kappa = 0.22 \pm 0.01$). Sensitivity and specificity of HER2/neu IHC were 99% and 100%, respectively, when measured against expert review and consensus score as a reference standard.

Conclusions.—There is substantial interlaboratory agreement in the interpretation of HER2/neu IHC despite variability in protocols. Although HER2/neu IHC is a highly sensitive and specific test, primary antibody selection may significantly affect IHC results. Furthermore, gastric tumors require a unique scoring system and expertise in interpretation. Intratumoral heterogeneity has a significant effect on HER2/neu scoring by IHC. Ongoing quality assurance exercises among laboratories will help ensure optimized HER2/neu testing (Fig 3).

▶ Sheffeld et al provide an excellent overview of inter-laboratory variation in HER2/neu testing in gastric cancer. Fig 3 compares expert review and consensus scoring with in situ hybridization. Analysis of interlaboratory reproducibility showed excellent agreement among positive cases, and very good agreement among negative cases, with less agreement among laboratories scoring

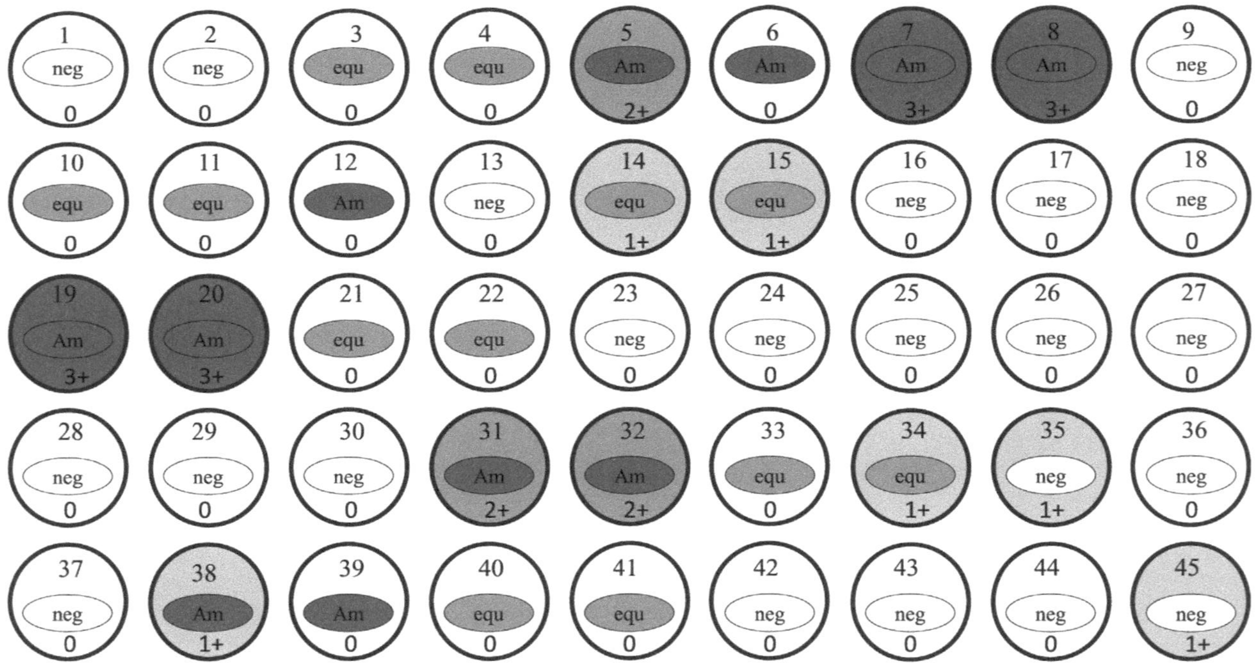

3

FIGURE 3.—HER2/neu status by expert review and in situ hybridization results for cores included in the tissue microarray (TMA). Each circle represents an individual core on the TMA. The top number indicates the core identification number (1–45); the central oval represents the in situ hybridization result for that tumor: amplified (Am) in red, equivocal (equ) in amber, and negative (neg) in white. The bottom number and the color of the entire circle represent the consensus immunohistochemical score at expert review: 0, white; 1^+, gray; 2^+, amber; and 3^+, red. For interpretation of the references to color in this figure legend, the reader is referred to web version of this article. (Reproduced with permission of College of American Pathologists from Sheffield BS, Garratt J, Kalloger SE, et al. HER2/neu testing in gastric cancer by immunohistochemistry: assessment of interlaboratory variation. *Arch Pathol Lab Med*. 2014;138:1495-1502; permission conveyed through Copyright Clearance Center, Inc.)

equivocal cases. Preanalytic variables may contribute to variable results, although the authors indicate that previous studies in breast cancer have shown that cold ischemic time, fixation time, and fixative type have less effect than originally thought on HER2/neu IHC.

S. Raab, MD

11 Hematolymphoid

Utility of bone marrow examination for workup of fever of unknown origin in patients with HIV/AIDS

Quesada AE, Tholpady A, Wanger A, et al (Univ of Texas Health Science Ctr at Houston)

J Clin Pathol 68:241-245, 2015

Aims.—The utility of bone marrow aspiration and biopsy (BMAB) as a diagnostic tool in patients with HIV/AIDS and fever of unknown origin (FUO) is a subject of debate. Because highly active antiretroviral therapy has reduced incidence of opportunistic infections, it is important to reassess the efficacy of BMAB for this diagnostic purpose. To our knowledge, no such studies have been performed in Harris County which has the highest incidence of HIV in the state of Texas.

Methods.—We reviewed all BMABs from patients with HIV/AIDS and FUO or persistent cytopenia(s) from 2007 to 2011.

Results.—Of 57 evaluable patients, BMAB was positive in 24 samples by acid fast bacilli (AFB) or Gomori methenamine silver (GMS) stains (17.5%), presence of granuloma and/or lymphohistiocytic aggregates (31.6%), culture (21.0%) or a combination. Cultures demonstrated *Mycobacterium avium/intracellulare* (4), *M tuberculosis* (2), *M gordonae* (1), *Histoplasma capsulatum* (3) and *Cryptococcus neoformans* (2). There were three cases in which a pathogen was grown in culture but that had a negative of 'direct examination' on tissue sections (negative AFB and GMS special stains, no morphological evidence of granuloma/ lymphohistiocytic infiltrates).

Conclusions.—This study supports the use of diagnostic BMAB as a rapid decision-making tool in patients with HIV and FUO in the proper clinical setting. BMAB demonstrated infection-related evidence prior to positive bone marrow culture in 75% of cases. Special stains and blood cultures had similar diagnostic yield, but BMAB offers faster results. Thus, this procedure assists in clinical decision making and the refinement of treatment in a more timely manner.

► Quesada et al provide data indicating the benefit of bone marrow examination in patients with human immunodeficiency virus/acquired immune deficiency syndrome and fever of unknown origin. Similar detection rates could be seen by other methods, but the authors indicate that the rapidity of detection is superior with bone marrow examination. For further reading, see reference list.[1,2]

S. Raab, MD

References

1. Keiser P, Rademacher S, Smith JW. Utility of bone marrow culture and biopsy in the diagnosis of disseminated infections in AIDS. *Am J Hematol.* 1997;56:1-4.
2. Benito N, Nunez A, de Gorgolas M, et al. Bone marrow biopsy in the diagnosis of fever of unknown origin in patients with the acquired immunodeficiency syndrome. *Arch Intern Med.* 1997;157:1577-1580.

Differentiating Benign From Malignant Bone Marrow B-Cell Lymphoid Aggregates: A Statistical Analysis of Distinguishing Features

Johnston A, Brynes RK, Naemi K, et al (Univ of California Irvine School of Medicine; Univ of Southern California Keck School of Medicine, Los Angeles; Univ of California San Francisco Med Ctr)

Arch Pathol Lab Med 139:233-240, 2015

Context.—Lymphoid aggregates are seen in a minority of bone marrow biopsy specimens, and when present, their neoplastic nature is often apparent by morphologic evaluation. However, the distinction between benign and malignant aggregates can be a diagnostic challenge when there are multiple aggregates with no documented history of lymphoma.

Objective.—To aid in the distinction between benign and malignant B-cell lymphoid aggregates.

Design.—Previously, we described specific distribution patterns for B and T lymphocytes within bone marrow aggregates. To statistically analyze the significance of these patterns as well as previously reported criteria, we examined 128 bone marrow specimens with benign aggregates and 78 specimens with documented malignant B-cell aggregates and calculated specific odds ratios (ORs) and 95% confidence intervals (CIs) to aid in differentiating between benign and malignant B-cell aggregates.

Results.—Aggregates with infiltrative edges (OR, 80.54; 95% CI, 31.76–204.21), a B-cell pattern (OR, 30.08; 95% CI, 13.28–68.10), paratrabecular location (OR, 10.17; 95% CI, 3.96–26.12), size greater than 600 μm (OR, 6.83: 95% CI, 3.61–12.93), or cytologic atypia correlated with malignancy.

Conclusions.—When taken collectively, the presence of more than 2 of these characteristic features was strongly predictive of malignancy.

▶ Johnston et al take an interesting statistical approach in histologic features of lymphoid aggregates in bone marrow specimens to determine if malignancy is present. This process helps standardize diagnostic interpretation. However, a large challenge, assuming a group or a panel of pathologists reaches precision and accuracy, is in teaching these criteria to others. This is important work, and the dissemination of photomicrographs (or whole slide images) of these criteria will be important in learning. For additional reading, please see reference list.[1,2]

S. Raab, MD

References

1. Thiele J, Zirbes TK, Kvasnicka HM, Fischer R. Focal lymphoid aggregates (nodules) in bone marrow biopsies: differentiation between benign hyperplasia and malignant lymphoma—a practical guideline. *J Clin Pathol.* 1999;52:294-300.
2. Nelson B. Bone marrow evaluation for lymphoma. In: Jaffe ES, Vardiman J, Campo E, Arber D, eds. *Hematopathology.* Philadelphia, PA: Elsevier Press; 2010:887-917.

Molecular Genetic Biomarkers in Myeloid Malignancies

Matynia AP, Szankasi P, Shen W, et al (Univ of Utah, Salt Lake City; ARUP Laboratories, Salt Lake City, UT)

Arch Pathol Lab Med 139:594-601, 2015

Context.—Recent studies using massively parallel sequencing technologies, so-called next-generation sequencing, have uncovered numerous recurrent, single-gene variants or mutations across the spectrum of myeloid malignancies.

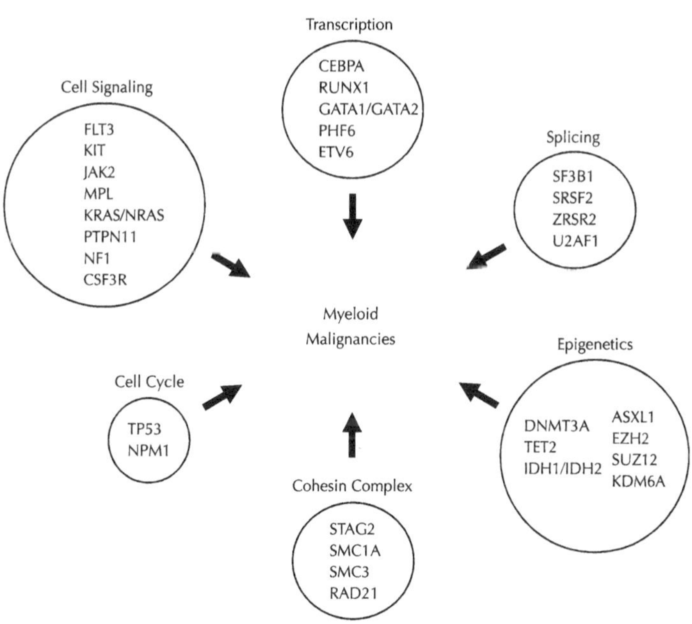

FIGURE 1.—Pathways affected by recurrent mutations in myeloid malignancies. (Reproduced with permission of College of American Pathologists from Matynia AP, Szankasi P, Shen W, et al. Molecular genetic biomarkers in myeloid malignancies. *Arch Pathol Lab Med.* 2015;139:594-601; permission conveyed through Copyright Clearance Center, Inc.)

Objectives.—To review the recent advances in the understanding of the molecular basis of myeloid neoplasms, including their significance for diagnostic and prognostic purposes and the possible implications for the development of novel therapeutic strategies.

Data Sources.—Literature review.

Conclusions.—The recurrent mutations found in myeloid malignancies fall into distinct functional categories. These include (1) cell signaling factors, (2) transcription factors, (3) regulators of the cell cycle, (4) regulators of DNA methylation, (5) regulators of histone modification, (6) RNA-splicing factors, and (7) components of the cohesin complex. As the clinical significance of these mutations and mutation combinations is established, testing for their presence is likely to become a routine part of the diagnostic workup. This review will attempt to establish a framework for understanding these mutations in the context of myeloproliferative neoplasms, myelodysplastic syndromes, and acute myeloid leukemia (Fig 1).

▶ Matynia and coworkers provide a good overview of molecular genetic biomarkers in myeloid malignancies. Fig 1 groups the mutations into cellular pathways. These biomarkers may be useful for diagnostic, prognostic, and therapeutic purposes. This review focuses on relatively recent discoveries and not on well-known chromosomal abnormalities and translocations.

S. Raab, MD

Specialist integrated haematological malignancy diagnostic services: an Activity Based Cost (ABC) analysis of a networked laboratory service model

Dalley C, Basarir H, Wright JG, et al (Sheffield Teaching Hosps NHS Foundation Trust, UK; Univ of Sheffield, UK)

J Clin Pathol 68:292-300, 2015

Aims.—Specialist Integrated Haematological Malignancy Diagnostic Services (SIHMDS) were introduced as a standard of care within the UK National Health Service to reduce diagnostic error and improve clinical outcomes. Two broad models of service delivery have become established: 'co-located' services operating from a single-site and 'networked' services, with geographically separated laboratories linked by common management and information systems. Detailed systematic cost analysis has never been published on any established SIHMDS model.

Methods.—We used Activity Based Costing (ABC) to construct a cost model for our regional 'networked' SIHMDS covering a two-million population based on activity in 2011.

Results.—Overall estimated annual running costs were £1 056 260 per annum (£733 400 excluding consultant costs), with individual running costs for diagnosis, staging, disease monitoring and end of treatment assessment components of £723 138, £55 302, £184 152 and £94 134 per annum, respectively. The cost distribution by department was 28.5% for haematology, 29.5% for histopathology and 42% for genetics laboratories. Costs of the diagnostic pathways varied considerably; pathways for myelodysplastic syndromes and lymphoma were the most expensive and the pathways for essential thrombocythaemia and polycythaemia vera being the least.

Conclusions.—ABC analysis enables estimation of running costs of a SIHMDS model comprised of 'networked' laboratories. Similar cost analyses for other SIHMDS models covering varying populations are warranted to optimise quality and cost-effectiveness in delivery of modern haemato-oncology diagnostic services in the UK as well as internationally.

► Dalley and colleagues provide an overview from a cost-based analysis of operating hematopathology subspecialty services in the United Kingdom. Subspecialty pathology is a growing trend in many countries based on improving accuracy and consistency. The models described by Dalley et al comprise crossover traditional clinical and anatomic pathology services and include not just diagnosis but other components of care, such as end-of-treatment assessments. I find the cost distribution allocation for the genetics branch (at 42%) interesting in that it is the largest cost component (higher than histopathology and hematology). The model of hematopathology care is generally divided in the United States into separate laboratories within single hospital systems. For additional reading, please see reference list.[1-3]

S. Raab, MD

References

1. Guidance for Commissioning Cancer Services. *Improving Outcomes in Haematological Cancers: The Manual.* London, UK: National Institute for Clinical Excellence; 2003.
2. Guidance for Commissioning Cancer Services. *Improving Outcomes in Haematological Cancers: The Research Evidence.* London, UK: National Institute for Clinical Excellence; 2003.
3. Ireland R. Haematological malignancies: the rationale for integrated haematopathology services, key elements of organization and wider contribution to patient care. *Histopathology.* 2011;58:145-154.

Systematic Review of the Effectiveness of Fine-Needle Aspiration and/or Core Needle Biopsy for Subclassifying Lymphoma

Frederiksen JK, Sharma M, Casulo C, et al (Univ of Rochester Med Ctr, NY)
Arch Pathol Lab Med 139:245-251, 2015

Context.—The World Health Organization system for lymphoma classification relies on histologic findings from excisional biopsies. In contradistinction to expert guidelines, practitioners increasingly rely on fine-needle aspiration cytology and core needle biopsies rather than excisional biopsies to diagnose lymphomas.

Objective.—To determine a rate at which fine-needle aspiration cytology and core needle biopsies, combined with flow cytometry and/or genetic techniques, can provide a diagnosis sufficient for optimal medical management of lymphoma.

Data Sources.—The English-language literature on fine-needle aspiration cytology and core needle biopsies for lymphoma was reviewed to identify studies that provided interpretations of all specimens regardless of whether these were deemed diagnostic.

Conclusions.—Forty-two studies (1989-2012) specified the lymphoma subtypes for each diagnosis or indicated a rate at which the methods failed to provide a diagnosis. The median rate at which fine-needle aspiration cytology and core needle biopsies yielded a subtype-specific diagnosis of lymphoma was 74%. Strictly adhering to expert guidelines, which state that follicular lymphoma cannot be graded by these techniques, decreased the diagnostic yield further to 66%. Thus, 25% to 35% of fine-needle aspirates and/or core biopsies of nodes must be followed by an excisional lymph node biopsy to fully classify lymphoma.

▶ Frederickson et al wrote a fascinating study determining the frequency of success (or failure, depending on how one looks at the data) of reaching a subtype-specific diagnosis of lymphoma using fine-needle aspiration (FNA)/core biopsy of lymph nodes. Currently, several organizations favor excisional tissue over FNA/core material for all cases. This study did not examine the accuracy of FNA/core diagnosis but only the reliability of making a definitive diagnosis. Those who favor the excisional approach may argue that the FNA/core method is less accurate. Individuals who favor the excisional approach also will argue that urgency and clinical instability are more important, as a 25% FNA/core failure frequency indicates longer waiting as the FNA/core results will not be actionable. The argument over method will continue, but at least this article puts these data out there for discussion. For additional reading, see reference list.[1-3]

S. Raab, MD

References

1. Hehn ST, Grogan TM, Miller TP. Utility of fine-needle aspiration as a diagnostic technique in lymphoma. *J Clin Oncol.* 2004;22:3046-3052.
2. Gong JZ, Snyder MJ, Lagoo AS, et al. Diagnostic impact of core-needle biopsy on fine-needle aspiration of non-Hodgkin lymphoma. *Diagn Cytopathol.* 2004;31: 23-30.
3. Senjug P, Ostovic KT, Miletic Z, et al. The accuracy of fine needle aspiration cytology and flow cytometry in evaluation of nodal and extranodal sites in patients with suspicion of lymphoma. *Coll Antropol.* 2010;34:131-137.

12 Neuropathology

Evaluation of simultaneous muscle and nerve biopsies for the diagnosis of neuromuscular diseases

Chen DJ, Prayson RA (Cleveland Clinic Dept of Pathology, OH)
Ann Diagn Pathol 18:282-285, 2014

Skeletal muscle and peripheral nerve are occasionally simultaneously biopsied with the goal of increasing diagnostic yield in patients with an uncertain clinical diagnosis or in cases where the pathology is known to be focal or multifocal (eg, vasculitis or amyloidosis). The purpose of the present study is to evaluate the diagnostic utility of performing simultaneous muscle and nerve biopsies. A surgical pathology database was searched from 1993 to 2011 to identify patients who had concomitant skeletal muscle and peripheral nerve biopsies. Demographic and pathologic findings were recorded for all cases. Two hundred eighty-seven patients were included for study. There were 161 (56%) males and 126 (44%) females with a mean age at the time of biopsy of 51 years. The most commonly sampled sites were gastrocnemius muscle (n = 186, 65%) and sural nerve (n = 264, 92%). Most cases (n = 166, 58%) were found to have a definitive diagnosis in either muscle or nerve. Of the cases with definitive diagnoses, 44 (27%) were based off the muscle only, 100 (60%) off the nerve only, and 22 (13%) had a definitive diagnosis in both the muscle and nerve. The most common diagnoses made on muscle biopsy alone were denervation atrophy (n = 34) and inflammatory myopathy (n = 7). The most common diagnosis made on nerve biopsy alone was a moderate or greater degree of axonal loss (n = 82). Vasculitis was found in muscle in 2 cases, in the nerve in 14 cases, and both muscle and nerve in 4 cases. Amyloidosis was exclusive to muscle in no cases, was seen in nerve only in 1 case, and was found in both muscle and nerve in 4 cases. Performing simultaneous muscle and nerve biopsies can improve diagnostic yield (from 8% to 58% in the current study).

▶ This highly informative article shows the diagnostic utility of evaluating both muscle and nerve specimens simultaneously from patients when their disease is known to be focal or multifocal or when their diagnosis is unclear. Performing simultaneous biopsies was found to increase the diagnostic yield, in this report, approximately 7 times, compared with that obtained with a single biopsy. A major challenge with translating this evidence into practice is the communication necessary between neuropathologists and surgeons, such that those surgeons who currently perform a single biopsy will be willing to change their practice with the confidence that they are improving patient care. See reference list for additional reading.[1,2]

D. M. Grzybicki, MD

References

1. Bennett DL, Groves M, Blake J, et al. The use of nerve and muscle biopsy in the diagnosis of vasculitis: a 5 year retrospective study. *J Neurol Neurosurg Psychiatry.* 2008;79:1376-1381.
2. Vital C, Lagueny A, Mercie P, Viallard JF, Delabrousse-Mayoux JP, Vital A. Usefulness of combined nerve and muscle biopsy in the diagnosis of amyloid neuropathy—a study of 6 new cases. *Clin Neuropathol.* 2010;29:59-64.

A Unique Four-Hub Protein Cluster Associates to Glioblastoma Progression

Simeone P, Trerotola M, Urbanella A, et al (Ce.S.I., Foundation Univ "G. d'Annunzio," Chieti, Italy; et al)
PLoS One 9:e103030, 2014

Gliomas are the most frequent brain tumors. Among them, glioblastomas are malignant and largely resistant to available treatments. Histopathology is the gold standard for classification and grading of brain tumors. However, brain tumor heterogeneity is remarkable and histopathology procedures for glioma classification remain unsatisfactory for predicting disease course as well as response to treatment. Proteins that tightly associate with cancer differentiation and progression, can bear important prognostic information. Here, we describe the identification of protein clusters differentially expressed in high-grade versus low-grade gliomas. Tissue samples from 25 high-grade tumors, 10 low-grade tumors and 5 normal brain cortices were analyzed by 2D-PAGE and proteomic profiling by mass spectrometry. This led to identify 48 differentially expressed protein markers between tumors and normal samples. Protein clustering by multivariate analyses (PCA and PLSDA) provided discrimination between pathological samples to an unprecedented extent, and revealed a unique network of deranged proteins. We discovered a novel glioblastoma control module centered on four major network hubs: Huntingtin, HNF4α, c-Myc and 14-3-3ζ. Immunohistochemistry, western blotting and unbiased proteome-wide meta-analysis revealed altered expression of this glioblastoma control module in human glioma samples as compared with normal controls. Moreover, the four-hub network was found to cross-talk with both p53 and EGFR pathways. In summary, the findings of this study indicate the existence of a unifying signaling module controlling glioblastoma pathogenesis and malignant progression, and suggest novel targets for development of diagnostic and therapeutic procedures.

▶ This article will be of interest primarily to neuropathologists who follow or perform molecular research focused on the identification of proteins that may associate with high specificity to malignant gliomas. The quest for a molecular association with malignancy is not new, but investigation in this area continues because the diagnosis and malignant potential of these tumors continues to be dependent on histopathology, which is highly subjective and, therefore, is limited in its prognostic usefulness. Importantly, these authors also describe additional protein interactions with the 4-hub protein cluster they have identified that provide interesting information regarding the pathogenesis of gliomas. See reference list for additional reading.[1,2]

D. M. Grzybicki, MD

References

1. Hanash SM, Bobek MP, Rickman DS, et al. Integrating cancer genomics and proteomics in the post-genome era. *Proteomics.* 2002;2:69-75.
2. Chumbalkar V, Sawaya R, Bogler O. Proteomics: the new frontier also for brain tumor research. *Curr Probl Cancer.* 2008;32:143-154.

13 Soft Tissue and Bone

Gastrointestinal stromal tumors with exon 8 c-*kit* gene mutation might occur at extragastric sites and have metastasis-prone nature

Ito T, Yamamura M, Hirai T, et al (Hyogo College of Medicine, Japan; Kawasaki Med School, Okayama, Japan; et al)

Int J Clin Exp Pathol 7:8024-8031, 2014

Gastrointestinal stromal tumors (GISTs) are the most common mesenchymal tumors of the human gut. Most sporadic GISTs have somatic gain-of-function mutations of the c-*kit* gene. The mutations are frequently found at exon 11, sometimes at exon 9 and rarely at exon 13 or 17. Recently, exon 8 c-*kit* gene mutations were reported in very minor proportion of sporadic GISTs. We also found 3 GISTs with exon 8 c-*kit* gene mutations in approximately 1,000 sporadic GISTs examined. In the present report, we showed the clinicopathological data of those GISTs. One case had a deletion of codon 419 of aspartate, and 2 cases had a substitution of 3 amino acids of codon 417 to codon 419 to tyrosine. The former was the same mutation recently reported in 2 GIST cases, but the latter has not been reported in any GISTs. All three cases occurred at extragastric sites and two of three showed distant metastasis. Since the remaining case was regarded as high risk for recurrence, imatinib adjuvant treatment has been done without evidence of metastasis. Our results confirmed the idea that exon 8 mutations are minor but actually existing abnormalities in sporadic GISTs, and suggested that such GISTs have a feature of extragastric development and a metastasis-prone nature. Since the exon 8 mutations appeared to be really sensitive to imatinib as shown in the present case study, accurate genotyping including exon 8 of the c-*kit* gene is necessary in GISTs to predict response to imatinib in both the unresectable/metastatic and adjuvant settings.

▶ The article by Ito et al highlights the potential importance of genetic testing for gastrointestinal stromal tumors (GISTs) for treatment and prognosis. This type of study helps to identify the boundaries of personalized medicine as anatomic pathology merges into molecular genetics and cybernetics. As pathologists, we are currently challenged on how to apply the latest genetic testing to our field. This concept is poorly defined, as a process method of scientific discovery is not fully integrated into clinical practice. As we know, this field has huge potential and will need pathology leadership to guide the integration. As practicing pathologists, we will need assistance in helping to understand when the science is sufficient to build these tests into the clinical domain. For further reading, see reference list below.[1,2]

S. Raab, MD

References

1. Hirota S, Isozaki K, Moriyama Y, et al. Gain-of-function mutations of c-*kit* in human gastrointestinal stromal tumors. *Science*. 1998;279:577-580.
2. Huss S, Kunstlinger H, Wardelmann E, et al. A subset of gastrointestinal stromal tumors previously regarded as wild-type tumors carries somatic activating mutations in KIT exon 8 (p.D419del). *Mod Pathol*. 2013;26:1004-1012.

Histopathological Diagnostic Discrepancies in Soft Tissue Tumours Referred to a Specialist Centre: Reassessment in the Era of Ancillary Molecular Diagnosis

Thway K, Wang J, Mubako T, et al (The Royal Marsden NHS Foundation Trust, London, UK)

Sarcoma 2014:686902, 2014

Introduction.—Soft tissue tumour pathology is a highly specialised area of surgical pathology, but soft tissue neoplasms can occur at virtually all sites and are therefore encountered by a wide population of surgical pathologists. Potential sarcomas require referral to specialist centres for review by pathologists who see a large number of soft tissue lesions and where appropriate ancillary investigations can be performed. We have previously assessed the types of diagnostic discrepancies between referring and final diagnosis for soft tissue lesions referred to our tertiary centre. We now reaudit this 6 years later, assessing changes in discrepancy patterns, particularly in relation to the now widespread use of ancillary molecular diagnostic techniques which were not prevalent in our original study.

Materials and Methods.—We compared the sarcoma unit's histopathology reports with referring reports on 348 specimens from 286 patients with suspected or proven soft tissue tumours in a one-year period.

Results.—Diagnostic agreement was seen in 250 cases (71.8%), with 57 (16.4%) major and 41 (11.8%) minor discrepancies. There were 23 cases of benign/malignant discrepancies (23.5% of all discrepancies). 50 ancillary molecular tests were performed, 33 for aiding diagnosis and 17 mutational analyses for gastrointestinal stromal tumour to guide therapy. Findings from ancillary techniques contributed to 3 major and 4 minor discrepancies. While the results were broadly similar to those of the previous study, there was an increase in frequency of major discrepancies.

Conclusion.—Six years following our previous study and notably now in an era of widespread ancillary molecular diagnosis, the overall discrepancy rate between referral and tertiary centre diagnosis remains similar, but there is an increase in frequency of major discrepancies likely to alter patient management. A possible reason for the increase in major discrepancies is the increasing lack of exposure to soft tissue cases in nonspecialist centres in a time of subspecialisation. The findings support the national guidelines in which all suspected soft tissue tumour pathology specimens should be referred to a specialist sarcoma unit.

▶ As reported previously with soft tissue tumors,[1] a high discordant frequency between a center of diagnostic expertise in soft tissue tumor diagnosis and community practices is reported by Thway et al.[2] Although it is not discussed in this article, experts also display a degree of imprecision in soft tissue tumor interpretation. Thway et al indicate that one potential cause of the discordant frequency between specialized centers and community practice may be secondary to the use of ancillary molecular diagnostic techniques used in specialized centers.

S. Raab, MD

References

1. Presant CA, Russell WO, Alexander RW, Fu YS. Soft-tissue and bone sarcoma histopathology peer review: the frequency of disagreement in diagnosis and the need for second pathology opinions. The southeastern cancer study group experience. *J Clin Oncol.* 1986;4:1658-1661.
2. Thway K, Fisher C. Histopathological diagnostic discrepancies in soft tissue tumours referred to a specialist centre. *Sarcoma.* 2009;2009:741975.

Clinical and morphological characteristics of osteoid osteoma and osteoblastoma: a retrospective single-center analysis of 204 patients

Yalcinkaya U, Doganavsargil B, Sezak M, et al (Uludag Univ Med School, Bursa, Turkey; Ege Univ Med School, Izmir, Turkey; et al)

Ann Diagn Pathol 18:319-325, 2014

Osteoid osteoma and osteoblastoma are histologically similar, benign bone-forming tumors. In this retrospective study, we aimed to evaluate the natural history; clinical, pathologic, and radiologic findings; and treatment results in 204 patients between 1959 and 2006 in a single institution. According to the World Health Organization's definition, tumors ≤1 cm in diameter were classified as osteoid osteoma, and those ≥2 cm, as osteoblastoma. For tumors between 1 cm and 2 cm, other criteria, such as the bone involved, the site, the presence of a nidus, and presence of peripheral sclerosis, were used for diagnosis. There were 131 patients with osteoid osteoma (93 male, 38 female) and 73 patients with osteoblastoma (40 male, 33 female). The mean age in the osteoid osteoma and osteoblastoma groups was 16.4 ± 7 and 19.6 ± 9.9 years, respectively. The osteoid osteoma cases were mostly localized in the extremities, whereas the osteoblastoma cases involved the vertebral column and sacrum. The nidus size varied between 0.2 and 1.5 cm in osteoid osteoma cases, and the tumor size range was 1.3–10 cm in the osteoblastoma cases. The pain was encountered in 89% of osteoid osteoma and 45% of osteoblastoma patients. Histopathology was similar in both cases. The treatment of choice was conservative surgery for both diagnoses. In conclusion, osteoblastoma is clinically and radiologically more aggressive than osteoid osteoma.

▶ This retrospective case series of 204 patients is useful for surgical pathologists who examine bone and soft tissue simply as a nice descriptive reinforcement of these 2 entities—how they compare and contrast and how their pathologic and radiologic features correlate with their clinical features, particularly their clinical aggressiveness. For further reading, see reference list.[1,2]

S. Raab, MD

References

1. Fletcher CDM, Unni KK, Mertens F. Osteoid osteoma and osteoblastoma. In: World Health Organization Classification of Tumors of Soft Tissue and Bone. 4th ed. Lyon France: IARC; 2013:277-280.
2. Barlow E, Davies AM, Cool WP, Barlow D, Mangham DC. Osteoid osteoma and osteoblastoma: novel histological and immunohistochemical observations as evidence for a single entity. *J Clin Pathol.* 2013;66:768-774.

An Update on the Application of Newly Described Immunohistochemical Markers in Soft Tissue Pathology

Lin G, Doyle LA (Geisinger Med Ctr, Danville, PA; Brigham and Women's Hosp, Boston, MA)
Arch Pathol Lab Med 139:106-121, 2015

Context.—During the last 5 to 10 years, significant progress has been made in the molecular characterization of soft tissue tumors, predominantly with the identification of recurrent translocations or amplification of certain genes in different tumor types. Alongside this, translational efforts have identified many novel and diagnostically useful immunohistochemical markers for many of these tumor types.

Objective.—This article reviews a select group of recently described immunohistochemical markers of particular use in the evaluation of mesenchymal neoplasms; the underlying biology of the protein product, practical utility, and limitations of each marker are discussed in detail.

Data Sources.—Literature review, authors' research data, and personal practice experience serve as sources.

Conclusions.—There are many diagnostically useful immunohistochemical markers to help confirm the diagnosis of many different soft tissue tumor types, some of which have reduced the need for additional, and more costly, studies, such as fluorescence in situ hybridization. However, no one marker is 100% specific for a given tumor, and knowledge of potential pitfalls and overlap in patterns of staining among other tumor types is crucial to ensure the appropriate application of these markers in clinical practice (Table 1).

▶ Lin and Doyle provide an important overview of the use of new immunohistochemical studies for soft tissue pathology. Table 1 provides a summary of

TABLE 1.—Recently Described Immunohistochemical Markers of Soft Tissue Tumors

Antibody	Expression Pattern	Main Use(s)	Comments
ERG	Nuclear	Confirm endothelial differentiation	Also stains a subset of epithelioid sarcomas, subset of Ewing sarcoma, and 45% of prostatic carcinomas (117 of 261 cases[17]; 30 of 66 cases[13])
MYC	Nuclear	Differentiate postradiation angiosarcoma from APRVP	Expressed in a small subset of primary angiosarcomas (usually head and neck)
MDM2/CDK4	Nuclear	Coexpressed in most well-differentiated and dedifferentiated liposarcomas Coexpressed in intimal sarcoma and parosteal and low-grade central osteosarcoma	MDM2 is positive in up to 64% of MPNSTs (21 of 33 cases[46]), 42% of myxofibrosarcomas (10 of 24 cases[46]), and 29% of embryonal rhabdomyosarcomas (12 of 41 cases[46]); MDM2 positivity is also seen in histiocytes
STAT6	Nuclear (+/− cytoplasmic)	Positive in >97% of SFTs (59 of 60 cases[60]; 54 of 54 cases[61]; 34 of 35 cases[62]; 49 of 49 cases[63])	Expressed in 15% of dedifferentiated liposarcomas (3 of 21 cases[60])
MUC4	Cytoplasmic	Expressed in vast majority of low-grade fibromyxoid sarcoma (49 of 49 cases[72]) and sclerosing epithelioid fibrosarcoma (32 of 41 cases[82]; 14 of 15 cases[83])	Focal positivity seen in synovial sarcoma, ossifying fibromyxoid tumors, and epithelioid GIST Expressed in many carcinomas
DOG1	Cytoplasmic + membranous	Positive in >87% of GISTs (136 of 139 cases[89]; 986 of 1040 cases[90]; 370 of 425 cases[91]) Useful to confirm a diagnosis of GIST in gastric KIT-negative tumors	Various other tumor types reported to show focal staining
SDHB/A	Cytoplasmic, granular	Loss of SDHB expression confirms diagnosis of SDH-deficient GIST Loss of SDHA expression indicative of *SDHA* mutations	Loss of SDHB staining also seen in pheochromocytoma/ paraganglioma and rare renal cell carcinomas associated with SDH complex dysfunction
INI1	Nuclear	Loss of expression in 93% of epithelioid sarcomas (127 of 136 cases[131]) and virtually all malignant rhabdoid tumors	Loss of staining also seen in 50% of epithelioid MPNSTs (12 of 24 cases[131]) and 40% of pediatric myoepithelial carcinomas (9 of 22 cases[133])
TLE1	Nuclear	Expression seen in >90% of synovial sarcomas (91 of 94 cases[150]; 249 of 259 cases[155]; 39 of 43 cases[156]; 35 of 35 cases[157]; 18 of 20 cases[158])	Expression often seen in MPNST and SFT (usually, but not always, less diffuse than in synovial sarcoma)
TFE3	Nuclear	Positive in virtually all ASPS	Also positive in Xp11 translocation–type renal cell carcinomas, subset of epithelioid hemangioendotheliomas (with *YAP1-TFE3* fusion gene), and a subset of PEComas
SOX10	Nuclear	Confirm neural crest differentiation—melanocytic tumors, clear cell sarcoma, most benign nerve sheath tumors and 27%–50% of MPNSTs (21 of 78 cases[179]; 38 of 77 cases[182])	Also stains a subset of myoepithelial and salivary gland tumors, and subset of carcinoid tumors and breast carcinomas
NY-ESO-1	Cytoplasmic and nuclear	Expressed in up to 80% of synovial sarcomas (20 of 25 cases[188]; 38 of 50 cases[189]) and 95% of myxoid liposarcomas (36 of 38 cases[192])	Positivity is also seen in melanoma and a variety of carcinomas

Editor's Note: Please refer to original journal article for full references.

Abbreviations: APRVP, atypical postradiation vascular proliferation; ASPS, alveolar soft part sarcoma; GIST, gastrointestinal stromal tumor; MPNST, malignant peripheral nerve sheath tumor; PEComa, perivascular epithelioid cell tumor; SDH, succinate dehydrogenase; SFT, solitary fibrous tumor.

these studies. Although many groups may not develop the in-house use of these studies, practices that see a significant number of soft tissue lesions most likely add some of these studies to their panels. The reference list contains an exhaustive and excellent source of information for specific tumor types and immunohistochemical use in the differential diagnoses.

S. Raab, MD

14 Pediatrics

Effect of interference from hemolysis, icterus and lipemia on routine pediatric clinical chemistry assays

Agarwal S, Vargas G, Nordstrom C, et al (Baylor College of Medicine and Texas Children's Hosp, Houston)

Clin Chim Acta 438:241-245, 2015

Background.—Clinical laboratory assays can be affected by interferents like hemoglobin (Hb), lipids and bilirubin. We evaluated the effect of these interferences on pediatric samples for different chemistry assays. Further we established cut-off indices above which these interferences confound sample results.

Methods.—Three separate serum pools were spiked with increasing concentrations of hemolysate or intralipid or bilirubin and different analytes were analyzed. The Hemolysis-(H), Lipemia-(T) and Icterus-(I) indices were measured on Vitros 5600. Analytes affected by lipemia were treated with LipoClear ® and re-analyzed. All the measured analytes were compromised by gross hemolysis (H-Index >1000).

Results.—Except lipase and magnesium (Mg^{++}), all other analytes were affected by moderate (H-Index >250) and significant hemolysis (H-Index >500). Low estradiol levels showed a significant effect at severe icterus (I-Index >20.0). C3, C4, Ceruloplasmin, Haptoglobin, Immunoglobulins (Ig) and Vitamin D were significantly affected by moderate (T-Index >100) and severe (T-Index >500) lipemia. LipoClear ® treatment significantly attenuated the lipemic interference on the above analytes except for C3, C4, and IgG.

Conclusions.—Accurate reporting of pediatric samples for the analytes affected by common interferences will lead to better clinical interpretation.

▶ Chemistry reference ranges on pediatric blood samples must be generated and validated because pediatric reference ranges for many analytes differ from adult ranges. These authors have focused on determining to what degree the presence of preanalytic factor has on multiple analyte measurements performed on pediatric blood samples because they identify potential interferences by these factors for the analytes measured. However, because this is a single-center study, the highly common occurrences of interlaboratory and interanalyzer variability means that readers will just be able to take away the general, nonspecific information provided here. Individual lab assessment of the preanalytic impact of these factors on their own pediatric samples will need to be performed, if not done already, to generate accurate clinically useful results for the analytes studied.

S. Raab, MD

Incidence and Outcome of Documented Fungal Endocarditis

Badiee P, Amirghofran AA, Ghazi Nour M, et al (Shiraz Univ of Med Sciences, IR Iran)

Int Cardiovasc Res J 8:152-155, 2014

Background.—Fungal endocarditis, the most severe form of infective endocarditis, is characterized by excessive mortality and morbidity.

Objectives.—The present study aimed to analyze the characteristics of fungal endocarditis to improve the management of these patients.

Materials and Methods.—In this cross-sectional study, vegetations on the mitral or tricuspid valves and embolic material surgically removed from the patients with suspected infective endocarditis between December 2009 and November 2011 were examined for fungal infection by direct smear and culture, and the susceptibility patterns of the isolated species were determined. Then, blood samples were cultured on BACTEC media and real-time PCR was done with blood and tissue samples.

Results.—Of the 31 patients with suspected infective endocarditis who did not respond to antibacterial therapy, 11 had confirmed fungal endocarditis. The most frequent predisposing risk factors were previous surgery and drug abuse. The organisms isolated were *Aspergillus spp.* and *Candida albicans*. Resistance to amphotericin B and itraconazole was observed in *Aspergillus* species, and to fluconazole in *Candida albicans*. Positive PCR results were obtained in blood and tissue samples.

Conclusions.—Fungal endocarditis should be considered in the patients not responsive to antimicrobials. Moreover, management of these patients can be improved with molecular diagnostic methods and by determining the susceptibility patterns of the etiologic agents.

▶ This article provides interesting contributory information related to the diagnosis and clinical management of patients with fungal endocarditis. The most common fungal organisms involved in their patient sample (*Candida* and *Aspergillus*) are not new information. However, they show the high utility of polymerase chain reaction for identification of the 2 organisms not only in tissue but also in blood from blood cultures that are commonly negative in patients with fungal endocarditis. In addition, they show a lack of timeliness for the administration of antifungals once patient nonresponsiveness to antibiotics occurs, thus emphasizing the need to culture and treat for fungal pathogens quickly when patients with endocarditis fail to respond to antibacterial therapy.

S. Raab, MD

Quantification of Sickle Cells in the Peripheral Smear as a Marker of Disease Severity

Alvarez O, Montague NS, Marin M, et al (Univ of Miami, FL; Jackson Memorial Hosp, Miami, FL)

Fetal Pediatr Pathol 34:149-154, 2015

Blinded readers examined peripheral smears of 108 children with steady sickle cell (SC) disease and controls by counting ten 100× microscope fields and calculating percent of irreversible and reversible SC from total red cell population SC index (SCI). SCI was correlated to disease severity, and transfusion, hydroxyurea, or neither. Controls had a mean of 0.28% SC (range 0–0.64). Children with hemoglobin SS had a mean SCI of 5.12% ± 5.37 (range 0–30). SCI increased 0.33% with each increasing year ($p < 0.0001$). Patients with SCI >0.64 were 3.32 times as likely to experience clinical complications ($p = 0.0124$). Although blood transfusions and hydroxyurea decreased percent of SC, 72% treated patients had SCI >0.64, correlating with persistent sickling. This standardized method quantifies SC in peripheral smears. Percent of SC increased with age and correlated with disease severity, especially hemolytic complications, providing readily available information with minimal or no extra cost.

▶ The title of this article suggests the potential clinical usefulness of quantitative examination of the peripheral smear as a correlate of sickle cell disease severity. However, the specificity of sickle cell counts on peripheral smears, as described by the authors, does not support its use for assessment of disease severity.

S. Raab, MD

15 Techniques/Molecular

Selective Pathology Fellowships: Diverse, Innovative, and Valuable Subspecialty Training

Iezzoni JC, Ewton A, Chévez-Barrios P, et al (Univ of Virginia Health System, Charlottesville; The Methodist Hosp, Houston, TX; et al)

Arch Pathol Lab Med 138:518-525, 2014

Context.—Although selective pathology fellowships have a long-standing history of developing trainees with advanced expertise in specific areas of pathology other than those of the American Board of Pathology-certified subspecialties, the widespread interest in this training continues to grow.

Objective.—To describe the historical background and current status of selective pathology fellowships, and to provide examples of 3 programs. In addition, Accreditation Council for Graduate Medical Education (ACGME)-accredited programs and nonaccredited programs in Selective Pathology are compared.

Data Sources.—ACGME data banks and publicly available online materials were used. Program directors of the fellowships examples in this paper provided program-specific information. Additionally, an online survey of the program directors and program coordinators of ACGME-accredited programs and nonaccredited programs in selective pathology was performed.

Conclusions.—There are currently 76 ACGME-accredited selective pathology programs. The programs are distributed between 3 major categories: surgical pathology, focused anatomic pathology, and focused clinical pathology. Although the vast majority of programs are concerned that their funding source may be cut in the next 3 years, most programs will not change the number of fellowship positions in their programs. Program requirements devoted specifically and solely to selective pathology have been developed and are in effect. The value of this training is recognized not only by pathologists, but by clinicians as well, in both academia and private practice. Importantly, the diversity and innovation inherent in selective pathology allow these programs to adeptly address new subspecialty areas and technologic advances in the current and evolving practice of pathology.

▶ This interesting article focuses on selective pathology fellowships and provides survey information about current training fellowships, emphasizing that there are multiple highly selective and focused fellowships available that pathologists and pathology trainees find highly valuable.

S. Raab, MD

Diagnosis of major cancer resection specimens with virtual slides: impact of a novel digital pathology workstation

Randell R, Ruddle RA, Thomas RG, et al (Univ of Leeds, UK; et al)
Hum Pathol 45:2101-2106, 2014

Digital pathology promises a number of benefits in efficiency in surgical pathology, yet the longer time required to review a virtual slide than a glass slide currently represents a significant barrier to the routine use of digital pathology. We aimed to create a novel workstation that enables pathologists to view a case as quickly as on the conventional microscope. The Leeds Virtual Microscope (LVM) was evaluated using a mixed factorial experimental design. Twelve consultant pathologists took part, each viewing one long cancer case (12-25 slides) on the LVM and one on a conventional microscope. Total time taken and diagnostic confidence were similar for the microscope and LVM, as was the mean slide viewing time. On the LVM, participants spent a significantly greater proportion of the total task time viewing slides and revisited slides more often. The unique design of the LVM, enabling real-time rendering of virtual slides while providing users with a quick and intuitive way to navigate within and between slides, makes use of digital pathology in routine practice a realistic possibility. With further practice with the system, diagnostic efficiency on the LVM is likely to increase yet more.

▶ One of the major issues that is a barrier to the adoption of digital imaging technology is the length of time to look at a digital image. Many pathologists believe they spend more time looking at a digital image compared with a glass slide. Randell et al provides data that efficiency may be improved in pathologist workflow with a different type of workstation.

S. Raab, MD

Interinstitutional Whole Slide Imaging Teleconsultation Service Development: Assessment Using Internal Training and Clinical Consultation Cases

Jones NC, Nazarian RM, Duncan LM, et al (Massachusetts General Hosp and Harvard Med School, Boston; et al)
Arch Pathol Lab Med 139:627-635, 2015

Context.—Assessment of accuracy and feasibility of whole slide imaging (WSI) for interinstitutional consultation in surgical pathology.

Objectives.—To train technical and pathologist staff in WSI technology, establish and evaluate a WSI workflow using training cases and second-opinion consultations, and assess diagnostic accuracy.

Design.—First, WSI training and evaluation using selected subspecialty service cases were performed and compared with the clinical glass slide (GS) diagnosis. Second, WSI and GS diagnoses of consecutive, second-opinion consultation cases were compared. Discrepancies underwent adjudication to determine a reference diagnosis. Participant observations on WSI initiation to practice were gathered.

Results.—There were 130 cases evaluated, with 123 correlations (94.6%) and 6 minor (4.6%) and 1 major (0.8%) discrepancies. The 74 consultation cases interpreted had 52 correlations (70.3%), and 18 minor (24.3%) and 4 major (5.4%) discrepancies. The WSI and GS adjusted major discrepancy rates in second-opinion consultations were 2.7% (2 of 74) and 4.1% (3 of 74), respectively. Statistical analysis showed that WSI was not inferior to GS interpretation. Pathologists agreed the software was easy to use and the images were adequate, but more time was spent rendering WSI interpretations.

Conclusions.—A significant learning curve was observed in the transition from the training set to clinical consultation cases associated both with WSI interpretation and adjustments to the digital analogs of routine GS workflow. Results from second-opinion consultations indicated that WSI interpretation was as accurate as GS interpretation among properly trained and experienced users. Overall, WSI-based practice appears feasible for second-opinion consultations.

▶ After a properly performed validation procedure, the interpretation of digital images, including whole-slide images, has been found to be as accurate as the interpretation of glass slide tissue sections. The article by Jones et al further explores several components of implementation beyond the establishment of whole-slide image validation. One use of whole-slide images in the United States is for secondary consultation services, especially in settings of subspecialty surgical pathology. The authors describe how the introduction of this technology affected workflow (predominantly an efficiency issue) and several issues of quality, which arose when interpreting whole-slide images. Lessons learned from this article include setting the intent for which whole-slide imaging will be used and designing an implementation plan based on the changes that will be made in laboratory process as a laboratory switches from glass to whole-slide images. For further reading, see reference list.[1,2]

S. Raab, MD

References

1. Wilbur DC, Madi K, Colvin RB, et al. Whole-slide imaging digital pathology as a platform for teleconsultation: a pilot study using paired subspecialist correlations. *Arch Pathol Lab Med.* 2009;133:1949-1953.

2. Graham AR, Bhattacharyya AK, Scott KM, et al. Virtual slide telepathology for an academic teaching hospital surgical pathology quality assurance program. *Hum Pathol.* 2009;40:1129-1136.

The College of American Pathologists Guidelines for Whole Slide Imaging Validation Are Feasible for Pediatric Pathology: A Pediatric Pathology Practice Experience

Arnold MA, Chenever E, Baker PB, et al (Nationwide Children's Hosp, Columbus, OH)

Pediatr Dev Pathol 18:109-116, 2015

Whole slide imaging (WSI) is rapidly transforming educational and diagnostic pathology services. Recently, the College of American Pathologists Pathology and Laboratory Quality Center (CAP-PLQC) published recommended guidelines for validating diagnostic WSI. We prospectively evaluated the guidelines to determine their utility in validating pediatric surgical pathology and cytopathology specimens. Our validation included varied pediatric specimen types, including complex or less common diagnoses, in accordance with the guidelines. We completed WSI review of 60 surgical pathology cases and attempted WSI review of 21 cytopathology cases. For surgical pathology cases, WSI diagnoses were highly concordant with glass slide diagnoses; a discordant diagnosis was observed in 1 of 60 cases (98.3% concordance). We found that nucleated red blood cells and eosinophilic granular bodies represented specific challenges to WSI review of pediatric specimens. Cytology specimens were more frequently discordant or failed for technical reasons, with overall concordance of 66.7%. Review of pediatric cytopathology specimens will likely require image capture in multiple focal planes. This study is the first to specifically evaluate WSI review for pediatric specimens and demonstrates that specimens representing the spectrum of pediatric surgical pathology practice can be reviewed using WSI. Our application of the proposed CAP-PLQC guidelines to pediatric surgical pathology specimens is, to our knowledge, the first prospective implementation of the CAP-PLQC guidelines.

▶ This article is an important reading for practices that are using or considering using digital pathology to examine pediatric specimens. The authors describe in great detail the methods they used to validate the use of whole-slide images for examination of pediatric cases, which follow the College of American Pathologists Guidelines for validation of the use of this technology for nonpediatric cases. For additional reading, please see reference list.[1,2]

D. M. Grzybicki, MD

References

1. Fine JL, Grzybicki DM, Silowash R, et al. Evaluation of whole slide image immunohistochemistry interpretation in challenging prostate needle biopsies. *Hum Pathol.* 2008;39:564-572.

2. Ho J, Parwani AV, Jukic DM, Yagi Y, Anthony L, Gilbertson JR. Use of whole slide imaging in surgical pathology quality assurance: design and pilot validation studies. *Hum Pathol.* 2006;37:322-331.

Diagnosis of major cancer resection specimens with virtual slides: impact of a novel digital pathology workstation

Randell R, Ruddle RA, Thomas RG, et al (Univ of Leeds, UK; et al)

Hum Pathol 45:2101-2106, 2014

Digital pathology promises a number of benefits in efficiency in surgical pathology, yet the longer time required to review a virtual slide than a glass slide currently represents a significant barrier to the routine use of digital pathology. We aimed to create a novel workstation that enables pathologists to view a case as quickly as on the conventional microscope. The Leeds Virtual Microscope (LVM) was evaluated using a mixed factorial experimental design. Twelve consultant pathologists took part, each viewing one long cancer case (12-25 slides) on the LVM and one on a conventional microscope. Total time taken and diagnostic confidence were similar for the microscope and LVM, as was the mean slide viewing time. On the LVM, participants spent a significantly greater proportion of the total task time viewing slides and revisited slides more often. The unique design of the LVM, enabling real-time rendering of virtual slides while providing users with a quick and intuitive way to navigate within and between slides, makes use of digital pathology in routine practice a realistic possibility. With further practice with the system, diagnostic efficiency on the LVM is likely to increase yet more.

▶ This interesting report describes a novel digital pathology workstation called the Leeds Virtual Microscope (LVM). The unique and significant characteristics of this workstation appear to allow pathologists to examine surgical pathology cases as efficiently as they currently can using light microscopy. Other digital pathology systems currently have not been widely adopted for daily use because of the longer time required to adequately view virtual slides. Although this study is limited by the small number of pathologists observed ($n = 12$), the mean slide viewing time, the total time taken, and diagnostic confidence were the same for the pathologists using LVM as for those using conventional light microscopy. This system has the potential for providing a platform whereby digital pathology may become widely used in day-to-day surgical pathology practice.

D. M. Grzybicki, MD, PhD

Practicing Pathology in the Era of Big Data and Personalized Medicine

Gu J, Taylor CR (Shantou Univ Med College, Guangdong, China; Univ of Southern California, Los Angeles)

Appl Immunohistochem Mol Morphol 22:1-9, 2014

The traditional task of the pathologist is to assist physicians in making the correct diagnosis of diseases at the earliest possible stage to effectuate the optimal treatment strategy for each individual patient. In this respect surgical pathology (the traditional tissue diagnosis) is but a tool. It is not, of itself, the purpose of pathology practice; and change is in the air. This January 2014 issue of *Applied Immunohistochemistry and Molecular Morphology* (AIMM) embraces that change by the incorporation of the agenda and content of the journal *Diagnostic Molecular Morphology* (DMP). Over a decade ago AIMM introduced and promoted the concept of "molecular morphology," and has sought to publish molecular studies that correlate with the morphologic features that continue to define cancer and many diseases. That intent is now reinforced and extended by the merger with DMP, as a logical and timely response to the growing impact of a wide range of genetic and molecular technologies that are beginning to reshape the way in which pathology is practiced. The use of molecular and genomic techniques already demonstrates clear value in the diagnosis of disease, with treatment tailored specifically to individual patients. Personalized medicine is the future, and personalized medicine demands personalized pathology. The need for integration of the flood of new molecular data, with surgical pathology, digital pathology, and the full range of pathology data in the electronic medical record has never been greater. This review describes the possible impact of these pressures upon the discipline of pathology, and examines possible outcomes. There is a sense of excitement and adventure. Active adaption and innovation are required. The new AIMM, incorporating DMP, seeks to position itself for a central role in this process (Fig 1).

▶ Gu and colleagues present an interesting overview of the future of anatomic pathology in the new era of "big data" and personalized medicine. The authors provide examples (shown in Fig 1) of lung adenocarcinoma, colonic adenocarcinoma, and melanoma, in which specific genetic mutations may receive targeted therapy. On a national level, the growth of personalized medicine will affect resident training, reimbursement for pathologist practice and laboratory services, and the role of a primary care pathologist, as described by Gu et al. This role has yet to be defined but most likely will include components of traditional anatomic pathology diagnostics, molecular medicine, and clinical consultation.

S. Raab, MD

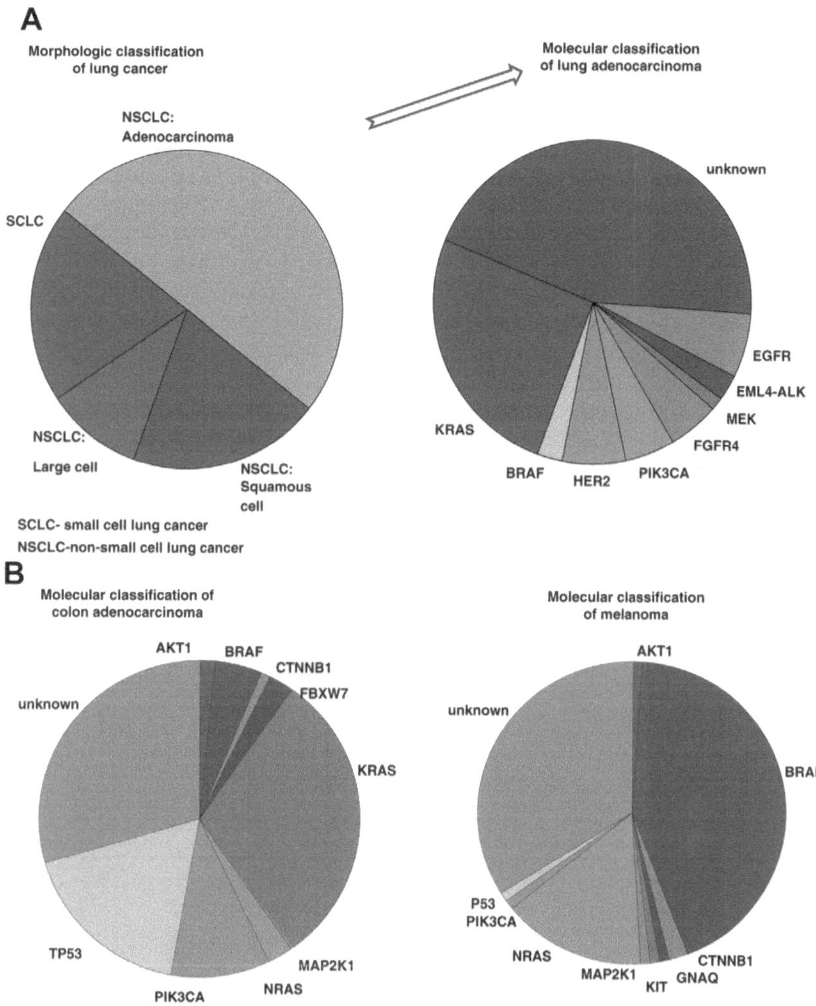

FIGURE 1.—A, Basic morphologic classification of lung cancer (L) is of no value in identifying "responders" to therapies that target a growing number of defined molecular subtypes (R). The exact proportion of tumors that manifest these mutations varies in different cancer populations. Data from Catalogue of Somatic Mutations in Cancer[4] and Beadling et al.[5] B, Other major tumor types show a range of molecular alterations, many of which have led to the generation of targeted therapies, as listed in Table 2. These therapies are targeted to the presence of the mutation, and thus have clinical application in tumor types that are distinct by morphology, provided that the mutation is present; for example, HER2, initially in breast cancer, but also in lung and stomach cancer, and BRAF in melanoma, colon and lung, as shown. Data from Catalogue of Somatic Mutations in Cancer[4] and Beadling et al.[5] *Editor's Note*: Please refer to original journal article for full references. (Reprinted from Gu J, Taylor CR. Practicing pathology in the era of big data and personalized medicine. *Appl Immunohistochem Mol Morphol.* 2014;22:1-9, with permission from Lippincott Williams & Wilkins.)

Validation of a whole slide imaging system for primary diagnosis in surgical pathology: A community hospital experience

Buck TP, Dilorio R, Havrilla L, et al (Manchester Memorial Hosp, CT)

J Pathol Inform 5:43, 2014

Guidelines for validating whole slide imaging (WSI) for primary diagnosis in surgical pathology have been recommended by an expert panel commissioned by the College of American Pathologists. The implementation of such a system using these validation guidelines has not been reported from the community hospital setting. The objective was to implement a WSI system, validate each pathologist using the system and run the system in parallel with routine glass slide interpretation. Six pathologists rereviewed approximately 300 previously diagnosed specimens each, divided equally between glass slides and digital images (scanned at ×20). Baseline intraobserver discordance rates (glass to glass) were calculated and compared to discordance rates between the original glass slide interpretation and the reviewed digital slide interpretation. A minimum of 3 months was used as the washout period. After validation, a subset

TABLE 2.—Parallel Case Review-List of Discordances

Pathologist	Type of Discordance	Discrepancy Type
Tech	Cropping error	Technical
Tech	Tissue float not scanned (seen on glass slide)	Technical
1	Missed intestinal metaplasia in gastroesophageal junction	Major
1	Missed increased intraepithelial lymphocytes in duodenum	Major
2	Missed neutrophils in upper gastrointestinal biopsy	Minor
2	Missed neutrophils in upper gastrointestinal biopsy	Minor
2	Missed neutrophils in upper gastrointestinal biopsy	Minor
4	Called no diagnostic abnormality instead of carcinoid tumor	Major
4	Called hyperplastic polyp instead of adenoma	Major
4	Missed neutrophils in upper gastrointestinal biopsy	Minor
4	Missed neutrophils in upper gastrointestinal biopsy	Minor
4	Missed neutrophils in upper gastrointestinal biopsy	Minor
4	Missed neutrophils in upper gastrointestinal biopsy	Minor
5	Missed neutrophils and paneth cells in colon biopsy	Major
5	Missed neutrophils and paneth cells in colon biopsy	Major
5	Missed neutrophils in upper gastrointestinal biopsy	Minor
5	Missed eosinophils in esophageal biopsy, insufficient in number for eosinophilic esophagitis	Minor
5	Missed eosinophils in esophageal biopsy, insufficient in number for eosinophilic esophagitis	Minor
5	Missed neutrophils in upper gastrointestinal biopsy	Minor
5	Missed neutrophils in upper gastrointestinal biopsy	Minor
6	Called adenoma with low grade dysplasia instead of high grade dysplasia	Major
6	Missed *H. pylori* on immunostain	Major
6	Missed *H. pylori* on immunostain	Major
6	Missed cryptitis in colon	Major
6	Missed neutrophils in upper gastrointestinal biopsy	Minor

H. pylori: Helicobacter pylori

Reprinted from Buck TP, Dilorio R, Havrilla L, et al. Validation of a whole slide imaging system for primary diagnosis in surgical pathology: a community hospital experience. *J Pathol Inform*. 2015;5:43, with permission from Buck TP.

of daily cases was diagnosed in parallel using traditional microscopy (TM) and WSI over an 8-month period. The TM and WSI discordance rates ranged from 3.3% to 13.3% and 2.1% to 10.1%, respectively. There was no statistically significant difference among the pathologists. The parallel study yielded similar rates of discordances. In our laboratory, after appropriate implementation and training, there was no difference between the WSI and TM methods (Table 2).

▶ In this report, Buck et al report on the validation of a whole-slide imaging system for primary diagnostic sign out. Currently, in the United States, digital imaging systems cannot be used for that purpose, although at some point in the future, digital imaging systems will be used for primary sign out. Table 2 is invaluable, as it shows the specific discordant cases seen in the validation phase of implementation. Understanding the underlying causes is critical to understanding how pathologists will initially use this system in the United States. For further reading, see reference list below.[1,2]

S. Raab, MD

References

1. Bauer TW, Schoenfield L, Slaw RJ, Yerian L, Sun Z, Henricks WH. Validation of whole slide imaging for primary diagnosis in surgical pathology. *Arch Pathol Lab Med.* 2013;137:518-524.
2. Pantanowitz L, Sinard JH, Henricks WH, et al. Validating whole slide imaging for diagnostic purposes in pathology: Guideline from the College of American Pathologists Pathology and Laboratory Quality Center. *Arch Pathol Lab Med.* 2013;137: 1710-1722.

16 Urinary Bladder and Male Genital Tract

Are *Ureaplasma* spp. a Cause of Nongonococcal Urethritis? A Systematic Review and Meta-Analysis

Zhang N, Wang R, Li X, et al (Tianjin Univ of Traditional Chinese Medicine, China; Tianjin Med Univ, China; et al)

PLoS One 9:e113771, 2014

Background.—Nongonococcal urethritis (NGU) is the most common male reproductive tract syndrome. *Ureaplasmas* spp. including *U. urealyticum* and *U. parvum*, have been increasingly reported to be implicated in NGU. However, there are still many contradictions about their pathogenic role in NGU.

Aims.—The goals of this study were to evaluate the association of *Ureaplasmas* spp. with NGU, and to compare the prevalence of *Ureaplasmas* spp. infection in China relative to the world average.

Methods.—A systematic review and meta-analysis was conducted following standard guidelines for meta-analysis. The quality of included studies was assessed by Newcastle-Ottawa scale.

Results.—A total of seven studies involving 1,507 NGU patients and 1,223 controls were eligible for meta-analysis. There was no significant difference in the *Ureaplasma* spp. positive rate between the NGU and control groups. However, the *U. urealyticum* positive rate was significantly higher in NGU patients compared to controls; the *U. parvum* positive rate was significantly higher in controls compared to NGU patients. Furthermore, within the NGU patient group, the positive rate of *U. urealyticum* was significantly higher than that of *U. parvum*, whereas within the control group, the opposite trend was observed. Compared to the world average, a significantly higher positive rate of *Ureaplasma* spp. was observed in both the NGU and control groups in China.

Conclusions.—Our analysis supports that *U. urealyticum*, but not *U. parvum*, is an etiological agent in NGU. More detailed studies of these two species in China and the world could contribute to a better understanding of the epidemiology and pathogenesis, and facilitate the development of better strategies for treatment and prevention of NGU.

▶ This article is a good example of the use of rigorous methods of literature review and analysis to confidently answer a clinically applied research question, and for that reason, it is worth reading. It answers a specific question about which of 2 species of ureaplasma, that are suspected to be pathogens for nongonococcal urethritis, is actually associated with clinical disease. In doing so, this report provides information about optimizing diagnosis and treatment for this common entity.

S. Raab, MD

The Critical Role of the Pathologist in Determining Eligibility for Active Surveillance as a Management Option in Patients With Prostate Cancer: Consensus Statement With Recommendations Supported by the College of American Pathologists, International Society of Urological Pathology, Association of Directors of Anatomic and Surgical Pathology, the New Zealand Society of Pathologists, and the Prostate Cancer Foundation

Amin MB, Lin DW, Gore JL, et al (Cedars-Sinai Med Ctr, Los Angeles, CA; Univ of Washington, Seattle; et al)

Arch Pathol Lab Med 138:1387-1405, 2014

Context.—Prostate cancer remains a significant public health problem. Recent publications of randomized trials and the US Preventive Services Task Force recommendations have drawn attention to overtreatment of localized, low-risk prostate cancer. Active surveillance, in which patients undergo regular visits with serum prostate-specific antigen tests and repeat prostate biopsies, rather than aggressive treatment with curative intent, may address overtreatment of low-risk prostate cancer. It is apparent that a greater awareness of the critical role of pathologists in determining eligibility for active surveillance is needed.

Objectives.—To review the state of current knowledge about the role of active surveillance in the management of prostate cancer and to provide a multidisciplinary report focusing on pathologic parameters important to the successful identification of patients likely to succeed with active surveillance, to determine the role of molecular tests in increasing the safety of active surveillance, and to provide future directions.

Design.—Systematic review of literature on active surveillance for low-risk prostate cancer, pathologic parameters important for appropriate stratification, and issues regarding interobserver reproducibility. Expert panels were created to delineate the fundamental questions confronting the clinical and pathologic aspects of management of men on active surveillance.

Results.—Expert panelists identified pathologic parameters important for management and the related diagnostic and reporting issues. Consensus recommendations were generated where appropriate.

Conclusions.—Active surveillance is an important management option for men with low-risk prostate cancer. Vital to this process is the critical role pathologic parameters have in identifying appropriate candidates for active surveillance. These findings need to be reproducible and

TABLE 9.—Summary of Key Recommendations From the College of American Pathologists, International Society of Urological Pathology, Association of Directors of Anatomic and Surgical Pathology, New Zealand Society of Pathologists, and the Prostate Cancer Foundation Consensus Statement Panelists

Overall, Including Sampling, Submission, and Processing Issues

- The Gleason score and tumor extent measurements are the most meaningful pathologic parameters in needle biopsies, determining eligibility for AS protocols.
- Sampling of the prostate gland, using contemporary biopsy templates that sample 12 to 16 areas within the prostate, including the midgland and lateral gland at the base, mid section, and apex of the prostate, is recommended; these may still miss detection of some prostate cancers.
- Samples for pathologic evaluation should ideally be separated and submitted according to biopsy sites targeted for appropriate reporting and documentation of the location and number of positive/negative cores.
- While submitting 1 core per container is optimal, if multiple cores are submitted in the same container, we recommend that no more than 2 cores be submitted per cassette.
- Although there is no definition for an optimal length of a prostatic needle core biopsy, the average length is 15 mm. When cancer involves a biopsy core less than 6 mm long, we recommend that the length of the core biopsy be specified, in addition to the extent of the needle core involvement.

Tumor Extent in Needle Biopsies

- Reporting should include in all cases:
  - Number of positive cores/total number of cores,
  - Linear percentage of prostatic tissue involved and/or total linear measurement of carcinoma and total core length,
  - Percentage of carcinoma in the most extensively involved core, and
  - Quantitation of these parameters should be based on the total amount of prostatic parenchyma; nonprostatic elements should not be included in the total core quantitation.
- Reporting biopsies with discontinuous foci:
  - Specify the presence of discontinuous foci, the linear extent in aggregate of the discontinuous foci, the percentage of involvement of the core (or the overall length of the core tissue), and the core length spanned by the discontinuous foci. An example of a report includes: Adenocarcinoma of prostate, Gleason score 3 + 3, involving 1 of 6 cores, with 2 discontinuous foci measuring 2 mm in aggregate, involving 10% of the core, and spanning 70% of the length of the core.
- Reporting biopsies with multiple cores in the same container:
  - Provide linear measurement (in millimeters) or linear extent (as a percentage) of prostatic tissue involved for the most-involved core and the overall linear percentage or measurement in millimeters of the tissue submitted from the site(s) with cancer.
- Reporting fragmented cores:
  - When assessment of the number of cores involved by carcinoma is difficult because of the extent of fragmentation and that determination is key for AS eligibility, a comment should be made suggesting that the urologist/physician obtaining the biopsy is in the best position to make the determination of the number of cores involved, based on the original submission of the number of cores; if necessary, undertake clinicopathologic correlation.
  - When an involved core is <6 mm long, reporting the percentage of the core involved by cancer and the core length information should be provided.

Gleason Score in Needle Biopsies

- Biopsy Gleason grade reclassification has emerged as one of the most meaningful intervention criteria for men on AS.
- Accurate distinction of Gleason pattern 3 from Gleason pattern 4 is critical for eligibility for most AS protocols. In cases with cusp histology between patterns 3 and 4:
    - Only poorly formed glands, not attributable to tangential sectioning and cribriform glands, should be classified as Gleason pattern 4,
    - Place these findings in the context of the overall company the carcinoma demonstrates (ie, predominantly Gleason pattern 3),
    - When there is doubt, default to the lower grade, follow the focus on the multiple levels and sections, and share such borderline cases with a colleague because the presence of Gleason pattern 4 may preclude the patient from AS.

Other Pathologic Considerations

- Pathologic findings in needle biopsies that would automatically exclude patients, irrespective of Gleason score, include prostatic adenocarcinoma with predominantly ductal features, intraductal carcinoma without invasive carcinoma, sarcomatoid, and small cell carcinoma, in addition to extraprostatic extension and vascular lymphatic invasion.
- Patients with prostate cancer with variant histology, such as atrophic, pseudohyperplastic, and foamy gland patterns, may be candidates for AS if the carcinoma is of an appropriate Gleason score and the extent in the needle biopsies with cancer is within guidelines.
- Perineural invasion in biopsies of patients who otherwise meet criteria for AS should not exclude patient for AS.
- Immunohistochemistry for atypical, small acinar proliferations in a patient with a cancer diagnosis should be performed only if the confirmation of cancer, or lack thereof, is important for AS or definitive treatment eligibility.

Precision Medicine Markers

- Currently, available data do not support a recommendation for any particular molecular tool or test for determining eligibility of patients into AS protocols. Several tests have recently been offered commercially and, although purported to be useful, need further clinical experience and prospective validation for consistent inclusion into clinical decision-making algorithms.

Abbreviation: AS, active surveillance.

consistently reported by surgical pathologists with accurate pathology reporting (Table 9).

▶ Amin and coauthors provide an excellent review article on the pathologist's role in clinical care of patients with prostate cancer and the critical importance of needle biopsy interpretation in determining the eligibility for active surveillance (AS) as a management option. Leading pathology societies identified 3 key issues: (1) clinical perspective on AS, (2) pathologic parameters critical to stratifying patients in AS protocols, and (3) the role of ancillary molecular diagnostic tests to increase the safety of AS. Table 9 is reproduced here and reports summary recommendations. The authors indicate that a number of sampling and tissue handling issues are critically important for the assessment and reporting of core biopsy specimens, and these are further discussed in the article.

S. Raab, MD

The Application of Immunohistochemical Biomarkers in Urologic Surgical Pathology

Wilkerson ML, Lin F, Liu H, et al (Geisinger Med Ctr, Danville, Pennsylvania; et al)

Arch Pathol Lab Med 138:1643-1665, 2014

Context.—Tumors of the genitourinary tract can be diagnostically challenging, particularly in core biopsies and cystoscopic biopsies with limited material. Immunohistochemistry is a valuable tool to use when morphology alone is insufficient for diagnosis.

Objectives.—To review tumors and benign lesions of the kidney, urinary bladder, prostate gland, testis, and paratesticular structures with an emphasis on difficult differential diagnoses, as well as staining patterns in normal tissue. Recommended immunohistochemical stain panels are discussed that can assist in the diagnostic workup.

Data Sources.—Review of current literature.

Conclusions.—Immunohistochemistry is a valuable tool, assisting in the diagnosis of problematic tumors and benign lesions of the genitourinary tract (Fig 1).

▶ Get a copy of this article if you sign out genitourinary or kidney tumors. Wilkerson et al provide an overview for immunohistochemical use in this subspecialty. Data are presented in tabular and flowchart formats. Fig 1 (reproduced here) is just one example indicating the authors' immunohistochemistry (IHC) panel recommendations for renal tumors. The challenge for the practicing pathologist lies in not having available all the antibodies listed and in cases in

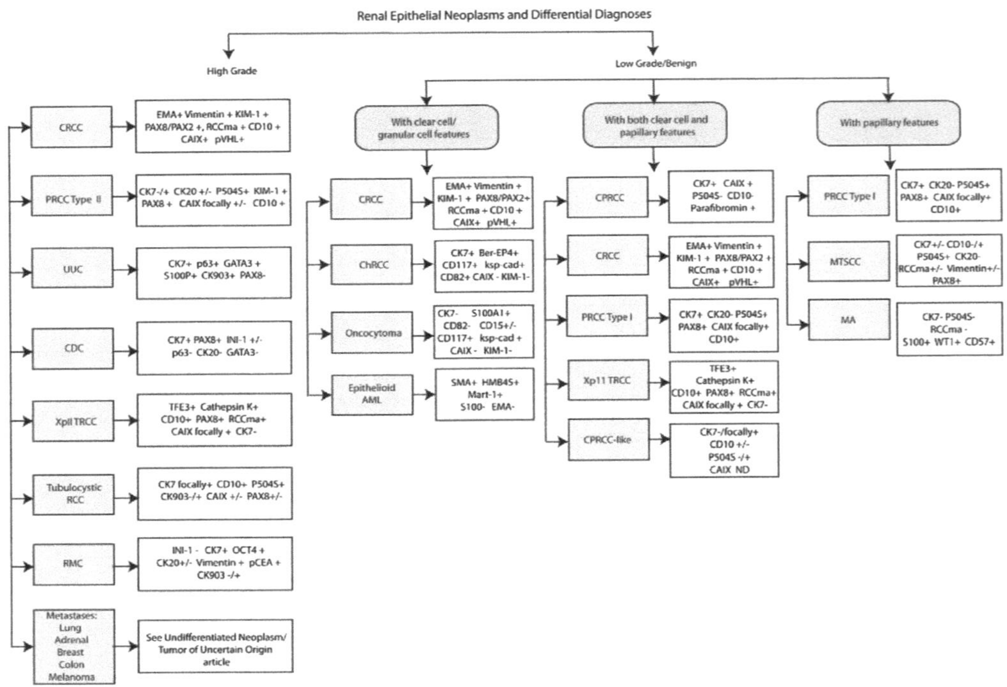

FIGURE 1.—Summary of the specific immunoprofile for each renal neoplasm. Abbreviations: AML, angiomyolipoma; Ber-EP4, epithelial cell adhesion molecule; CAIX, carbonic anhydrase IX; CD, cluster of differentiation; CDC, collecting duct carcinoma; ChRCC, chromophobe renal cell carcinoma; CK, cytokeratin; CPRCC, clear cell papillary renal cell carcinoma; CRCC, clear cell renal cell carcinoma; EMA, epithelial membrane antigen; GATA3, GATA-binding protein 3; HMB-45, human melanoma black 45; INI-1, integrase interactor 1; KIM-1, kidney injury molecule–1; ksp-cad, kidney-specific cadherin; MA, metanephric adenoma; Mart-1, melanoma-associated antigen recognized by T cells 1; MTSCC, mucinous tubular and spindle cell carcinoma; ND, no data; OCT4, octamer-binding transcription factor 4; PAX, paired box gene; pCEA, polyclonal carcinoembryonic antigen; PRCC, papillary renal cell carcinoma; pVHL, von Hippel–Lindau tumor suppressor; P504S, a-methylacyl-CoA racemase; RCC, renal cell carcinoma; RCCma, renal cell carcinoma marker; RMC, renal medullary carcinoma; SMA, smooth muscle actin; S100P, placental S100; TFE3, transcription factor E3; UUC, upper urinary tract urothelial carcinoma; WT1, Wilms tumor 1; Xp11 TRCC, Xp11 translocation renal cell carcinoma. (Reproduced with permission of College of American Pathologists from Wilkerson ML, Lin F, Liu H, et al. The application of immunohistochemical biomarkers in urologic surgical pathology. *Arch Pathol Lab Med.* 2014;138:1643-1665; permission conveyed through Copyright Clearance Center, Inc.)

which the IHC results do not line up with the classifications in the tables. Nonetheless, this is an excellent reference article to keep handy.

S. Raab, MD

Recurrent papillary urothelial neoplasm of low malignant potential. Subtle architectural disorder detected by quantitative analysis in DAXX-immunostained tissue sections

Castellini P, Montironi MA, Zizzi A, et al (Polytechnic Univ of the Marche Region, Ancona, Italy; et al)

Hum Pathol 45:745-752, 2014

The aim of the study was to identify subtle changes in the so-called architectural predominant order in nonrecurrent and recurrent papillary urothelial neoplasm of low malignant potential (PUNLMP). Quantitative analysis was performed with a software package written in LabVIEW (National Instruments, Austin, TX) in DAXX-immunostained tissue sections. Twelve cases of PUNLMP with papillary fronds sectioned lengthwise through the core were investigated and subdivided as follows: 7 nonrecurrent and 5 recurrent PUNLMP cases. Six cases of normal urothelium (NU) were included. When an epithelial thickness threshold is set at 108 μm (ie, 400 pixels), there is a complete separation between NU and PUNLMP; however, nonrecurrent and recurrent cases fall in the same range of thickness. In setting a nuclear elongation factor threshold at 2.1, there are differences between the 2 PUNLMP groups, recurrent PUNLMP and NU cases, showing a somewhat similar proportion of elongated nuclei. The nuclear orientation separates nonrecurrent from recurrent PUNLMP groups; however, NU cases do not appear as a separate group from the 2 PUNLMP groups. In combining epithelial thickness, nuclear elongation, and orientation in a multivariate analysis, the 2 PUNLMP groups appear separate between them and from NU. NU is less thickened than the 2 PUNLMP groups and shows a combination of elongated and less elongated nuclei. Elongated nuclei are more numerous in nonrecurrent PUNLMP, whereas the nuclei in recurrent PUNLMP are less elongated and less polarized than in the other group. Such finding can be used routinely to identify those PUNLMP patients who will have recurrence.

▶ One of the basic principles of neoplasia is that the cellular architecture becomes disordered, although this disorder may require quantitative analysis to demonstrate. For Castellini et al, quantitative analysis was used to determine a subcategory of papillary urothelial neoplasm of low malignant potential (PUNLMP) that may recur. The data indicate that up to 47% of PUNLMPs recur, so quantitative analysis could play an important role in patient management. For further reading, see reference list.[1,2]

S. Raab, MD

References

1. Montironi R, Mazzucchelli R, Scarpelli M, Lopez-Beltran A, Cheng L. Morphological diagnosis of the urothelial neoplasms. *J Clin Pathol.* 2008;61:3-10.
2. Montironi R, Lopez-Beltran A, Scarpelli M, Mazzucchelli R, Cheng L. Morphological classification and definition of benign, preneoplastic and non-invasive neoplastic lesions of the urinary bladder. *Histopathology.* 2008;53:621-633.

PART II

LABORATORY MEDICINE

17 Clinical Chemistry

Clinical biochemistry laboratory rejection rates due to various types of preanalytical errors

Atay A, Demir L, Cuhadar S, et al (Katip Celebi Univ, Izmir, Turkey)

Biochem Med (Zagreb) 24:376-382, 2014

Introduction.—Preanalytical errors, along the process from the beginning of test requests to the admissions of the specimens to the laboratory, cause the rejection of samples. The aim of this study was to better explain the reasons of rejected samples, regarding to their rates in certain test groups in our laboratory.

Materials and Methods.—This preliminary study was designed on the rejected samples in one-year period, based on the rates and types of inappropriateness. Test requests and blood samples of clinical chemistry, immunoassay, hematology, glycated hemoglobin, coagulation and erythrocyte sedimentation rate test units were evaluated. Types of inappropriateness were evaluated as follows: improperly labelled samples, hemolysed, clotted specimen, insufficient volume of specimen and total request errors.

Results.—A total of 5,183,582 test requests from 1,035,743 blood collection tubes were considered. The total rejection rate was 0.65%. The rejection rate of coagulation group was significantly higher (2.28%) than the other test groups ($P < 0.001$) including insufficient volume of specimen error rate as 1.38%. Rejection rates of hemolysis, clotted specimen and insufficient volume of sample error were found to be 8%, 24% and 34%, respectively. Total request errors, particularly, for unintelligible requests were 32% of the total for inpatients.

Conclusions.—The errors were especially attributable to unintelligible requests of inappropriate test requests, improperly labelled samples for inpatients and blood drawing errors especially due to insufficient volume of specimens in a coagulation test group. Further studies should be performed after corrective and preventive actions to detect a possible decrease in rejecting samples.

▶ This study provides detailed information regarding reasons for various specimen rejections. It is useful reading for 2 reasons. First, it provides information useful for other laboratories investigating their own reasons for specimen rejection. This information is not new, but it emphasizes that rejection is an ongoing and significant problem in clinical laboratories. Second, it emphasizes the limitation of this and other studies like it, which is that no follow-up quality improvement plan that is actually initiated is discussed. Although it is necessary to understand the details of a clinical problem, equally, if not more important, is to embark on meaningful and feasible actions to improve it.

S. Raab, MD

Harmonization: the Sample, the Measurement, and the Report

Miller WG, Tate JR, Barth JH, et al (Virginia Commonwealth Univ, Richmond; Royal Brisbane and Women's Hosp, Brisbane, Queensland, Australia; et al)
Ann Lab Med 34:187-197, 2014

Harmonization of clinical laboratory results means that results are comparable irrespective of the measurement procedure used and where or when a measurement was made. Harmonization of test results includes consideration of pre-analytical, analytical, and post-analytical aspects. Progress has been made in each of these aspects, but there is currently poor coordination of the effort among different professional organizations in different countries. Pre-analytical considerations include terminology for the order, instructions for preparation of the patient, collection of the samples, and handling and transportation of the samples to the laboratory. Key analytical considerations include calibration traceability to a reference system, commutability of reference materials used in a traceability scheme, and specificity of the measurement of the biomolecule of interest. International organizations addressing harmonization include the International Federation for Clinical Chemistry and Laboratory Medicine, the World Health Organization, and the recently formed International Consortium for Harmonization of Clinical Laboratory Results (ICHCLR). The ICHCLR will provide a prioritization process for measurands and a service to coordinate global harmonization activities to avoid duplication of effort. Post-analytical considerations include nomenclature, units, significant figures, and reference intervals or decision values for results. Harmonization in all of these areas is necessary for optimal laboratory service. This review summarizes the status of harmonization in each of these areas and describes activities underway to achieve the goal of fully harmonized clinical laboratory testing.

▶ This report is extremely important, because it deals with standardization of clinical laboratory testing not just on a regional or national level, but on a global level, as a necessity for patient safety. An interesting aspect of this report is that it discusses all phases of the testing cycle, including the pre-preanalytic as well as the post-postanalytic, phases that are uncommonly discussed in the laboratory medicine literature.

S. Raab, MD

Measurements for 8 Common Analytes in Native Sera Identify Inadequate Standardization among 6 Routine Laboratory Assays

Stepman HCM, on behalf of the participating laboratories (Ghent Univ, Belgium; et al)

Clin Chem 60:855-863, 2014

Background.—External quality assessment (EQA) with commutable samples is essential for assessing the quality of assays performed by laboratories, particularly when the emphasis is on their standardization status and interchangeability of results.

Methods.—We used a panel of 20 fresh-frozen single-donation serum samples to assess assays for the measurement of creatinine, glucose, phosphate, uric acid, total cholesterol, HDL cholesterol, LDL cholesterol, and triglycerides. The commercial random access platforms included: Abbott Architect, Beckman Coulter AU, Ortho Vitros, Roche Cobas, Siemens Advia, and Thermo Scientific Konelab. The assessment was done at the peer group level and by comparison against the all-method trimmed mean or reference method values, where available. The considered quality indicators were intraassay imprecision, combined imprecision (including sample—matrix interference), bias, and total error. Fail/pass decisions were based on limits reflecting state-of-the-art performance, but also limits related to biological variation.

Results.—Most assays showed excellent peer performance attributes, except for HDL- and LDL cholesterol. Cases in which individual assays had biases exceeding the used limits were the Siemens Advia creatinine (−4.2%), Ortho Vitros phosphate (8.9%), Beckman Coulter AU triglycerides (5.4%), and Thermo Scientific Konelab uric acid (6.4%), which lead to considerable interassay discrepancies. Additionally, large laboratory effects were observed that caused interlaboratory differences of >30%.

Conclusions.—The design of the EQA study was well suited for monitoring different quality attributes of assays performed in daily laboratory practice. There is a need for improvement, even for simple clinical chemistry analytes. In particular, the interchangeability of results remains jeopardized both by assay standardization issues and individual laboratory effects.

► Although these authors confirm what has been accepted for a long time, that interlaboratory and interinstrument variability is significantly high, precluding generalization of results across laboratories, it serves to emphasize this critical limitation in diagnostic and screening testing. These findings also have important implications related to proficiency testing. Hopefully, this long-standing problem in all clinical chemistry testing will be addressed to improve the quality of testing information.

S. Raab, MD

18 Clinical Microbiology

Emerging Rapid Resistance Testing Methods for Clinical Microbiology Laboratories and Their Potential Impact on Patient Management

Frickmann H, Masanta WO, Zautner AE (Bundeswehrkrankenhaus Hamburg, Germany; Universitätsmedizin Göttingen, Germany; et al)

Biomed Res Int 2014:375681, 2014

Atypical and multidrug resistance, especially ESBL and carbapenemase expressing Enterobacteriaceae, is globally spreading. Therefore, it becomes increasingly difficult to achieve therapeutic success by calculated antibiotic therapy. Consequently, rapid antibiotic resistance testing is essential. Various molecular and mass spectrometry-based approaches have been introduced in diagnostic microbiology to speed up the providing of reliable resistance data. PCR- and sequencing-based approaches are the most expensive but the most frequently applied modes of testing, suitable for the detection of resistance genes even from primary material. Next generation sequencing, based either on assessment of allelic single nucleotide polymorphisms or on the detection of nonubiquitous resistance mechanisms might allow for sequence-based bacterial resistance testing comparable to viral resistance testing on the long term. Fluorescence *in situ* hybridization (FISH), based on specific binding of fluorescence-labeled oligonucleotide probes, provides a less expensive molecular bridging technique. It is particularly useful for detection of resistance mechanisms based on mutations in ribosomal RNA. Approaches based on MALDI-TOF-MS, alone or in combination with molecular techniques, like PCR/electrospray ionization MS or minisequencing provide the fastest resistance results from pure colonies or even primary samples with a growing number of protocols. This review details the various approaches of rapid resistance testing, their pros and cons, and their potential use for the diagnostic laboratory.

▶ Although this is a review article, I believe it is highly important reading because it addresses a critical issue in clinical microbiology—the increasing need for clinically effective and timely resistance testing in a global environment in which an increasing number of bacterial pathogens are gaining unpredictable multidrug resistance rapidly. The authors give a detailed description of the multiple rapid methods available and the advantages and disadvantages of each. Microbiologists will need to strongly consider the eventual adoption of one or more of these methods if they haven't already in order to provide timely resistance testing that will be increasing in demand.

S. Raab, MD

Evaluation of the decision support system for antimicrobial treatment, TREAT, in an acute medical ward of a university hospital

Arboe B, Laub RR, Kronborg G, et al (Copenhagen Univ Hosp, Hvidovre, Denmark)

Int J Infect Dis 29:156-161, 2014

Objectives.—TREAT, a decision support system for antimicrobial therapy, was implemented in an acute medical ward.

Methods.—Patients admitted on suspicion of infection were included in the study. The evaluation of TREAT was done both retrospectively and prospectively. Coverage of empirical antimicrobial treatments was compared to recommendations from TREAT and the optimal use of local guidelines.

Results.—Five hundred and eleven patients were included, of whom 162 had a microbiologically documented infection. In the retrospective part of the study, TREAT, physician, and guideline antimicrobial coverage rates were 65%, 51%, and 79%, respectively, and in the prospective part, 68%, 62%, and 77%, respectively. TREAT provided lower coverage than local guidelines ($p < 0.001$), but was similar to the performance of physicians in a university hospital ($p = 0.069$). No differences were found in length of hospital stay, or hospital or 30-day mortality. Direct costs were significantly higher for TREAT advice than for local guidelines or the physician prescriptions ($p < 0.001$), but the ecological costs were lower for TREAT advice than for both local guidelines ($p < 0.001$) and physician prescriptions ($p = 0.247$). The coverage of TREAT advice for the bacteraemia patients was non-inferior to the physicians ($p = 1.00$).

Conclusions.—TREAT can potentially improve the ecological costs of empirical antimicrobial therapy for patients in acute medical wards, but provided lower coverage than local guidelines.

▶ This article is highly valuable reading for 2 major reasons. First, it illustrates that the incorporation of an information technology tool designed to improve practice does not always produce the expected positive outcomes. As a consequence, it also illustrates the absolute need for pilot testing of new information technology tools before full implementation. Second, it confirms that use of clinical practice guidelines by physicians and other health care practitioners will produce superior outcomes, when applied appropriately and assuming the guidelines are of high quality.

S. Raab, MD

Fungal Infections in Liver Transplant Patients Admitted to the Intensive Care Unit

Marzaban R, Salah M, Mukhtar AM, et al (Cairo Univ, Egypt; et al)

Ann Transplant 19:667-673, 2014

Background.—Fungal infections have a significant impact on patient survival after liver transplantation, mostly caused by *Candida* and *Aspergillus*. The clinical manifestations vary, and range from colonization, active local infection, to severe invasive form. A high degree of suspicion is required for the early diagnosis and, accordingly, the optimal management of these infections. This study aimed to evaluate fungal infection in the Intensive Care Unit (ICU) in admitted liver transplant patients, focussing of etiologic agent, clinical/laboratory presentation (including mortality), and risk factors.

Material/Methods.—This retrospective study included living related liver transplanted patients admitted to the ICU. Clinical data was collected, thorough clinical evaluation was done, and laboratory tests were performed. Microbiological examination detecting the presence of fungus in various samples, using cultures and serology, and imaging investigations were carried out in all patients.

Results.—This study included 23 cases of ICU-admitted liver transplant patients who were diagnosed with fungal infection. *Candida* was the most common fungal infection and occurred at a mean of 2 months after transplantation; while *Aspergillus* was less common and occurred later with worse laboratory findings. Invasive fungal infection constituted 43% of the diagnosed cases. Difference in mortality between *Aspergillus* and *Candida* was insignificant, as was difference between patients with and without fungal infection.

Conclusions.—Fungal infection among LT patients was common, including the invasive forms.

▶ This article is a useful reading because it gives a good literature review and institutional description of *Candida* and *Aspergillus* infections in liver transplant patients in the intensive care setting. The descriptions are detailed and may be informative for hepatologists and clinical microbiologists who care for these patients. The limitation of the study, in my view, is the statistics-based conclusions of the authors that there was no difference in mortality between patients with fungal infections and those without. To my reading, the authors do not perform the most appropriate statistical analysis to answer this question, seemingly not considering the many demographic and clinical variables they describe for the patients included in the study. Therefore, despite the wealth of description related to these patients and their course, they do not provide a convincing answer to their question regarding the effect of fungal infection on mortality in this group of patients.

S. Raab, MD

Pathogenesis of Necrotizing Enterocolitis: Modeling the Innate Immune Response

Tanner SM, Berryhill TF, Ellenburg JL, et al (Univ of Alabama at Birmingham; et al)

Am J Pathol 185:4-16, 2015

Necrotizing enterocolitis (NEC) is a major cause of morbidity and mortality in premature infants. The pathophysiology is likely secondary to innate immune responses to intestinal microbiota by the premature infant's intestinal tract, leading to inflammation and injury. This review provides an updated summary of the components of the innate immune system involved in NEC pathogenesis. In addition, we evaluate the animal models that have been used to study NEC with regard to the involvement of innate immune factors and histopathological changes as compared to those seen in infants with NEC. Finally, we discuss new approaches to studying NEC, including mathematical models of intestinal injury and the use of humanized mice.

▶ This review is worth reading, as it provides detailed information about the immunopathology of necrotizing enterocolitis. This information is highly valuable to clinical microbiologists and immunologists who may not recall or be aware of the general pathology and current research related to this pediatric disease with a significantly high morbidity and mortality.

S. Raab, MD

The aetiology of pharyngotonsillitis in adolescents and adults – *Fusobacterium necrophorum* is commonly found

Hedin K, Bieber L, Lindh M, et al (Lund Univ, Malmö, Sweden; Central Hosp, Växjö, Sweden; Sahlgrenska Univ Hosp, Gothenburg, Sweden)

Clin Microbiol Infect 21:263.e1-263.e7, 2015

Sore throat is common in primary healthcare. Aetiological studies have focused on the presence of a limited number of pathogens. The aim of the present study was to investigate the presence of a wide range of bacteria and viruses, including *Fusobacterium necrophorum*, in patients with pharyngotonsillitis and in asymptomatic controls. A prospective case control study was performed in primary healthcare in Kronoberg County, Sweden. Patients ($n = 220$) aged 15 to 45 years with a suspected acute pharyngotonsillitis, and controls ($n = 128$), were included. Nasopharyngeal and throat swabs were analysed for β-hemolytic streptococci, *F. necrophorum*, *Mycoplasma pneumoniae*, and *Chlamydophila pneumoniae*, and 13 respiratory viruses. Serum samples were analysed for antibodies to Epstein-Barr virus. The patient history and symptoms, including Centor score, were analysed in relation to pathogens. In 155/220 (70.5%) of the patients, as compared to 26/128 (20.3%) of the controls ($p < 0.001$), at least one microorganism was found. Group A streptococci, *F. necrophorum*, and influenza B virus were the three most common findings, and all significantly more common in patients than in controls ($p < 0.001$, p 0.001, and p 0.002, respectively). Patients with *F. necrophorum* only ($n = 14$) displayed a lower Centor score than patients with Group A streptococcus only ($n = 46$), but a higher score than patients with influenza B, other viruses, or no potential pathogen (Kruskal-Wallis $p < 0.001$). A pathogen was detected in 70% of the patients, displaying a wide range of pathogens contributing to the aetiology of pharyngotonsillitis. This study supports *F. necrophorum* as one of the pathogens to be considered in the aetiology of pharyngotonsillitis.

▶ This report is highly valuable, as it describes a very comprehensive investigation into the multiple bacterial and viral organisms that may be cultured from nonpediatric patients with pharyngotonsillitis. One of its major strengths is that the authors were able to include many clinical factors in their analysis, which allowed them to conclude that *Fusobacterium* is the second most common organism cultured, after group A *Streptococcus*, particularly in patients who smoke or have tonsillar coating. Because pharyngotonsillitis is a common clinical complaint that often results in throat culture, this information is important for both clinicians and microbiologists.

S. Raab, MD

Testing quality of a self-monitoring blood glucose sensor with an auto-coding mechanism when used by patients versus technicians

Hsu C-T, Wu M-H, Kuo C-Y, et al (Chung Shan Med Univ, Taichung, Taiwan; Min Sheng Hosp, Taoyuan, Taiwan; Tai An Hosp, Taichung, Taiwan; et al)
Clin Chim Acta 437:62-65, 2014

Background.—In response to the problem of erroneous readings due to miscoding when performing self-monitoring blood glucose (SMBG), this study introduces a user-friendly SMBG biosensor with an innovative auto-coding module on the meter and strip. Actual users characterized the performance of the SMBG systems.

Methods.—A total of 105 patients were incorporated in the study and Clarke error grid analysis (EGA) was administered to evaluate the clinical accuracy of the results obtained by the patients versus the technicians. All patients used the questionnaires to comment on the use of the auto-coding sensor.

Results.—In the imprecision test, the total CV of the 5 BG levels was 2.1%. In the EGA plot, the results of the auto-coding sensor were 96.2%, both lots A and B, in zone A for the patients and 99.0% and 97.1% for the technician. The paired t-test demonstrated no statistically significant difference between the patient and technician measurements. Regression analysis also demonstrated that the measurements taken by the patients agreed with those obtained using the laboratory method.

Conclusions.—The patients achieved satisfactory performance using the auto-coding SMBG sensor and derived similar results with both laboratory reference and operation by a technician.

▶ Patient self-monitoring of blood glucose and health practitioner monitoring of patients' glucose levels have the potential of being inaccurate for both. These hand-held glucose meters are found to have the potential for being highly inaccurate. One source of inaccuracy that is not uncommon is user failure to input the correct calibration code for the particular test strips being used. This article describes the increased accuracy by both patients and health care personnel when using a self-monitoring blood glucose system with an innovative auto-coding component on the meter and test strip. Large-scale production and distribution of this system, which at this stage appears to be in an early testing phase, is not discussed; however, use of the system would significantly improve the accuracy of glucose point-of-care testing.

S. Raab, MD

19 Cytogenetics and Molecular Pathology

Practicing Pathology in the Era of Big Data and Personalized Medicine

Gu J, Taylor CR (Shantou Univ Med College, Guangdong, China; Univ of Southern California, Los Angeles)

Appl Immunohistochem Mol Morphol 22:1-9, 2014

The traditional task of the pathologist is to assist physicians in making the correct diagnosis of diseases at the earliest possible stage to effectuate the optimal treatment strategy for each individual patient. In this respect surgical pathology (the traditional tissue diagnosis) is but a tool. It is not, of itself, the purpose of pathology practice; and change is in the air. This January 2014 issue of *Applied Immunohistochemistry and Molecular Morphology* (AIMM) embraces that change by the incorporation of the agenda and content of the journal *Diagnostic Molecular Morphology* (DMP). Over a decade ago AIMM introduced and promoted the concept of "molecular morphology," and has sought to publish molecular studies that correlate with the morphologic features that continue to define cancer and many diseases. That intent is now reinforced and extended by the merger with DMP, as a logical and timely response to the growing impact of a wide range of genetic and molecular technologies that are beginning to reshape the way in which pathology is practiced. The use of molecular and genomic techniques already demonstrates clear value in the diagnosis of disease, with treatment tailored specifically to individual patients. Personalized medicine is the future, and personalized medicine demands personalized pathology. The need for integration of the flood of new molecular data, with surgical pathology, digital pathology, and the full range of pathology data in the electronic medical record has never been greater. This review describes the possible impact of these pressures upon the discipline of pathology, and examines possible outcomes. There is a sense of excitement and adventure. Active adaption and innovation are required. The new AIMM, incorporating DMP, seeks to position itself for a central role in this process.

▶ This article enthusiastically describes the rapid changes in surgical pathology and traditional diagnosis by the abundance of information provided by molecular pathology and digital pathology. Both of these enhancements are leading to the long-time goal of molecular pathologists and geneticists—personalized medicine.

S. Raab, MD

20 Hematology and Immunology

Verification and Standardization of Blood Cell Counters for Routine Clinical Laboratory Tests

Verbrugge SE, Huisman A (Univ Med Ctr Utrecht, The Netherlands)

Clin Lab Med 35:183-196, 2015

Verification of an automated blood cell counter (hematology analyzer) can be done according to the Clinical and Laboratory Standards Institute or the International Committee for Standardization in Haematology guidelines depending on the preference of the laboratory professional. For complete blood count parameters, a limited number of partially outdated reference methods is available; there is a need for updated methods for established parameters and reference methods for new parameters. International standardization of reporting units is desirable.

▶ The content of this article may seem very straightforward to clinical hematologists working in hematology laboratories. However, validation of current and new tests is an essential quality assurance process that some laboratories do not perform accurately or completely simply because of a need for educational refreshment of the details of the process or a lack of original comprehensive training. This article serves as a good reminder of the validation process that laboratories can use to ensure the quality of their own practices.

S. Raab, MD

21 Laboratory Management and Outcomes

Risk Management in the Clinical Laboratory

Njoroge SW, Nichols JH (Vanderbilt Univ School of Medicine, Nashville, TN)

Ann Lab Med 34:274-278, 2014

Clinical laboratory tests play an integral role in medical decision-making and as such must be reliable and accurate. Unfortunately, no laboratory tests or devices are foolproof and errors can occur at pre-analytical, analytical and post-analytical phases of testing. Evaluating possible conditions that could lead to errors and outlining the necessary steps to detect and prevent errors before they cause patient harm is therefore an important part of laboratory testing. This can be achieved through the practice of risk management. EP23-A is a new guideline from the CLSI that introduces risk management principles to the clinical laboratory. This guideline borrows concepts from the manufacturing industry and encourages laboratories to develop risk management plans that address the specific risks inherent to each lab. Once the risks have been identified, the laboratory must implement control processes and continuously monitor and modify them to make certain that risk is maintained at a clinically acceptable level. This review summarizes the principles of risk management in the clinical laboratory and describes various quality control activities employed by the laboratory to achieve the goal of reporting valid, accurate and reliable test results.

▶ This review is valuable reading because it describes risk management as an integral component of daily laboratory quality assurance and continuous quality improvement. In the United States, risk management is commonly associated with the management of organizational risk in the event of patient harm likely to result in litigation. However, the role of risk management has evolved into a day-to-day practice that seeks to ensure the quality of laboratory practice. This shifting role of risk management is a topic all laboratorians should be aware of and integrate into their thinking and practice.

S. Raab, MD

The quality of laboratory aspects of troponin testing in clinical practice guidelines and consensus documents needs to be improved

Aakre KM, Langlois MR, Barth JH, et al (Haukeland Univ Hosp, Bergen, Norway; AZ St-Jan Hosp, Bruges, Belgium; et al)

Clin Chim Acta 437:58-61, 2014

Objective.—The European Federation of Laboratory Medicine (EFLM) and the Union of European Medical Specialists (UEMS) joint Working Group on guidelines recently proposed a checklist to help standardize the description of laboratory investigations in clinical practice guidelines (CPG).

Methods.—Nine CPGs or consensus documents published from 2011 to 2013 describing the investigation of chest pain, diagnosis of acute coronary syndrome, or myocardial infarction were evaluated against the published checklist.

Results.—Clinical use of troponin analysis are commonly dealt with but the publications present variable, vague and sometimes conflicting information regarding this laboratory test being very much relied on upon making a diagnosis of acute coronary syndrome. Most of the laboratory related checklist items are not considered or need to be updated; e.g. suggested analytical quality goals are not applicable for the high sensitive assays and important interferences that may lead to false positive or negative diagnoses are commonly not mentioned.

Conclusion.—The current paper sums up important analytical and biological issues related to troponin assays and gives suggestions for analytical quality goals that could be included in CPGs.

▶ This important article investigates the consistency of published clinical guidelines related to troponin diagnostic testing for patients with acute chest pain. Not surprisingly, the authors find a great deal of variation, which may lead to suboptimal management. Both clinicians and clinical laboratory professionals need to collaborate to standardize guidelines and improve patient safety.

S. Raab, MD

Clinical Consequences of Specimen Rejection: A College of American Pathologists Q-Probes Analysis of 78 Clinical Laboratories

Karcher DS, Lehman CM (The George Washington Univ Med Ctr, DC; University of Utah School of Medicine, Salt Lake City)

Arch Pathol Lab Med 138:1003-1008, 2014

Context.—Clinical laboratory specimens may be rejected as unsuitable for analysis for a variety of reasons and specimen rejection may have significant clinical consequences.

Objective.—To quantify the clinical consequences of specimen rejection and determine the impact of laboratories' policies and practices on these consequences.

Design.—Participants prospectively reviewed consecutive blood and urine specimens submitted to the chemistry and/or hematology laboratories to identify rejected specimens. For each rejected specimen, the patient's age, specimen type, testing priority, rejection reason, time from specimen receipt to receipt of recollected/relabeled specimen, recollection method, and test result time were recorded. Specimen/test abandonment was determined by failure to recollect or relabel a rejected specimen. Each laboratory's policy regarding relabeling of incorrectly labeled specimens was recorded, along with how many relabeled specimens were subsequently discovered to be mislabeled.

Results.—Specimen rejection led to a (1) high rate of specimen recollection, (2) delay in result availability (median of 65 minutes), and (3) high rate of specimen/test abandonment. Longer test result delay was associated with higher hospital bed size; and higher test abandonment rate, with failure of the laboratory to request specimen recollection. Relabeling of incorrectly labeled specimens was found to be of little benefit and was associated with a substantial percentage of subsequently mislabeled specimens.

Conclusions.—Specimen rejection has significant clinical consequences, including patient discomfort, significant delay in result availability, and high rate of specimen/test abandonment. Allowing routine relabeling of incorrectly labeled specimens is a dangerous practice, with little measureable benefit and with an increased risk to patient safety.

▶ This Q-Probes report is interesting and important reading. The authors investigated laboratory and clinical consequences of specimen rejection, a common practice in all areas of the clinical laboratory. The definition of rejection they used was rejection of an original specimen (primarily caused by mislabeling) with a request for proper labeling before processing. They found that specimen rejection with relabeling had no benefit to either the laboratory and, in fact, had negative effects on laboratories and patients. Laboratories may want to seriously consider these findings when generating or renewing their own specimen rejection policies.

S. Raab, MD

Immunohistochemistry Practices of Cytopathology Laboratories: A Survey of Participants in the College of American Pathologists Nongynecologic Cytopathology Education Program

Fischer AH, Schwartz MR, Moriarty AT, et al (Univ of Massachusetts Memorial Health Care, Worcester; The Methodist Hosp, Houston, TX; AmeriPath Indiana, Indianapolis; et al)

Arch Pathol Lab Med 138:1167-1672, 2014

Context.—Immunohistochemistry (IHC) is important for cytology but poses special challenges because preanalytic conditions may differ from the conditions of IHC-positive controls.

Objectives.—To broadly survey cytology laboratories to quantify preanalytic platforms for cytology IHC and identify problems with particular platforms or antigens. To discover how validation guidelines for HER2 testing have affected cytology.

Design.—A voluntary survey of cytology IHC practices was sent to 1899 cytology laboratories participating in the College of American Pathologists Nongynecologic Cytopathology Education Program in the fall of 2009.

Results.—A total of 818 laboratories (43%) responded to the survey by April 2010. Three hundred forty-five of 791 respondents (44%) performed IHC on cytology specimens. Seventeen different fixation and processing platforms prior to antibody reaction were reported. A total of 59.2% of laboratories reported differences between the platforms for cytology specimens and positive controls, but most (155 of 184; 84%) did not alter antibody dilutions or antigen retrieval for cytology IHC. When asked to name 2 antibodies for which staining conditions differed between cytology and surgical samples, there were 18 responses listing 14 antibodies. A total of 30.6% of laboratories performing IHC offered HER2 testing before publication of the 2007 College of American Pathologists/American Society of Clinical Oncologists guidelines, compared with 33.6% afterward, with increased performance of testing by reference laboratories. Three laboratories validated a nonformalin HER2 platform.

Conclusions.—The platforms for cytology IHC and positive controls differ for most laboratories, yet conditions are uncommonly adjusted for cytology specimens. Except for the unsuitability of air-dried smears for HER2 testing, the survey did not reveal evidence of systematic problems with any antibody or platform.

▶ This interesting and important report from the College of American Pathologists focuses on describing current practice regarding the use of immunocytohistochemical methods on cytology specimens. Not surprisingly, the authors report a large degree of variability among the participating laboratories in the methods they use in the analytical phase of testing; specifically in the preparation of samples for staining and in the use of control material. Two of the conclusions of the study are: (1) there does not appear to be any problems with the preanalytical phase of testing, and (2) despite the degree of practice variability, there also do not appear to be any current problems in general with the diagnostic performance of this testing in the participating laboratories. It is generally accepted, however, in all medical practice, that a high level of variability indicates that not all practices are performing at the optimum level of quality. Variability signals a need for investigation into standardization, the development of clinical practice guidelines that represent best practice. The authors do acknowledge the need for standardization and offer suggestions on methods that may be used to achieve this end.

S. Raab, MD

Clinical Consequences of Specimen Rejection: A College of American Pathologists Q-Probes Analysis of 78 Clinical Laboratories

Karcher DS, Lehman CM (The George Washington Univ Med Ctr, DC; Univ of Utah School of Medicine, Salt Lake City)

Arch Pathol Lab Med 138:1003-1008, 2014

Context.—Clinical laboratory specimens may be rejected as unsuitable for analysis for a variety of reasons and specimen rejection may have significant clinical consequences.

Objective.—To quantify the clinical consequences of specimen rejection and determine the impact of laboratories' policies and practices on these consequences.

Design.—Participants prospectively reviewed consecutive blood and urine specimens submitted to the chemistry and/or hematology laboratories to identify rejected specimens. For each rejected specimen, the patient's age, specimen type, testing priority, rejection reason, time from specimen receipt to receipt of recollected/relabeled specimen, recollection method, and test result time were recorded. Specimen/test abandonment was determined by failure to recollect or relabel a rejected specimen. Each laboratory's policy regarding relabeling of incorrectly labeled specimens was recorded, along with how many relabeled specimens were subsequently discovered to be mislabeled.

Results.—Specimen rejection led to a (1) high rate of specimen recollection, (2) delay in result availability (median of 65 minutes), and (3) high rate of specimen/test abandonment. Longer test result delay was associated with higher hospital bed size; and higher test abandonment rate, with failure of the laboratory to request specimen recollection. Relabeling of incorrectly labeled specimens was found to be of little benefit and was associated with a substantial percentage of subsequently mislabeled specimens.

Conclusions.—Specimen rejection has significant clinical consequences, including patient discomfort, significant delay in result availability, and high rate of specimen/test abandonment. Allowing routine relabeling of incorrectly labeled specimens is a dangerous practice, with little measureable benefit and with an increased risk to patient safety.

▶ This Q-Probes study from the College of American Pathologists gives a comprehensive description of specimen rejection practices provided by the participants in this program. Notably, it also provides detailed information about the clinical consequences of rejection, which are significant. Some interesting and important results of this study include the finding that the practice of allowing relabeling of specimens does not result in significant benefits for the laboratory or the patient; in fact, in this study, relabeling resulted in more mislabeling errors. One limitation of the study is that it does not specify which particular laboratory staff members reported; this is likely important because, under hectic laboratory conditions, accessioners often fail to report every mislabeled or otherwise defective specimen that was rejected, making current estimates of proportions of rejected specimens artificially low. Also, although the authors give us an extremely good idea of the current state regarding specimen rejection and some of its consequences, they do not offer or hypothesize about ways to start remedying this significant gap in laboratory quality. For further reading, please view reference list.[1,2]

D. M. Grzybicki, MD

References

1. Stark A, Jones BA, Chapman D, et al. Clinical laboratory specimen rejection—association with the site of patient care and patients' characteristics: findings from a single health care organization. *Arch Pathol Lab Med.* 2007;131:588-592.
2. Jones BA, Calam RR, Howanitz PJ. Chemistry specimen acceptability: a college of American pathologists Q-Probes study of 453 laboratories. *Arch Pathol Lab Med.* 1997;121:19-26.

Article Index

Chapter 1: Outcomes Analysis

The Modern Pathologist: Lab Data Deliverer, Interpreter, and Diagnostician 3

Anatomic and Clinical Pathology Boot Camps: Filling Pathology-Specific Gaps in Undergraduate Medical Education 4

A clinician's perspective on laboratory utilization management 5

Cancer Tracking: Clinician Compliance and Program Outcome 6

RP Implementation: Specimen Management 7

Are Amended Surgical Pathology Reports Getting to the Correct Responsible Care Provider? 8

Analysis of Addenda in Anatomic Pathology as a Quality Monitoring Initiative 9

Communicating diagnostic uncertainty in surgical pathology reports: Disparities between sender and receiver 10

Surgical pathology and the patient: a systematic review evaluating the primary audience of pathology reports 11

A Team-Based Approach to Autopsy Education: Integrating Anatomic and Clinical Pathology at the Rotation Level 12

Recognition and Discrimination of Tissue-Marking Dye Color by Surgical Pathologists: Recommendations to Avoid Errors in Margin Assessment 14

Q-Probes Studies in Anatomic Pathology: Quality Improvement Through Targeted Benchmarking 15

A systematic analysis of commonly used antibodies in cancer diagnostics 16

Interpretive Diagnostic Error Reduction in Surgical Pathology and Cytology: Guideline From the College of American Pathologists Pathology and Laboratory Quality Center and the Association of Directors of Anatomic and Surgical Pathology 19

Utilization management in anatomic pathology 21

The Wonderful Colors of the Hematoxylin–Eosin Stain in Diagnostic Surgical Pathology 22

Variable fidelity of tissue-marking dyes in surgical pathology 23

Turnaround Time for Large or Complex Specimens in Surgical Pathology: A College of American Pathologists Q-Probes Study of 56 Institutions 24

Chapter 2: Hepatobiliary System and Pancreas

Acute Liver Allograft Antibody-Mediated Rejection: An Inter-Institutional Study of Significant Histopathological Features 27

SALL4 Immunoreactivity Predicts Prognosis in Western Hepatocellular Carcinoma Patients but Is a Rare Event: A Study of 236 Cases 28

Update on the New Classification of Hepatic Adenomas: Clinical, Molecular, and Pathologic Characteristics 30

Diagnostic utility and limitations of glutamine synthetase and serum amyloid-associated protein immunohistochemistry in the distinction of focal nodular hyperplasia and inflammatory hepatocellular adenoma. 32

Different collagen types show distinct rates of increase from early to late stages of hepatitis C-related liver fibrosis 34

Quantification of portal–bridging fibrosis area more accurately reflects fibrosis stage and liver stiffness than whole fibrosis or perisinusoidal fibrosis areas in chronic hepatitis C 35

Discrepancy rates in liver biopsy reporting 37

Poorly differentiated neuroendocrine carcinomas of the pancreas: a clinicopathologic analysis of 44 cases 39

Congestive hepatic fibrosis score: a novel histologic assessment of clinical severity 41

Immunohistochemical distinction between intrahepatic cholangiocarcinoma and pancreatic ductal adenocarcinoma 44

Aberrant Centrizonal Features in Chronic Hepatic Venous Outflow Obstruction: Centrilobular Mimicry of Portal-based Disease 45

Automatic classification of white regions in liver biopsies by supervised machine learning 48

Chapter 3: Cytopathology

Increasing the sensitivity of endocervical curettings by performing ThinPrep® Pap on transport container fluid: is diagnostic material going down the drain? 51

Role of endoscopic ultrasound fine-needle aspiration evaluating adrenal gland enlargement or mass 52

Making Mock-FNA Smears from Fresh Surgical Pathology Specimens to Improve Smear Preparation Technique and to Create Cytohistological Correlation Series 53

'Suspicious for Papillary Thyroid Carcinoma' before and after The Bethesda System for Reporting Thyroid Cytopathology: Impact of Standardized Terminology 54

Investigating MicroRNA Expression Profiles in Pancreatic Cystic Neoplasms 55

An Assessment of Gynecological Cytology Screening Practices Among Health Care Providers Nationwide 57

The Utility of Liquid-Based Cytology in Salivary Gland Fine-Needle Aspirates: Experience of an Academic Institution 59

Chapter 4: Head and Neck

Epidemiological Trends in Head and Neck Cancer and Aids in Diagnosis 61

Lymphoepithelial-like carcinomas of the head and neck 61

Papillary Thyroid Carcinoma in a Branchial Cleft Cyst without a Thyroid Primary: Navigating a Diagnostic Dilemma 66

Polymorphous Low Grade Adenocarcinoma has a Consistent p63+/p40– Immunophenotype that Helps Distinguish it from Adenoid Cystic Carcinoma and Cellular Pleomorphic Adenoma 67

Multifocal Fibrosing Thyroiditis and Its Association with Papillary Thyroid Carcinoma Using BRAF Pyrosequencing 70

SMARCB1 (INI-1)-deficient Carcinomas of the Sinonasal Tract 71

Prognostic features in mucoepidermoid carcinoma of major salivary glands with emphasis on tumour histologic grading 75

Pediatric sinonasal tumors in the United States: incidence and outcomes 79

Basal Cell Adenocarcinoma and Basal Cell Adenoma of the Salivary Glands: A Clinicopathological Review of Seventy Tumors with Comparison of Morphologic Features and Growth Control Indices 83

A Prospective Assessment Defining the Limitations of Thyroid Nodule Pathologic Evaluation 85

Malignant triton tumour of the sinonasal tract: Case report and literature review 89

Cerebellopontine Angle and Intracanalicular Masses Mimicking Vestibular Schwannomas 92

Recent advances in the diagnostic pathology of salivary carcinomas 94

Chapter 5: Kidney

Defining the spectrum of immunoglobulin A–dominant/codominant glomerular deposition in diabetic nephropathy 97

Focal and segmental glomerulosclerosis: clinical and kidney biopsy correlations 98

Tuberous Sclerosis–associated Renal Cell Carcinoma: A Clinicopathologic Study of 57 Separate Carcinomas in 18 Patients 100

Validation of a histopathologic classification scheme for antineutrophil cytoplasmic antibody–associated glomerulonephritis 101

Granulomatosis With Polyangiitis Presenting as a Renal Tumor 103

Rhabdoid Differentiation is Associated With Aggressive Behavior in Renal Cell Carcinoma: A Clinicopathologic Analysis of 76 Cases With Clinical Follow-up 105

Diagnostic Approach to Eosinophilic Renal Neoplasms 106

Biopsy-Proven Acute Interstitial Nephritis, 1993-2011: A Case Series 108

Membranous-like glomerulopathy with masked IgG kappa deposits 110

The reproducibility and predictive value on outcome of renal biopsies from expanded criteria donors 113

Best Practices Recommendations in the Application of Immunohistochemistry in the Kidney Tumors: Report From the International Society of Urologic Pathology Consensus Conference 115

Chapter 6: Female Genital Tract

The role of immunohistochemistry in the evaluation of gynecologic pathology: a single institutional experience 121

Endometrial stromal tumours revisited: an update based on the 2014 WHO classification 122

The Utility of Immunohistochemistry in the Differential Diagnosis of Gynecologic Disorders 122

Low Grade Serous Ovarian Carcinoma: From the molecular characterization to the best therapeutic strategy 123

Assessment of endometrial sampling as a predictor of final surgical pathology in endometrial cancer 124

Chapter 7: Breast

Concomitant Detection of HER2 Protein and Gene Alterations by Immunohistochemistry (IHC) and Silver Enhanced In Situ Hybridization (SISH) Identifies HER2 Positive Breast Cancer with and without Gene Amplification 129

Second opinion in breast pathology: policy, practice and perception 130

Effects of tissue decalcification on the quantification of breast cancer biomarkers by digital image analysis 132

Breast cancer detection in axillary sentinel lymph nodes: the impact of the method of pathologic examination 134

A Targetable Androgen Receptor–Positive Breast Cancer Subtype Hidden Among the Triple-Negative Cancers 135

Estrogen Receptor Expression Is High but Is of Lower Intensity in Tubular Carcinoma Than in Well-Differentiated Invasive Ductal Carcinoma 136

Chapter 8: Lung and Mediastinum

Pulmonary Adenocarcinoma With Signet Ring Cell Features: A Comprehensive Study From 3 Distinct Patient Cohorts 139

Interobserver Variability for the WHO Classification of Pulmonary Carcinoids 140

Immunohistochemical study of 36 cases of pulmonary sarcomatoid carcinoma—sensitivity of TTF-1 is superior to napsin 141

Pulmonary Large Cell Carcinoma Lacking Squamous Differentiation Is Clinicopathologically Indistinguishable From Solid-Subtype Adenocarcinoma 143

ALK Rearrangement in a Large Series of Consecutive Non–Small Cell Lung Cancers: Comparison Between a New Immunohistochemical Approach and Fluorescence In Situ Hybridization for the Screening of Patients Eligible for Crizotinib Treatment 145

Surgical pathology of pleural coccidioidomycosis: a clinicopathological study of 36 cases 147

The Presence of Anti-HLA Donor-Specific Antibodies in Lung Allograft Recipients Does Not Correlate With C4d Immunofluorescence in Transbronchial Biopsy Specimens 149

Lung Tumors Masquerading as Desquamative Interstitial Pneumonia (DIP): Report of 7 Cases and Review of the Literature 150

Approach to Lung Biopsies From Patients With Pneumothorax 153

Clinicopathologic features associated with relapse in cryptogenic organizing pneumonia 155

Prognostic Significance of Adenocarcinoma In Situ, Minimally Invasive Adenocarcinoma, and Nonmucinous Lepidic Predominant Invasive Adenocarcinoma of the Lung in Patients With Stage I Disease 157

Banff 2013 Meeting Report: Inclusion of C4d-Negative Antibody-Mediated Rejection and Antibody-Associated Arterial Lesions 158

p16 FISH Deletion in Surface Epithelial Mesothelial Proliferations Is Predictive of Underlying Invasive Mesothelioma 163

Chapter 9: Cardiovascular

Sudden Cardiac Death: A Modern Pathology Approach to Hypertrophic Cardiomyopathy 165

Pathologic diagnosis of antibody-mediated rejection in endomyocardial biopsy after heart transplantation based on renewed International Society for Heart and Lung Transplantation criteria 166

Chapter 10: Gastrointestinal System

Diagnosis of inflammatory bowel disease: Potential role of molecular biometrics 167

Challenges Posed to Pathologists in the Detection of *KRAS* Mutations in Colorectal Cancers 168

Association between *Helicobacter pylori* and Barrett's Esophagus: A Case–Control Study 169

Guidelines for Diagnosis and Treatment of Carcinoma of the Esophagus April 2012 edited by the Japan Esophageal Society 170

Utility of ancillary stains for *Helicobacter pylori* in near-normal gastric biopsies 172

Traditional serrated adenomas (TSAs) admixed with other serrated (so-called precursor) polyps and conventional adenomas: a frequent occurrence 174

HER2/neu Testing in Gastric Cancer by Immunohistochemistry: Assessment of Interlaboratory Variation 175

Chapter 11: Hematolymphoid

Utility of bone marrow examination for workup of fever of unknown origin in patients with HIV/AIDS 179

Differentiating Benign From Malignant Bone Marrow B-Cell Lymphoid Aggregates: A Statistical Analysis of Distinguishing Features 180

Molecular Genetic Biomarkers in Myeloid Malignancies 181

Specialist integrated haematological malignancy diagnostic services: an Activity Based Cost (ABC) analysis of a networked laboratory service model 182

Systematic Review of the Effectiveness of Fine-Needle Aspiration and/or Core Needle Biopsy for Subclassifying Lymphoma 183

Chapter 12: Neuropathology

Evaluation of simultaneous muscle and nerve biopsies for the diagnosis of neuromuscular diseases 185

A Unique Four-Hub Protein Cluster Associates to Glioblastoma Progression 186

Chapter 13: Soft Tissue and Bone

Gastrointestinal stromal tumors with exon 8 c-*kit* gene mutation might occur at extragastric sites and have metastasis-prone nature 189

Histopathological Diagnostic Discrepancies in Soft Tissue Tumours Referred to a Specialist Centre: Reassessment in the Era of Ancillary Molecular Diagnosis 190

Clinical and morphological characteristics of osteoid osteoma and osteoblastoma: a retrospective single-center analysis of 204 patients 191

An Update on the Application of Newly Described Immunohistochemical Markers in Soft Tissue Pathology 192

Chapter 14: Pediatrics

Effect of interference from hemolysis, icterus and lipemia on routine pediatric clinical chemistry assays 195

Incidence and Outcome of Documented Fungal Endocarditis 196

Quantification of Sickle Cells in the Peripheral Smear as a Marker of Disease Severity 197

Chapter 15: Techniques/Molecular

Selective Pathology Fellowships: Diverse, Innovative, and Valuable Subspecialty Training 199

Diagnosis of major cancer resection specimens with virtual slides: impact of a novel digital pathology workstation 200

Interinstitutional Whole Slide Imaging Teleconsultation Service Development: Assessment Using Internal Training and Clinical Consultation Cases 200

The College of American Pathologists Guidelines for Whole Slide Imaging Validation Are Feasible for Pediatric Pathology: A Pediatric Pathology Practice Experience 202

Diagnosis of major cancer resection specimens with virtual slides: impact of a novel digital pathology workstation 203

Practicing Pathology in the Era of Big Data and Personalized Medicine 204

Validation of a whole slide imaging system for primary diagnosis in surgical pathology: A community hospital experience 206

Chapter 16: Urinary Bladder and Male Genital Tract

Are *Ureaplasma* spp. a Cause of Nongonococcal Urethritis? A Systematic Review and Meta-Analysis 209

The Critical Role of the Pathologist in Determining Eligibility for Active Surveillance as a Management Option in Patients With Prostate Cancer: Consensus Statement With Recommendations Supported by the College of American Pathologists, International Society of Urological Pathology, Association of Directors of Anatomic and Surgical Pathology, the New Zealand Society of Pathologists, and the Prostate Cancer Foundation 210

The Application of Immunohistochemical Biomarkers in Urologic Surgical Pathology 213

Recurrent papillary urothelial neoplasm of low malignant potential. Subtle architectural disorder detected by quantitative analysis in DAXX-immunostained tissue sections 215

Chapter 17: Clinical Chemistry

Clinical biochemistry laboratory rejection rates due to various types of preanalytical errors 219

Harmonization: the Sample, the Measurement, and the Report 220

Measurements for 8 Common Analytes in Native Sera Identify Inadequate Standardization among 6 Routine Laboratory Assays 221

Chapter 18: Clinical Microbiology

Emerging Rapid Resistance Testing Methods for Clinical Microbiology Laboratories and Their Potential Impact on Patient Management 223

Evaluation of the decision support system for antimicrobial treatment, TREAT, in an acute medical ward of a university hospital 224

Fungal Infections in Liver Transplant Patients Admitted to the Intensive Care Unit 225

Pathogenesis of Necrotizing Enterocolitis: Modeling the Innate Immune Response 226

The aetiology of pharyngotonsillitis in adolescents and adults – *Fusobacterium necrophorum* is commonly found 226

Testing quality of a self-monitoring blood glucose sensor with an auto-coding mechanism when used by patients versus technicians 227

Chapter 19: Cytogenetics and Molecular Pathology

Practicing Pathology in the Era of Big Data and Personalized Medicine 229

Chapter 20: Hematology and Immunology

Verification and Standardization of Blood Cell Counters for Routine Clinical Laboratory Tests 231

Chapter 21: Laboratory Management and Outcomes

Risk Management in the Clinical Laboratory 233

The quality of laboratory aspects of troponin testing in clinical practice guidelines and consensus documents needs to be improved 234

Clinical Consequences of Specimen Rejection: A College of American Pathologists Q-Probes Analysis of 78 Clinical Laboratories 234

Immunohistochemistry Practices of Cytopathology Laboratories: A Survey of Participants in the College of American Pathologists Nongynecologic Cytopathology Education Program 235

Clinical Consequences of Specimen Rejection: A College of American Pathologists Q-Probes Analysis of 78 Clinical Laboratories 237

Author Index

A

Aakre KM, 234
Agarwal S, 195
Al-Haddad M, 52
Alì G, 145
Ali RH, 122
Ali S, 75
Alvarez O, 197
Ambuzs JM, 110
Amin MB, 210
Amirghofran AA, 196
Antonescu CR, 71
Arboe B, 224
Argani P, 106
Arnold MA, 202
Atay A, 219
Atlinboga AA, 54
Aubry MC, 141
Azancot MA, 113

B

Babwah JP, 9
Badiee P, 196
Baker PB, 202
Baloch ZW, 51, 70, 85
Barrios R, 149
Barth JH, 220, 234
Basarir H, 182
Basturk O, 39
Bellamy C, 27
Bergman J, 16
Bernheim OE, 172
Berryhill TF, 226
Bieber L, 226
Bishop JA, 67, 71
Black-Schaffer S, 21
Blair JE, 147
Bockhorst J, 48
Boland JM, 139
Bonsib SM, 110
Boonyaarunnate T, 54
Boursier J, 35
Brat DJ, 3
Brynes RK, 180
Buck TP, 206

C

Cagle PT, 149
Calhoun BC, 134
Calzada AP, 92
Can B, 45
Carney PA, 130
Castellini P, 215
Casulo C, 183
Chaigneau J, 35
Chamberlain BK, 121
Chambers K, 134
Chan JKC, 22
Chapman WC, 28
Chen DJ, 185
Chen L, 44
Chen W, 34
Chenever E, 202
Chetty R, 174
Chévez-Barrios P, 199
Cibas ES, 85
Cohen P, 8
Colasacco C, 19
Colling R, 37
Contac A, 53
Cossey LN, 97
Covens A, 124
Crum CP, 122
Cuhadar S, 219

D

Dai D-F, 41
Dakin Haché K, 23
Dalley C, 182
Dalurzo ML, 150
Darwish-Yassine M, 57
Della Pepa C, 123
Demir L, 219
den Bakker MA, 140
Desouki MM, 121
Dhingra S, 30
Di Palma S, 94
Dilorio R, 206
Djureinovic D, 16
Doganavsargil B, 191
Domfeh A, 8
Doyle LA, 192
Dudley J, 168
Duncan LM, 200

E

Ellenburg JL, 226
Ewton A, 199

F

Fadare O, 121
Fellegara G, 85
Fernandes J, 165
Ferrell L, 45
Ferrell LD, 32
Fiel MI, 30
Fischbach LA, 169
Fischer AH, 235
Flippo-Morton T, 134
Frank R, 70
Frederiksen JK, 183
Frickmann H, 223
Fryer E, 37

G

Garratt J, 175
Garvin AD, 57
Geller BM, 130
Gentile C, 70
Gerth DJ, 79
Gertych A, 132
Ghazi Nour M, 196
Ghossein R, 75
Gillies EM, 10
Girard L, 101
Go JL, 92
Gore JL, 210
Graham DY, 169
Grajkowska W, 166
Graybill-D'Ercole P, 7
Gremel G, 16
Gu J, 204, 229
Guo J, 100

H

Haas M, 158
Hache KD, 14
Hafezi-Bakhtiari S, 174
Hammad F, 89
Hassell LA, 10
Havrilla L, 206
Healy PN, 136
Hébert TM, 12
Hedin K, 226
Helpman L, 124
Hirai T, 189
Hruban RH, 39

Hsu C-T, 227
Huisman A, 231
Hwang DH, 143
Hwang H, 163

I

Iacob A, 53
Idowu MO, 24
Iezzoni JC, 199
Ito T, 189

J

Jain D, 32
James M, 101
Jang JS, 139
Johnston A, 180
Johnston CM, 57
Jones NC, 200
Jorda M, 106
Jorns JM, 136
Joseph NM, 32

K

Kadota K, 157
Kalloger SE, 175
Karcher DS, 234, 237
Kaspar HG, 122
Katabi N, 75
Ketterer J, 150
Khalifa M, 9
Kocovski L, 165
Komorowski R, 48
Konya C, 103
Kramer JR, 169
Krieger EV, 41
Krings G, 45
Kronborg G, 224
Kryvenko ON, 106
Kuo C-Y, 227
Kupets R, 124
Kuwano H, 170

L

Langlois MR, 234
Langlois O, 89
Larsen CP, 110
Lastra RR, 51
Laub RR, 224
Layfield LJ, 6
LeBlanc J, 52
Lee LS, 55
Lehman CM, 234, 237
Leung N, 108
Lewandrowski K, 21
Li X, 209
Lin DW, 210
Lin F, 44, 213
Lin G, 192
Lindh M, 226
Lindley SW, 10
Liu H, 213
Liu T-C, 28
Lok T, 44

M

Maclary S, 132
Maleki S, 12
Marin M, 197
Mark EJ, 103
Martinez M, 52
Marzaban R, 225
Masanta WO, 223
Mathai SK, 155
Matynia AP, 181
McCall SJ, 15
McKenney JK, 105
Messias E, 97
Messias N, 97
Meykler SE, 51
Mezei T, 53
Michael CW, 59
Michelle Shiller S, 27
Miller WG, 220
M'Koma AE, 167
Moch H, 129
Mohan S, 132
Montague NS, 197
Montironi MA, 215
Moreso F, 113
Moriarty AT, 235
Mossanen M, 11
Mubako T, 190
Mukhtar AM, 225
Murali R, 153
Muriithi AK, 108

N

Naemi K, 180
Nakhleh RE, 19
Naritoku WY, 4
Nasr SH, 98
Nazarian RM, 200
Nelson HD, 130
Nichols JH, 233
Nishimura Y, 170
Nishino M, 155
Njoroge SW, 233
Nohr E, 101
Nordstrom C, 195
Nosé V, 19

O

O'Leary JG, 27
Olson MT, 54
Oyama T, 170

P

Panarelli NC, 172
Parkash V, 8
Pelliccioni S, 145
Perry AS, 143
Prayson RA, 185
Proietti A, 145
Pronicki M, 166
Przybycin CG, 105

Q

Quesada AE, 179

R

Randell R, 200, 203
Raparia K, 150
Rarick JM, 59
Reuter VE, 115
Reynolds JP, 105
Ricciotti RW, 147
Roberts JA, 149
Robinson RA, 83
Rock JB, 34
Rodriguez S, 163
Rooper L, 67, 168
Ross DS, 172
Rouzbahman M, 122
Rowsell C, 9
Ruddle RA, 200, 203
Ruhl DS, 66

S

Safarpour D, 135
Salah M, 225
Salcedo M, 113

Sandrini J, 35
Santini D, 123
Schnabel JL, 6
Schneider F, 153
Schoenfeld D, 155
Schwartz MR, 235
Serra S, 174
Sethi S, 98
Sezak M, 191
Sharma M, 183
Sharma R, 67
Sheffield BS, 175
Shekhel TA, 147
Shen W, 181
Sheridan MF, 66
Simeone P, 186
Simpson RHW, 94
Skálová A, 94
Sniezek JC, 66
Souers RJ, 24
Steinberg JJ, 4
Stepman HCM, 221
Swanson PE, 41
Swarts DRA, 140
Szafranska-Schwarzbach AE, 55
Szankasi P, 181
Szeto DP, 143
Szymańska S, 166

T

Tang L, 39
Tanner SM, 226
Tashiro J, 79
Tate JR, 220
Tavassoli FA, 135
Taylor CR, 204, 229
Terra SBSP, 141
Thaller SR, 79
Tholpady A, 179
Thomas DG, 136
Thomas RG, 200, 203
Thway K, 190
Tonini G, 123
Trerotola M, 186
Tretiakova MS, 100
Troxell ML, 100
True LD, 11
Tschirhart DL, 92
Tse C, 163
Tseng L-H, 168
Tubbs RR, 129
Tworek JA, 15

U

Urbanella A, 186

V

Vachharajani N, 28
Valeri AM, 108
van Suylen R-J, 140
Vanderbeck S, 48
Varga Z, 129
Vargas G, 195
Vasovic L, 4
Vasovic LV, 12
Veraldi KL, 153
Verbrugge SE, 231
Verrill C, 37
Vigneswaran N, 61
Villena-Vargas J, 157
Volmar KE, 15, 24

W

Wampfler JA, 139
Wang J, 190
Wang R, 209
Wanger A, 179
Ward A, 103
Wasman J, 59
Wenig BM, 61
Westra WH, 71
Wilkerson ML, 213
Williams AS, 14, 23
Williams MD, 61
Wilson TC, 83
Wright JG, 182
Wright JL, 11
Wu M-H, 227
Wylie D, 55

Y

Yalcinkaya U, 191
Yamamura M, 189
Yearsley MM, 34
Yeh DD, 5
Yi ES, 141
Yoshizawa A, 157

Z

Zakzouk A, 89
Zand L, 98
Zautner AE, 223
Zhang N, 209
Zizzi A, 215

FSC
www.fsc.org
MIX
Papier | Fördert gute Waldnutzung
FSC® C083411

Kolibri 360 GmbH
Ferdinand-Jühlke-Straße 7
99095 Erfurt, Deutschland
produktsicherheit@kolibri360.de